Mechanisms of Invasion in Cancer

UICC Monograph Series · Volume 6

Mechanisms of Invasion in Cancer

Edited by

Pierre Denoix

With 62 figures

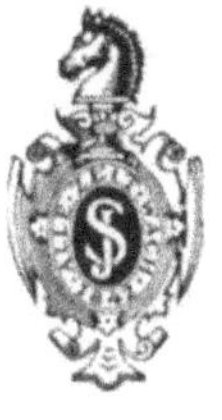

Springer-Verlag Berlin Heidelberg New York 1967

Professor Dr. Pierre Denoix,
Institut Gustave Roussy, 94 Villejuif, France

ISBN-13: 978-3-642-87460-4   e-ISBN-13: 978-3-642-87458-1
DOI: 10.1007/978-3-642-87458-1

Title-No. 7517

Contents

Participants

Dr. M. ABERCROMBIE, University College London, Dower Street, London W.C. 1, Great Britain

Dr. E. J. AMBROSE, Chester Beatty Research Institute, Institute of Cancer Research, Royal Cancer Hospital, Fulham Road, London S.W. 3, Great Britain

Dr. G. BARSKI, Laboratoire de Culture de Tissus et de Virologie, Institut Gustave-Roussy, 94 Villejuif, France

Dr. Z. BRADA, Cancer Research Institute, Department of Biochemistry, Brno, Czechoslovakia

Professor O. COSTACHEL, Oncological Institute, B-dul 1 Mai 11, Bucharest, Rumania

Professor P. DENOIX, Institut Gustave-Roussy, 94 Villejuif, France

Dr. M. FELDMAN, Section of Cell Biology, Weizmann Institute of Science, Rehovoth, Israel

Professor B. N. HALPERN, Centre de recherches allergiques et immunologiques, 96 Rue Didot, Paris, France

Professor H. HAMPERL, Pathologisches Institut der Universität, Venusberg, 5300 Bonn, Deutschland

Professor B. KELLNER, Research Institute of Oncopathology, Ráth Gy.-u. 5, Budapest, Hungary

Dr. F. LACOUR, Institut Gustave-Roussy, 94 Villejuif, France

Dr. J. LEIGHTON, Department of Pathology, School of Medicine, University of Pittsburgh, Pittsburgh 152, Pa., U.S.A.

Dr. O. M. LEJNEVA, Department of Immunology and Oncology of Gamaleya Institute, Moscow, USSR

Dr. R. E. MADDEN, Department of Surgery, New York Medical College, Flower and Fifth Avenue Hospitals, 1249 Fifth Avenue, New York 29, N.Y., U.S.A.

Dr. R. A. MALMGREN, Pathologic Anatomy Branch, National Cancer Institute, National Institutes of Health, Public Health Service, US Department of Health, Education and Welfare, Bethesda 14, Md. U.S.A.

Dr. P. MORI-CHAVEZ, Laboratorio de Investigación de Cancer, Instituto de Investigationes de la Altura, Universidad Peruana "Cayetano Heredia", Union 1146, Lima Peru

Professor M. STOKER, Institute of Virology, University of Glasgow, Church Street, Glasgow, Great Britain

Dr. P. STRÄULI, Department of Cancer Research and Experimental Pathology, Institute of Pathology, University of Zürich, Schmelzbergstraße 12, Zürich, Switzerland

Dr. B. SYLVÉN, The Cancer Research Division of Radiumhemmet, Karolinska Institute, Stockholm 60, Sweden

Dr. G. A. VOISIN, Centre d'Immuno-Pathologie de l'Association Claude-Bernard, Hôpital Saint-Antoine, Paris 12ème, France

Professor E. WOLFF, Laboratoire d'Embryologie Experimentale, 49 bis Av. de la Belle Gabrielle, 94 Nogent sur Marne, France

Dr. S. WOOD, jr., Department of Pathology, John Hopkins Hospital, Baltimore, Md. 21205, U.S.A.

Appreciation de l'Invasion dans les Cancers Humains

Pierre Denoix

Institut Gustave Roussy, Villejuif (Val de Marne), France

Au début de ce colloque qui va étudier le mécanisme de l'invasion de l'organisme par la cellule cancéreuse, il m'a paru utile de rappeler que le cancer contre lequel nous combattions étant le cancer humain, il pouvait être intéressant de considérer si, du dehors, nous pouvions avoir quelque idée des conséquences de cette invasion chez les malades.

La notion de relations hôte-tumeur est une des acquisitions récentes les plus importantes pour les cliniciens; elle a modifié pour eux la conception classique qui faisait du cancer un parasite se développant de façon inexorable sur un hôte passif, le raisonnement thérapeutique qui en découlait était dominé jusque là par la notion de lutte avec le temps de façon à espérer pouvoir intervenir avant que l'extension ait dépassé les possibilités d'action, seulement loco-régionales, de nos moyens de traitement. On sait maintenant que la notion de temps est secondaire et relative, car lorsque le malade manifeste pour la 1ère fois les symptômes qui attirent l'attention, il y a plus ou moins longtemps que le cancer luimême existe, se développe et a déjà diffusé des cellules à partir de la tumeur principale.

Le degré d'extension au moment du premier symptome est le résultat de l'interaction hôte-tumeur. Pour un grand nombre de cas bien des choses sont déjà en place contre lesquelles la lutte contre le temps seul, s'il elle ne permet de gagner que quelques mois pour se rapprocher de ce premier symptome ne peut être la méthode efficace car bien souvent c'est depuis des années que ces différents éléments ont été mis en place.

C'est dans la cadre des relations hôte-tumeur que «la loi de progression» proposée par Leslie Foulds (1964), permet d'expliquer un certain nombre des phénomènes constatés par les cliniciens.

La notion d'évolution discontinue comportant de plus ou moins longues périodes de stabilité entrecoupées de périodes d'accroissement ou phases évolutives, se révèle être d'une grande importance quant aux conséquences qu'elle peut entraîner dans l'établissement d'un plan thérapeutique. C'est en particulier à l'IGR que l'on a depuis longtemps (Huguenin, 1946) insisté sur cette notion de phase évolutive en considérant qu'il était nécessaire d'éviter à ce moment d'aggraver le déséquilibre qui s'est constitué aux dépens de l'hôte. Une thérapeutique agressive telle que la chirurgie doit être repoussée jusqu'au moment où une stabilisation aura pu être obtenue.

Il a été également constaté par les cliniciens (Denoix, 1955) qu'il y avait une différence dans le comportement des tumeurs et dans la probabilité d'apparition de complications ultérieures, selon qu'il s'agissait d'une forme sans envahissement des ganglions lymphatiques, forme N- ou d'une forme avec envahissement des ganglions lymphatiques, forme N+. Dans les formes N— lorsque l'examen histologique des ganglions a été suffisamment précis pour que l'on puisse être sûr qu'il s'agissait vraiment d'une forme N—, la probabilité de récidive dans la zone où siège la tumeur, à condition que celle-ci ait été enlevée complètement, est pratiquement inexistante. Par contre on observe des recidives locales, dans les formes N+.

Il n'y a pas de différence dans la possibilité de métastases à distances, sauf sur le plan quantitatif, car les formes N— ont un avenir nettement plus favorable.

C'est ainsi que dans une série récemment publiée (VOGT-HOERNER, 1964) par l'Institut Gustave Roussy, concernant des tumeurs malignes du sein ayant fait l'objet d'une intervention chirurgicale préalable et complétée ou non par de la radiothérapie, selon qu'il y avait ou non envahissement ganglionnaire, les formes N— chirurgicales pures avaient un taux de survie à 5 ans de 91% sans que soit observée parmi les échecs la moindre récidive locale, les seuls échecs étaient liés à des métastases à distance, par contre dans les formes N+, dont le traitement avait été complété par une radiothérapie loco-régionale, la survie à 5 ans avait été de 64% les échecs comportant des récidives locales associées aux métastases à distance. Signalons que dans cette même série il y eut 29 malades classés en phase évolutive et que la survie à cinq ans de ce groupe ne fut que de 41%.

Ces diverses constatations ont conduit (DENOIX, 1954) au démembrement des cancers en 3 groupes, un premier T, N—, Mo, comportant une tumeur s'étendant lentement et de façon inégale, sans envahissement des ganglions et sans métastase à distance, un 2ème groupe, T, N+, Mo avec envahissement progressif du système lumphatique mais sans métastase à distance et enfin un 3ème groupe M+ quel que soit T et N où l'existence des métastases à distance domine la situation et l'avenir des malades.

Ces 3 groupes d'événements représentant 3 formes différentes de l'invasion du processus malin à travers l'ensemble de l'organisme sont le témoin des relations hôte-tumeur. Chacune de ces éventualités ne constituant pas une étape dans une succession d'événements appartenant à une même forme, mais trois résultats différents des relations hôte-tumeur.

Il est pour le clinicien fort important de pouvoir comprendre ce qui se passe dans ces 3 éventualités. Pourquoi dans les formes purement locales n'y-a-t-il rien à distance étant donné qu'il est admissible de penser que ce n'est pas parce que rien n'est parti de la tumeur, mais parce que ce qui en est parti a été détruit? ou stabilisé?

Pourquoi dans les formes N+ les cellules malignes sont-elles acceptées par les ganglions qu'elles vont envahir, puis, à partir d'un certain moment pourquoi vont-elles déborder les limites de ce système lymphatique et passer dans la grande circulation?

Pourquoi enfin dans les formes diffusées y a-t-il acceptation des cellules qui sont parties de la tumeur et maintien de celles-ci non decelables pendant un temps plus ou moins long jusqu'à ce qu'un jour ces métastases à distance se développent. Ces foyers à distance sont la raison principale et essentielle de nos échecs actuels.

Nous devons guérir les formes T, N-, Mo si l'on n'a pas attendu que ce soit produite une extension trop importante, cela est du domaine du possible et du journalier. Ilest encore possible de guérir les formes T, N+, Mo si l'on n'a pas permis à l'extension ganglionnaire de dépasser un certain seuil. Nous sommes, par contre, incapables, avec nos seules méthodes actuelles: la chirurgie et les radiations, puisqu'elles n'ont d'effet que loco-régional, de guérir les formes diffusées M. Nous sommes actuellement désarmés devant les métastases à distance.

Afin d'étayer ces différentes réflexions basées sur l'observation clinique, nous avons étudié le comportement dans le temps d'un certain nombre de cancers. Il apparaissait souhaitable de pouvoir évaluer l'expansion du processus tumoral, ce qui nous a conduit à l'appréciation de sa «vitesse d'accroissement». Cet ac-

tableau I, ils montrent que la vitesse de développement ainsi définie a une signification certaine, car quel que soit le délai au bout duquel le diagnostic a été pratiqué, le taux de survie baisse regulièrement en fonction des 3 catégories de tumeurs: stationnaire, à développement lent et à developpement rapide et dans tous les cas la différence observée est significative à 1 pour 1.000.

Tableau I. *Tumeur maligne du sein. Taux de survie en fonction de la rapidité de développement tumoral*

Développement	Taux de survie à				
	1an	2ans	3ans	4ans	5ans
T. Stationnaire	(269) 91%	(268) 81%	(245) 76%	(222) 72%	(150) 67%
D. Lent	(150) 83%	(148) 63%	(136) 49%	(117) 38%	(70)27%
D. Rapide	(62) 61%	(62 39%)	(52) 27%	(39) 21%	(25) 16%
Signification	***	***	***	***	***

— $*p = 0,05$ — $**p = 0,01$ — $***p = 0,001$ —.

— Les effectifs sont indiqués entre parenthèses.

croissement est relativement facile à reconnaître lorsqu'il concerne la tumeur elle-même et lorsqu'il s'agit d'une tumeur accessible; c'est la raison pour laquelle le plus grand nombre de renseignements ont été recueillis dans les tumeurs malignes du sein.

C'est ainsi que sur une série de 497 cas de tumeur du sein (LALANNE, 1962), nous avons pu procéder à une répartition en «groupes selon le temps mis par la tumeur pour atteindre un certain volume».

— tumeurs stationnaires: 273 cas soit 55%,

— tumeurs d'accroissement lent: 159 cas soit 32%,

— tumeurs d'accroissement rapide: 65 cas soit 13%.

Sur ce total de 497 cas nous avons alors étudié quelle était la relation entre le taux de survie en fonction de la rapidité du développement tumoral. Les renseignements recueillis apparaissent sur le

Nous avons utilisé la survie comme test d'appréciation pour juger des éléments étudiés, car ce n'est pas l'expansion de la seule tumeur qui a un sens, et nous avons pensé que la survie pouvait être le témoin du processus d'extension de l'ensemble de la maladie maligne dont la tumeur n'était qu'un des aspects. Nous savons que les causes d'échecs sont liées à la diffusion et essentiellement aux foyers à distance beaucoup plus qu'au développement de la tumeur elle-même.

La survie peut donc être considérée comme le témoin du résultat des relations hôte-tumeur.

Si nous essayons de serrer de plus près le phénomène, nous pouvons étudier comment évolue le taux de survie en fonction de la vitesse d'accroissement de la tumeur et du délai qui s'écoule entre le premier symptome et le premier traitement. C'est ce qui apparaît sur le tableau IIa et b, concernant successivement le taux de survie à 2 ans et le taux de survie à 4 ans en fonction de la vitesse de développement et pour des délais entre le premier symptome et le moment du diagnostic de moins de 6 mois ou bien supérieurs ou égaux à 6 mois.

On constate à l'étude de ce tableau que la vitesse d'accroissement de la tumeur conserve une valeur indicative de gravité quel que soit le délai écoulè

c'est pourquoi il nous a paru interessant de la détailler en quelque sorte, et d'étudier les relations que l'on pouvait observer entre le délai et la survie, étant admis que cette notion de délai n'avait qu'une importance relative et qu'elle devait être associée à la notion de taille de la tumeur pour en déduire celle de vitesse d'accroissement.

Tableau IIa. *Tumeur maligne du sein. Taux de survie en fonction de la vitesse d'accroissement de la et tumeur du délai qui s'écoule entre le 1er symptôme et le 1er traitement. Taux de survie à 2 ans*

Développement	Délai		
	< 6 mois	> 6 mois	Signification
T. Stationnaire	(163) 81%	(86) 80%	
D. Lent	(50) 74%	(69) 57%	*
D. Rapide	(32) 53%	(22) 18%	**
Signification	**	***	

Tableau IIb. *Taux de survie à 4 ans*

Développement	Délai		
	< 6 mois	> 6 mois	Signification
T. Stationnaire	(127) 69%	(79) 73%	
D. Lent	(47) 45%	(54) 31%	
D. Rapide	(18) 22%	(17) 18%	
Signification	***	***	

— *$p = 0,05$ — **$p = 0,01$ — ***$p < 0,001$ —.
—Les effectifs sont indiqués entre parenthéses.

entre le 1er symptôme et le 1er traitement. Plus complexe, cependant, est le rôle du délai sur la survie pour des vitesses données, les tumeurs stationnaires conservent un bon pronostic, que le délai soit long ou court; les tumeurs à développement lent voient leur pronostic se détériorer légèrement au fur et à mesure que le délai croît, il en va de même pour les tumeurs à développement rapide, mais les taux de survie s'égalisent à peu près à 4 ans, quel que soit le délai.

Cette relation n'a pu, pour le moment, être appréciée pour d'autres cancers,

Quoi qu'il en soit, si l'on ne se réfère qu'aux relations entre délai et survie, on peut pour les tumeurs malignes du sein faire apparaître les données qui sont notées dans le tableau IIIa, b où l'on a successivement étudié les taux de survie en fonction du 1er délai pour les tumeurs de faible extension T 1 et T 2, ou de forte extension T 3 et T 4, on y constate que les cancers de faible extension ont une survie comparable quelle que soit la durée qui s'écoule entre le 1er symptôme et le 1er traitement, les taux de survie étant même légèrement supérieurs lorsque le délai dépasse 12

Tableau IIIa. *Tumeur maligne du sein. Taux de survie en fonction du délai pour les tumeurs de faible extension (T 1 T 2 de la nomenclature de l'U.I.C.C.)*

Délai	Taux de survie à				
	1 an	2 ans	3 ans	4 ans	5 ans
< 2 mois	(131) 91%	(113) 84%	(92) 74%	(70) 66%	(41) 59%
2 à 5 mois	(127) 93%	(111) 77%	(93) 67%	(76) 63%	(48) 65%
6 à 12 mois	(73) 97%	(69) 86%	(52) 79%	(40) 70%	(32) 66%
> 12 mois	(46) 98%	(40) 93%	(33) 91%	(31) 81%	(18) 72%
Signification			*		

— *$p = 0,05$ — **$p = 0,01$ — ***$p < 0,001$ —.
— Les effectifs sont indiqués entre parenthèses.

Tableau IIIb. *Tumeur maligne du sein Taux de survie en fonction du délai pour les tumeurs de forte extension (T 3 T 4 de la nomenclature de l'U.I.C.C.)*

Délai	Taux de survie à				
	1 an	2 ans	3 ans	4 ans	5 ans
< 2 mois	(71) 80%	(56) 61%	(37) 49%	(24) 46%	(12) 25%
2 à 5 mois	(79) 75%	(63) 62%	(54) 48%	(41) 37%	(26) 31%
6 à 12 mois	(87) 71%	(69) 51%	(57) 37%	(41) 34%	(32) 28%
> 12 mois	(91) 64%	(77) 43%	(63) 33%	(49) 24%	(29) 24%
Signification					

Tableau IV. *Tumeur maligne du col utérin. Relation délai — survie à 3 ans pour des cancers d'extension donnée*

Extension	Délai				
	< 2 mois	2 à 5 mois	6 à 11 mois	≧ 12 mois	Signification
T 1	(48) 88%	(73) 81%	(26) 96%	(32) 97%	*
T 2	(101) 71%	(161) 71%	(65) 71%	(63) 70%	
T 3	(139) 45%	(203) 31%	(114) 40%	(102) 46%	*
T 4	(18) 17%	(35) 9%	(21) 10%	(33) 18%	

— *$p = 0,05$ — **$p = 0,01$ — ***$p = 0,001$ —.
— Les effectifs sont indiqués entre parenthèses.

mois. Ceci correspond au fait, facile à comprendre, qu'un cancer resté limité pendant longtemps est un cancer de moindre gravité. Nous retrouvons donc ici la notion de taux d'accroissement.

Pour les cancers plus étendus T 3, T 4, les taux de survie sont un peu plus faibles pour les longs délais et la différence n'est pas significative.

Ce que nous avons indiqué jusqu'ici ne concerne que les tumeurs malignes du sein, il est interessant de vérifier si l'on retrouve les mêmes notions dans d'autres localisations où la vérification du volume de la tumeur et de son extension se révele pratiquement impossible et où nous devons nous contenter d'étudier la relation délai et survie. Mais nous avons vu par les exemples donnés à propos des tumeurs malignes du sein que la notion de délai n'était pas liée à la notion de rythme d'accroissement.

Pour les tumeurs malignes du col utérin (WOLFF, G. P., 1963), le tableau IV donne la relation délai-survie à 3 ans pour des cancers de différentes extensions allant de T 1 à T 4. Ce tableau appel les commentaires suivants:

Tableau V. *Tumeur maligne des Bronches. Taux de survie à 6 mois en fonction du délai 1er symptôme — 1er bilan portant sur 1118 malades*

Délai	Taux de survie à 6 mois
1 mois	55%
2 mois	54%
3 mois	48%
4 mois	47%
5 mois	47%
6 mois	53%
7 à 12 mois	51%
12 mois	60%
24 mois	56%
Signification	N.S.

Pour les T 1, en particulier, les taux de survie les plus élevés s'observent pour les femmes ayant attendu plus de 12 mois avant de consulter. On s'explique d'ailleurs aisément qu'un cancer qui reste limité au col pendant 12 mois, représente une forme favorable.

Pour les T 2 les taux de survie sont identiqués quel que soit le délai.

Pour les T 3 et les T 4 ils s'abaissent pour les délais moyens et s'élèvent pour les délais égaux ou supérieurs à 12 mois.

Le phénomène est particulièrement net pour les T 3 (différence significative au seuil de 5 p. 100). Dans ces dernières formes l'explication est plus complexe.

— Il est évident que les femmes qui consultent au bout d'un an représentent une sélection, puisque sont éliminées toutes celles qui sont mortes moins d'un an après leur premier symptôme.

— En outre, ces femmes présentent sans doute des formes moins évolutives dont les symptômes plus discrets leur ont permis de différer la consultation.

Ces faits expliquent que l'avenir des femmes ayant consulté tardivement est aussi bon que celui des femmes ayant consulté tôt, bien qu'il y ait parmi elles plus de cancers étendus (T 4), mais parmi ces femmes il existe un nombre non négligeable de cancers limités au col (T 1) dont le pronostic est d'autant meilleur que le délai est plus long.

Une autre localisation a fait l'objet de nos études (FLAMANT, 1966). Elles concernent 1.118 cas de tumeurs malignes des bronches. Etant donné la localisation profonde de cette tumeur, il n'a pas non plus été possible d'apprécier les limites de la tumeur elle-même dont l'opacité est habituellement noyée dans l'opacité liée à l'effet de la tumeur sur la ventilation pulmonaire, quoi qu'il en soit, dans un premier tableau, tableau V, nous avons établie une relation entre le taux de la survie à 6 mois en fonction du délai 1er symptôme et 1er bilan clinique. On constate qu'il existe une légère baisse des taux de survie pour les délais compris entre 3 et 5 mois, mais que cette différence n'est pas significative et qu'elle n'existe plus pour les délais les plus élevés. Si par ailleurs, on classe les malades selon ce que nous avons appelé la note de gravité, qui est un ensemble d'éléments basés sur l'observation clinique et qui témoigne d'une certaine agressivité traduite par la symptomatologie plus importante de la tumeur elle-méme, on peut considérer que cette note de gravité a une certaine relation avec l'invasion maligne. Nous avons établi le tableau VI, qui établit le relation entre délai-1er symptôme survie à 6 mois pour des cancers de note de gravité donnée, il n'existe pas non plus de relation entre le délai 1er symptôme 1er bilan et la survie à 6 mois.

Comme on le voit, le délai seul est sans valeur dans certaines localisations, tuels. C'est de l'étude des raisons de ces différences et du mécanisme même de cette action que devrait pour le clinicien découler l'accroissement de ses moyens

Tableau VI. *Tumeur maligne des Bronches (1118 cas). Relation entre délai 1er symptôme — 1er bilan et survie à 6 mois pour des cancers de'note de gravité donnée*

Note de gravité	Délai moyen en mois des sujets vivants à 6 mois	Délai moyen en mois des sujets décédés à 6 mois
0, 1, 2	5,7 (67 sujets)	5,4 (15 sujets)
3	7,1 (60 sujets)	4,5 (18 sujets)
4	7,3 (76 sujets)	4,8 (36 sujets)
5	7,3 (88 sujets)	5,9 (33 sujets)
6	6,6 (73 sujets)	6,1 (49 sujets)
7	6,9 (43 sujets)	7,3 (53 sujets)
8	5,2 (45 sujets)	5,9 (53 sujets)
9	5,7 (24 sujets)	9,3 (53 sujets)
10	8,4 (14 sujets)	8,3 (61 sujets)
11, 12, 13	9,5 (13 sujets)	7,3 (77 sujets)
14 à 19	5 (2 sujets)	7,3 (24 sujets)

ou d'une valeur très relative dans d'autres. Le délai apparait donc comme une composante assez indirecte de la gravité d'une tumeur maligne, tandis que nous l'avons vu, ce qui est essentiel c'est la vitesse d'accroissement. Les différences dans les vitesses d'accroissement avec la signification qu'elles ont pour l'avenir des malades sont pour nous le témoin des relations hôte-tumeur.

Les conséquences des relations hôte-tumeur vont des formes aisément curables jusqu'aux formes que nous ne pouvons espérer guérir par nos moyens ac-

d'action. Dès maintenant, même avant d'avoir tout compris de ce phénomène, certaines des constatations que nous venons de signaler et en particulier l'absence de récidive locale dans les formes N— ont eu une influence sur la thérapeutique et ont pu permettre de la simplifier sans diminuer les chances de guérison des malades. Chaque fois que nous comprenons mieux tel ou tel aspect du mécanisme de l'invasion dans le cancer, nos malades en bénéficient, puisse ce colloque nous permettre un nouveau progrès.

Summary

The concept of host-tumour relationship in cancer is beginning to be taken into account by clinicians in their choice of treatment.

A reflection of this can be seen in man, in the study of the mean "mode of evolution" in groups of patients. It is found the rate of growth, i.e. the time taken for the tumour to reach a certain size, has prognostic significance, whereas the time which has elapsed before treatment, considered alone, has little or no prognostic significance.

Examples are given which relate to tumours of the breast, uterus and bronchii.

Sommaire

La notion de relations Hôte-Tumeur dans le cancer est progressivement reconnue par les cliniciens qui commencent à en tenir compte pour le choix des thérapeutiques.

Il est possible chez l'homme d'en observer un reflet dans l'étude du mode évolutif moyen de groupes de malades. On constate alors que le taux d'accroissement, c'est-à-dire le temps mis pour attendre une certaine extension, a une signification pronostique alors que le délai écoulé avant le traitement considéré isolément en a peu ou pas du tout.

Des exemples sont donnés qui concernent les tumeurs du sein, de l'utérus et des bronches.

Discussion

P. Sträuli: When you speak of the rhythm of growth of a malignant breast tumour, what in your view is the importance of possible changes in the rate of growth such a tumour? A tumour may change from a slow to a fast rate of growth. How is the rate of growth (that is to say, the relationship between size and time) evaluated in such a case?

B. Kellner: Is there any relationship between the rapidity of tumour growth and the histological picture?

Our investigations have shown that the rate of growth is not constant but changes at certain periods, a rapid rate of growth being invariably associated with the formation of pericarcinomatous metastases. Have you made any observations of this kind?

H. Hamperl: When assessing the speed of growth of a given human tumour, one should bear in mind that very definite changes may occur in the lifetime of the tumour: for unknown reasons, it may sometimes grow fast, then slow down for a while or stop growing altogether, and finally resume its original or even a higher speed of growth. The description "slow-growing" or "fast-growing" can therefore only be applied to a tumour in respect of a limited space of time, moreover, even the same tumour may grow at different speeds at the *same* time in different localizations: a small primary tumour sometimes grows very slowly, whereas its metastases grow very fast, forming huge masses. Hence, it is doubtful if the growth rate can successfully be assessed by measuring a single metastasis at different times — a procedure now often used for the characterization of certain human tumours.

G. Barski: In your paper, you said that the host-tumour relationships follow the law of "progression", as formulated by Foulds. What, then, are the roles played, respectively, by the host and by the tumour — i.e. by the cancer cell in the course of its development?

G. Vogt-Hoerner: Histological examination of biopsy material obtained by puncture from breast cancers at an acute clinical stage in the development of the tumour do not reveal any morphological signs characteristic of this acute stage.

R. A. Malmgren: I would like to contribute some data related to the rhythm of growth which Prof. Denoix spoke about.

Dr. Romsdahl and his associates (Romsdahl, *et al.*, 1960) studied malignant melanoma in the human as part of an investigation of factors associated with the finding of cancer cells in the blood. The melanoma is a very appropriate tumour to study for this purpose because one may evaluate its growth by X-ray measurement of skin or lung metastasis. These studies demonstrated a close relationship between the presence of cells in the blood and the rate of growth of the metastasis. The studies also showed that the rate of growth changed at various times in the progress of the disease.

P. Denoix: The paper that I read was based on a statistical study relating to a single group of patients. The results, therefore, can only reflect the average situation for each type of cancer concerned. The usual rhythm of growth of a malignant tumour may be said to be discontinuous, alternating between periods of stability and phases of development (change of speed). These phases of development are as a rule progressive — i.e. the tumour spreads — and only in exceptional cases regressive.

Each site of the disease (tumour, lymph-node, or metastasis) has its own rate of growth.

At the end of a certain time, the extent of the tumour is found to have changed. The relationship between the time that has elapsed and the extent to which the tumour has spread (average rate of growth) is of importance in that, as far as the clinician is concerned, it determines the survival time. Viewed in isolation, however, the terms "spread" or "time elapsed" have little significance.

We attach a great deal of importance to the progressive phases of tumour growth because, for us, they reflect a loss of equilibrium in the host-tumour relationship — an imbalance which is to the detriment of the host. As regards the human subject, we are not yet in a position to say where the responsibility for this imbalance lies — with the tumour for becoming more agressive or with the host for relaxing its control. However this may be, we believe that the inherent instability of the situation should be carefully borne in mind when treating a patient in a progressive phase and that every effort should be made to avoid aggravating matters. Treatment should be directed first of all at restoring the balance and then, once the progressive phase is over, at suppressing, if possible, the manifestations of the malignant disease.

Mrs. VOGT-HOERNER has stated that, at least as far as malignant breast tumours are concerned, no correlation has been observed between histological findings and the various phases of tumour growth. At the Gustave-Roussy Institute we have been looking, so far without success, for biological signs which might help us to pinpoint the moment at which a tumour progresses.

We hope that this Colloquium will produce some new ideas which may enable us to direct our research along more fruitful lines.

Bibliographie

DENOIX, P., De la diversité de certains cancers. A propos de 33.784 observations de cancers du sein, du col de l'utérus, de la langue, de la peau, du larynx, de l'oesophage et du rectum. Inst. Nat. d'Hygiène. Monographie No 5, 257 (1954).

—, and GELLE, X., Mode de décès des malades atteintes de tumeurs malignes du sein en fonction de l'envahissement microscopique du système lymphatique. *Bull. Ass. franç. Cancer* **42**, 548—555 (1955).

FLAMANT, R., Cancers bronchiques à petites cellules. Résultats d'une enquête pronostique inter-hospitalière. *Rev. Tubérc. (Paris)* (1966) **30**, No. 7—8, 819—824.

FOULDS, L., Tumour progression and neoplastic development. In: P. EMMELOT and O. MÜHLBOCK (eds.), *Cellular control mechanisms and cancer*, p. 242—258. Amsterdam: Elsevier Publ. Co. 1964.

Huguenin, R., *Quelques vérités premieres (ou soidisant telles) sur le cancer*, vol. 1, Paris: Masson & Cie. 1946.

Lalanne, C. M., Taux d'accroissement et pronostic des tumeurs malignes du sein. In: Symposium on the prognosis of malignant tumours of the breast, Paris, 11—13 July, 1962 *Acta Un. int. Cancer*. **18**, 807—809 (1962).

Vogt-Hoerner, G., Lalanne, C. M., Juret, P., Lacour, J., Hourtoulle, F., Roujeau, J., Rouquette, C., Survie à la cinquième année d'une série de 237 cancers du sein opérés d'emblée. *Mém. Acad. Chir.* **90**, 653—659 (1964).

Wolff, J. P., Rouquette, C., and Danon, J., Valeur de l'extension clinique dans le pronostic du cancer du col. *Bul. Cancer* **50**, 481—484 (1963).

The Significance of Pericarcinomatous Metastases in Local Growth

B. Kellner

Research Institute of Oncopathology Budapest, Hungary

Various explanations have been suggested for the detachment of tumour-cells. The author's investigations seem to prove that the release of cells occurs following necrobiotic processes. Even under physiological conditions aged and degenerated cells escape from their cell-to-cell connection and desquamate. With the progression of the tumour, ever more and increasingly viable cells become detached from it and find their way into the surrounding tissue spaces and for distant parts. Studying the fate of the cells which escape from the primary tumour into the immediate surroundings, round cancer cells can be identified in nearby tissue spaces, in the lumen of lymphatic and blood vessels, showing the well-known cytodiagnostic criteria of atypia, or they degenerate exactly as tumour cells do in the blood or lymph stream. Initially cancer cells in small numbers are present, later they disseminate over an ever widening area, ever fewer degenerated cells may be seen and more, seemingly viable cells with retained structures occur.

Mitoses are quite exceptional, but round cells with two or more nuclei gradually grow in number until every second or third cell becomes binuclear or multinuclear.

In my opinion the multinuclear cells indicate the first phase of metastasis formation. I propose for them the term "micrometastases". Many workers doubt the viability of multinuclear cells, but histological and cinematographical evidence shows their capacity to multiply later. Soon after clumps of epithelial cells make their appearence which, although giving the impression of isolated processes, are generally believed to represent cross sections of more or less bulky epithelial pegs out from the cancer. We made and photographed true serial sections: it could be shown in each case with certainty that the seemingly isolated epithelial cell clumps near the cancer were definitely independent bodies: pericarcinomatous metastases.

In some cancers the thiniest epithelial cell groups immediately break down to individual cells; this is how round cell-groups and round-cell tumours arise, and this characterizes linitis plastica, and gelatiniform cancer consisting of signet-ring cells. Sometimes the cells of this thiniest metastases become elongated and their growth is of the reticular type of the connective tissue. All this causes a good deal of difficulty proving pericarcinomatous development of metastases in scirrhous and round cell cancers. Nevertheless in most cases no true serial sections are needed to decide the presence or absence of tiny metastases; it suffices to work up several parts of the cancer, and the sections have to include a wider than immediate pericarcino-

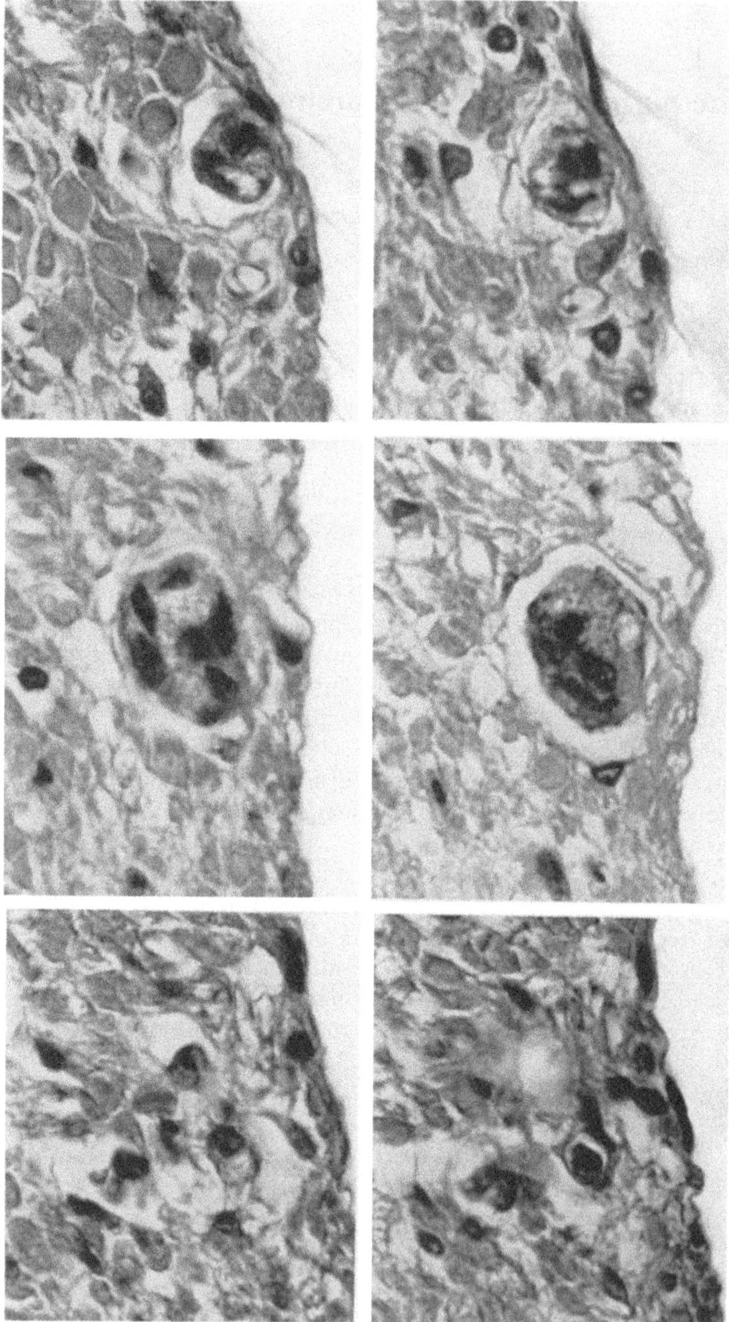

Fig. 1. Carcinoma gelatinosum ventriculi. Small group of tumour cells in

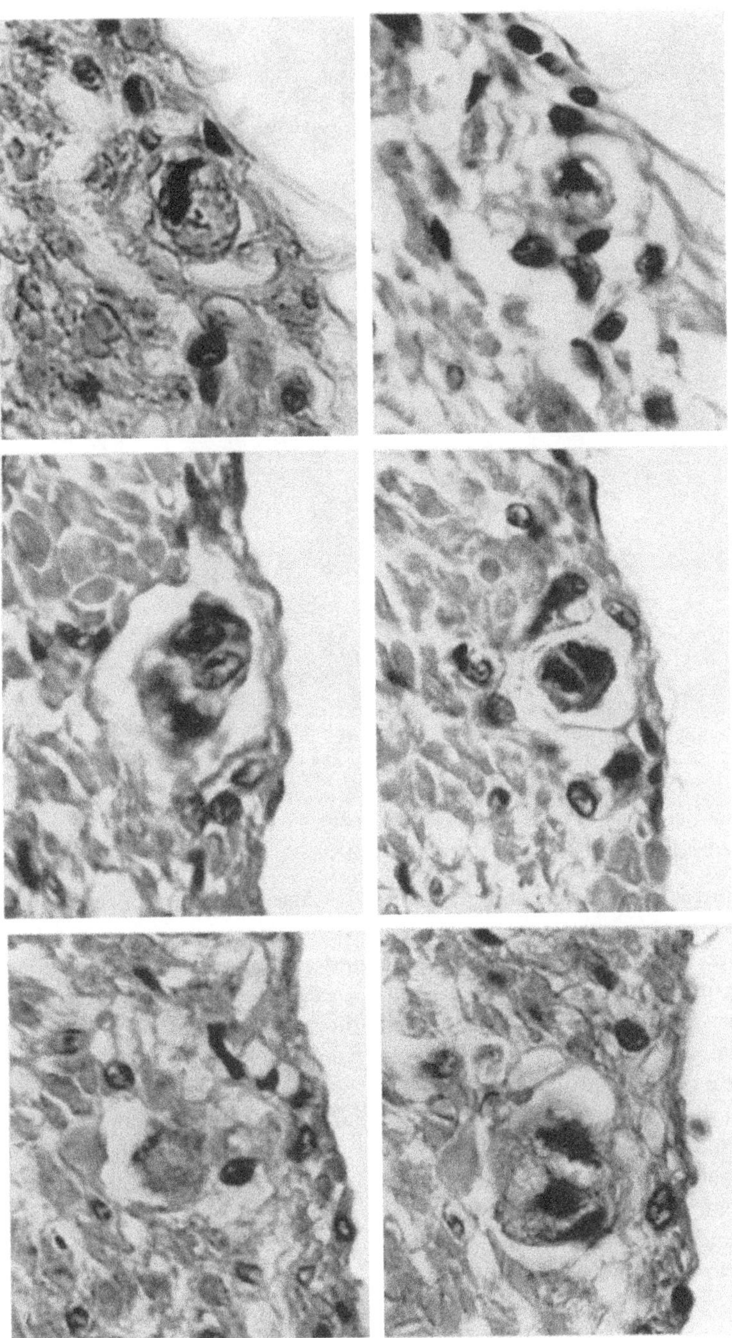

the muscular layer. Their independence is demonstrated in serial sections

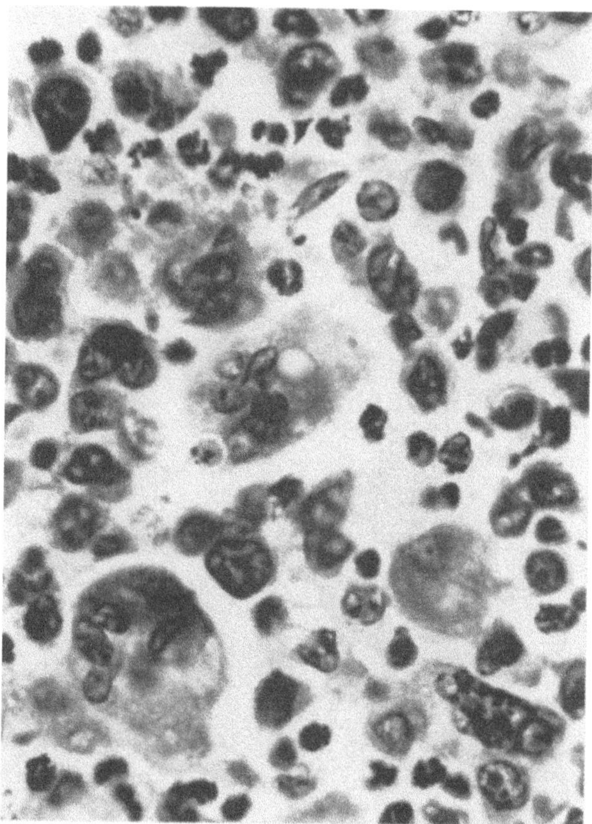

Fig. 2. Methylcholanthrene-induced skin cancer in a mouse. Rounded and multinuclear tumour cells

matous area. The dispersion of pericarcinomatous metastases is uneven: in some spaces they appear sporadically in others rather densely; as is to be expected their number is greatest within lymphatic channels. Most readily recognizable are the multinuclear epithelial cells and those thiniest islands consisting of several cells.

Clinical and histopathological findings seem to prove that pericarcinomatous metastasis formation causes the tumour to burst into eruptive growth.

Many data support the assumption that pericarcinomatous and remote metastases are formed simultaneously with or even somewhat earlier than metastases in the surroundings of the original tumour.

It seems that reliable information about the presence or absence of pericarcinomatous metastases might be a suitable tool for predicting remote metastases. I have found that it actually offers a usable new grading system.

Discussion

B. Kellner: I should like to illustrate some of the statements contained in my paper.

First, I shall try to show that, at a certain phase of its growth, cancer begins to form pericarcinomatous metas-

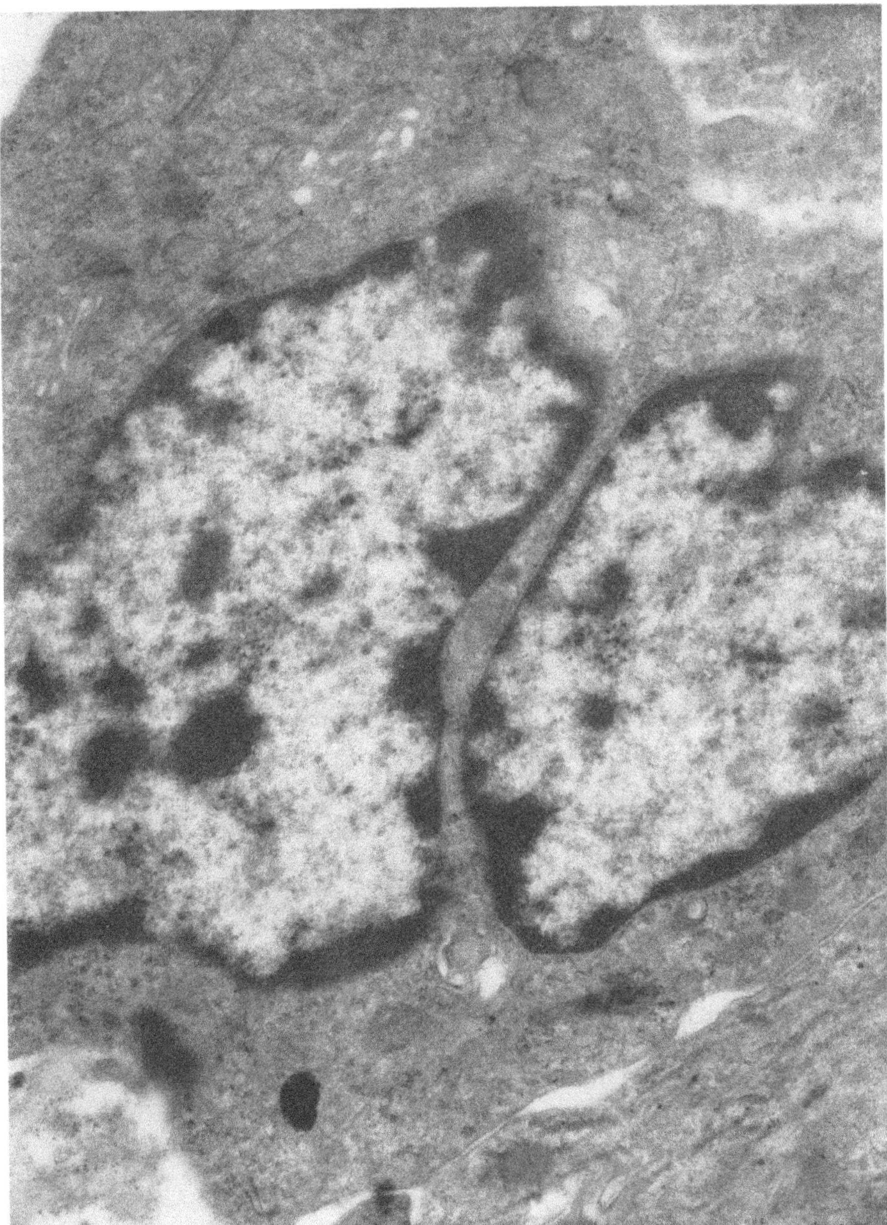

Fig. 3. Binuclear tumour cell from the vicinity of a solid mammary cancer (10,100 × 3.5)

tases. This development can be demonstrated by carefully examining the smallest cell groups in serial sections of tissue taken from the immediate vicinity of the cancer.

The first case seems to be particularly suitable for this purpose: a mucinous carcinoma showing diffuse, infiltrative growth. In the gastric wall, and even in the serosa, epithelial pegs of varying sizes can be seen. One of these I will show in larger magnification, and then in serial sections. The beginning and the end of the multicellular group can also be demonstrated, so that there does not seem to be any connection with the bulk of the cancer. We would thus appear to be dealing here with the smallest kind of metastasis (Fig. 1).

The same findings can be demonstrated in tissue taken from the immediate vicinity of a mouse skin carcinoma induced by means of methylcholanthrene. In this slide, for example, a fairly large area is occupied by a tumourous infiltrate consisting of rounded single cells, with a large number of giant cells among them (Fig. 2). The picture displays a rich array of details, each visual field and preparation changing in appearance. The discontinuity of the cell groups consisting of 2—3 cells can already be seen in some of these sections.

Secondly, in the centre of every epithelial peg and lumen degenerated necrobiotic cells and masses accumulate. At the same time, cells with a less well-preserved structure may be found in the lumina; their number increase during phases of tumour growth.

The necrobiotic area is massively packed with lipids, mucopolysaccharides, and phosphatases. After the breakthrough, inhibition of all these substances occurs in the connective tissue, and it is highly probable that this circumstance has a considerable influence on the alteration of the stroma.

It is rather difficult to obtain definite proof as to whether all these tumour cells are eventually broken down or whether they are capable of forming metastases. My investigations seem to suggest that the steady invasion of the necrobiotic mass containing viable tumour cells into the connective tissue plays an important role not only in the change in chemical composition of the connective tissue but also in the formation of metastases.

Thirdly, I should like to demonstrate the fate of those tumour cells which reach areas adjacent to the tumour. For this purpose, we selected in frozen sections and in half-thin preparations suitable cells and cell groups from around the tumour, and from these we made electron-microscope pictures.

Our results can be summarized as follows: 1. Most of the tumour cells are broken down. Some of them settle in the connective tissue. 2. A close functional interrelationship seems to exist between the tumour cells and connective tissue. 3. The tumour cells, both in the vicinity of the tumour and in the lungs, quite often become transformed into multinuclear cells (Fig. 3). I consider it probable that the surviving cell type is represented mainly by multinuclear cells. 4. The fate of the tumour cells which reach the connective tissue is similar to that of the tumour cells which are transported by the blood-stream to the lung.

Early Invasive Growth as Seen in Uterine Cancer and the Role of the Basal Membrane

H. HAMPERL

Department of Pathology, University of Bonn; Bonn, Germany

In the course of the "progression" of an *in situ* carcinoma of the human uterine cervix towards the typical carcinoma there is a stage called "early stromal invasion" or "early stromal infiltration" (Fig. 1). It is characterized by prong-like fibers, which in their turn are connected with the reticulin network of the deeper layers of connective tissue. This basal membrane is not to be confused with the basal membrane of the electronmicroscopist: This is about 300—400 Å thick

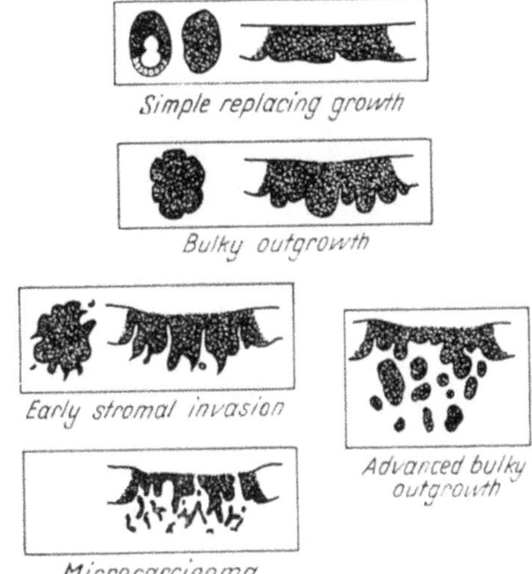

Fig. 1. Different stages of *in situ* carcinoma of the cervix (after HAMPERL)

protrusions of the surface epithelium into the stroma, comparable to the claws of a crayfish. This stage has repeatedly been used for studying at its very beginning, the infiltrating growth which is so characteristic of malignant neoplasms. Such an undertaking was favored by the fact that the border between the surface epithelium and the underlying stroma is clearly marked by a basal membrane composed of or reinforced by reticulin and intimately follows the basal cells and even their foot processes; it is not visible with the light microscope (ZWILLENBERG 1959). The basal membrane, however, to which I shall refer in the following, lies 5,000 Å deeper and is easily stained with the different silver methods. Its content of acid mucopolysaccharides is indicated by rather delicate staining with PAS (PAHLKE, 1954).

H. HAMPERL

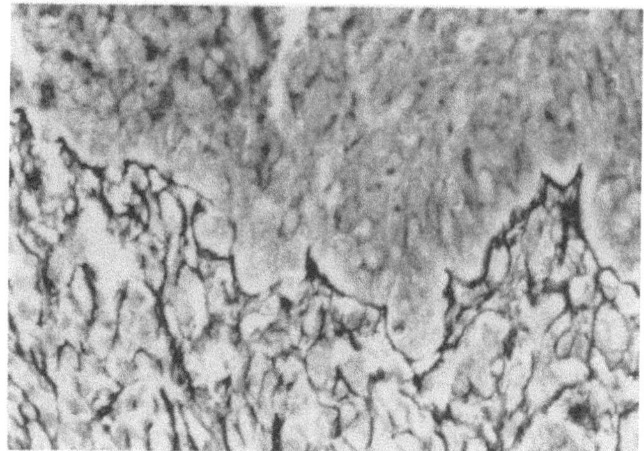

Fig. 2. Rounded protrusions of the epithelium towards the stroma covered by a definite basal membrane. Foote Silver stain. Kernechtrot. × 300

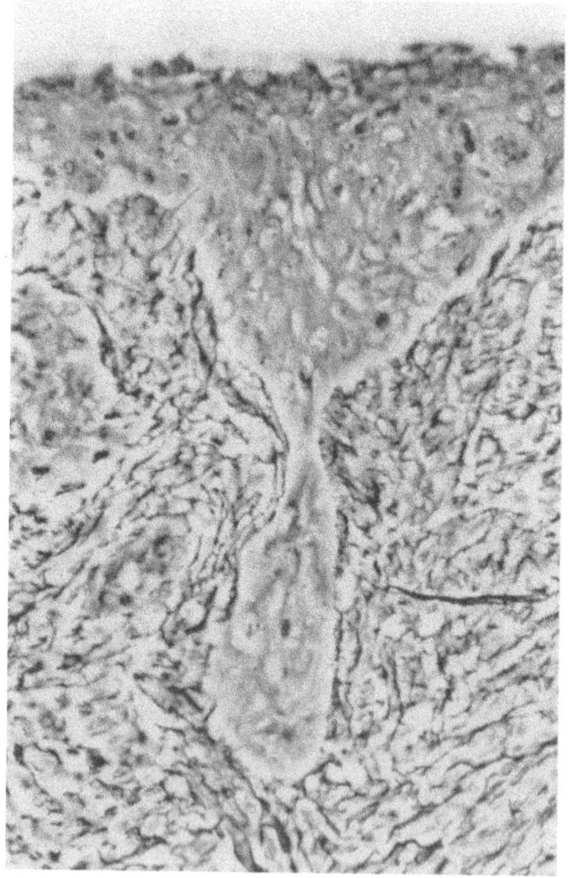

Fig. 3. Deeper-reaching protrusion still covered by basal membrane. Staining as Fig. 2. × 300

On several occasions the assumption has been made (CLAUSS and BERIC, 1958; FIDLER and BOYES, 1959) that the very beginning of malignant growth consists in a break-through or a perforation of this basal membrane by the growing carcinomatous epithelium. Recognition of this perforation would therefore be not only of theoretical but of practical value smallest bulgings (Fig. 2) as well as for the outgrowths which penetrate deeper into the stroma (Fig. 3). Furthermore, the basal membrane is continuous to the basal membrane of the other surface epithelium and does not differ from it in any way. One has the impression that the reticular fibrous structures connected with the basal membrane are somewhat

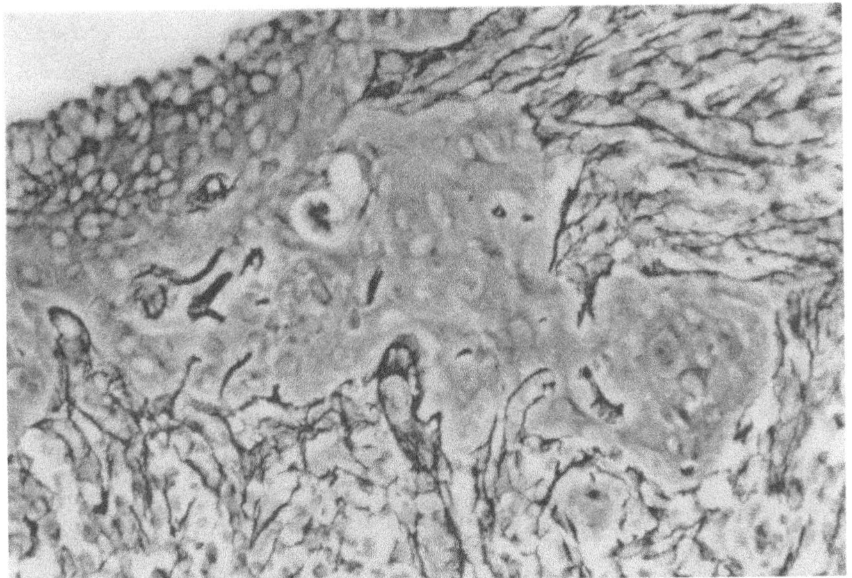

Fig. 4. Discontinuities of the basal membrane filled by infiltrating epithelium. Staining as Fig. 2. ×300

in the diagnosis of early cancer. However, this role of the basal membrane was doubted by others (ULM, 1954; LAX, 1955). An investigation of this question therefore seemed warranted, using the huge material of *in situ* carcinoma cases seen and recorded during the last ten years by our group. The results thereof will now be presented briefly.

Roughly speaking, one can distinguish between two forms of behaviour of the basal membrane in these cases of early stromal invasion by a carcinoma *in situ*.

1. The prong-like epithelial outgrowths are surrounded by an intact basal membrane. This is true for the compressed by the sprouting epithelium, but not visibly damaged.

2. Less frequently one encounters areas where a continuous basal membrane is missing and only the reticulin fibers reaching towards the surface from the depth of the stroma are left behind — as if one had taken away the leaf of a table leaving behind only the supporting structures. The epithelium spreads between and surrounds these reticulin fibers (Fig. 4) and finally encloses them altogether. They are then to be found in a slightly degenerated shape in the middle of the cancerous epithelium (Fig. 5). Findings like these were without doubt considered as a break-through by the proliferating epi-

thelium through the basal membrane. To split the latter open merely physical forces e.g. pressure or some enzymatic activity of the epithelium were considered substantial enough.

I would like to give another explanation of how this picture may originate. It is not all difficult to find in a cancer *in situ* and, even under simply hyper-

ed with the invasion of the stroma by cancerous epithelium: the tendency of the epithelium to grow and to spread how and where ever it is possible: if the basal membrane is intact, it is pushed forward and obviously adapts itself to the growing mass it surrounds by stretching and taking on a new formation; if the basal membrane is lacking, the grow-

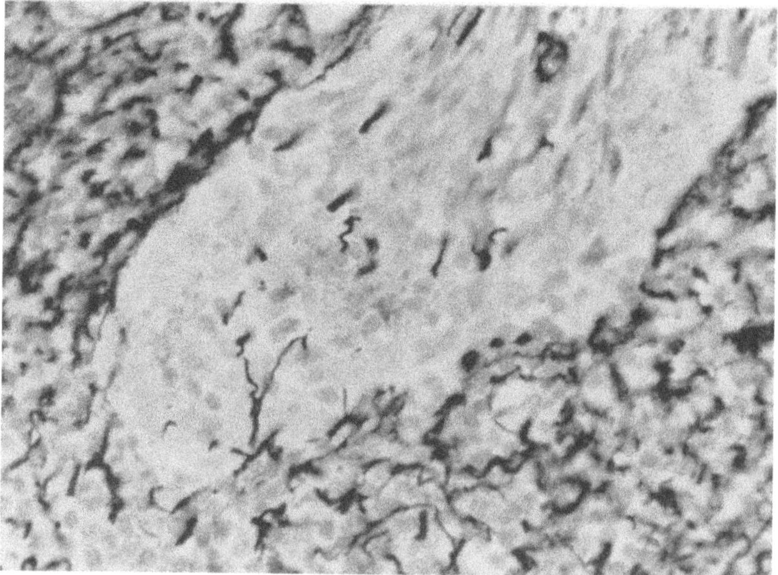

Fig. 5. Desintegrating reticulin fibers enclosed in a peg of cancer cells which is almost entirely surrounded by a (new) basal membrane. Staining as Fig. 2. ×480

plastic epithelium, gaps in the basal membrane of the same shape as described as breakthrough. They occur in areas where there is some chronic inflammation and emigration of leukocytes and lymphocytes through the surface epithelium as Limburg (1956) and Bajardj and Burghardt (1956), have already pointed out. It is most probable that precisely this stream of migrating cells passing through the basal membrane finally causes its temporary disintegration (Cartier, 1959) rather than any influence originating from the growing epithelium itself.

There is one fact common to both occurrences described here and connect-

ing epithelium fills the gaps between the reticulin fibers, in other words: it uses the gaps but does not create them. The reason for the infiltrating growth as it presents itself in our model of early stromal invasion is evidently the internal pressure of the epithelial tissue caused by the higher mitotic rate of the tumour cells.

There is no indication of any lytic enzymatic action of tumour cells directed against any component of the normal tissue and there is no indication of ameboid motility of the tumour cells which would carry single tumour cells far into the normal tissue (Fasske and

THEMANN, 1960). Undeniably, in some tumours there are lytic enzymes present which may favor the infiltrative growth of an existing tumour (SYLVÉN, 1961). This quality is, however, not a general one present in all infiltrating tumours and it therefore cannot explain the infiltrating growth in general. The same may be true for the ameboid motility (ENTERLINE and COMAN, 1950) and migration of single tumour cells so convincingly demonstrated in tissue cultures by BARSKI and BELEHRADEK (1965). Only the internal pressure of the tumour tissue thus remains as an active force on a general plan: The tumour cells do not infiltrate actively by themselves but are rather infiltrated like a mass forcefully injected into a foreing medium. YOUNG (1959) has duplicated these conditions very convincingly in an experiment with gelatine.

We have every reason to assume that the conditions present in "early stromal invasion" and the behaviour of the tumor tissue towards the normal one are repeated later during the invasive growth of the typical malignant tumour: pushing aside normal structures and using existing gaps in them for expansion.

There remains only one last question to be answerd: Are these patterns of the infiltrative growth, once established, maintained during the lifetime of a given tumour or may they interchange? By studying the established tumours it becomes evident that such changes do occur: there are areas of cancer cells which still contain remnants of reticulin fibers they engulfed, but are again surrounded by a typical basal membrane as is usually the case in cervical cancers (FASSKE, 1956; ZWILLENBERG and BERGER, 1957; GLATTHAAR and VOGEL, 1961). Here the shift went obviously in the direction of establishing a basal membrane around a cluster of cancer cells, which primarily filled gaps in the reticulin network (LUIBEL, 1960). The opposite may occur here and there, when the opportunity for such a spread arises locally.

The presence or absence of a basal membrane around normal developing or established cancer cells is therefore to be considered as a purely secondary feature without significance in any theoretical or diagnostic respect.

Discussion

Questions put to H. HAMPERL

J. Leighton: What is your concept of the relationship between carcinoma *in situ* and early invasive carcinoma? in either case, the basement membrane as illustrated in your preparation with reticulum stains was probably intact. Do you make a distinction between the two — i.e. between early invasive carcinoma and carcinoma *in situ*?

H. Hamperl: The stage of early stromal invasion is an intermediate stage between typical carcinoma *in situ* and microcarcinoma of the cervix. From our clinical experience I would rather consider the early stromal invasion as belonging to carcinoma *in situ*, as we have never seen recurrences following local treatment. The presence or absence of the basement membrane does not influence diagnosis or prognosis.

D. F. H. Wallach: Would you expand your concept of pressure within tumours?

H. Hamperl: The internal pressure of a tumour has been measured by ascertaining the resistance of the tumour to the injection of saline: this resistance was distinctly higher than that of the surrounding normal tissue.

P. Mori Chavez: I was impressed by the elegant silver-stained sections shown by Prof. HAMPERL to illustrate his paper on early invasive growth. I should like to question what he calls his paradoxical interpretation — namely, that epithelial tumour cells do not really infiltrate the stromal tissue but are rather infiltrated by the stromal fibres.

I wonder if this interpretation is in conflict with the new ideas about a local immune reaction that prevents or allows tumour cells to infiltrate and grow?

H. Hamperl: There is a misunderstanding here. To make my point clear, I used an exaggeration (or paradox) when I said: the epithelial cells do not infiltrate actively, but are rather infiltrated passively like a mass forcefully injected into a tissue. I have never held that the internal pressure of a growing cell mass is the one and only factor responsible for invasive growth. There may be immunological factors involved, among others. I know, however, of no immunological investigations concerning or correlated with the development of cancer *in situ* of the cervix.

P. Mori Chavez: There are some clinical and pathological reports to the effect that carcinoma of the uterine cervix may remain in the *in situ* stage for many years. Also, there are well-known, and well-proven cases of a spontaneous cure in the literature. One of these papers is by Dr. FRED STEWART, the former pathologist at the Memorial Hospital, New York (Texas Medical Report). It is supposed that tumour cells might be subject to some mechanism of control — either in the early stage of *in situ* carcinoma, or later on in well-developed and invasive cancers — which prevents or allows them to infiltrate and grow.

H. Hamperl: The papers quoted by Dr. MORI CHAVEZ are familiar to me, but they concern tumours other than carcinoma *in situ*. It still has to be proved whether or not these immunological explanations hold true for all tumours and especially for carcinoma *in situ* of the cervix. It would, of course, be a most fascinating subject for study.

I. Petra: Professor HAMPERL, do you consider that the mechanism of invasion involves merely a mechanical factor — i.e. the pressure exerted on the basement membrane, leading to its destruction — or do the tumour cells perhaps contain enzymes which might contribute to the destruction of the basement membrane?

Have you also made use of histochemical and biochemical tests in your histological studies?

In our experience, tumour cells display certain histochemical changes which might reflect an additional biochemical or hormonal action capable of influencing the local mechanism of cancer invasion.

H. Hamperl: I do not think that the growing epithelium destroys the basement membrane either by pressure or by enzymatic action. On the contrary, it can easily be demonstrated that the basement membrane disappears even in places where there is no epithelial outgrowth, but only an emigration of leucocytes and lymphocytes. I myself have not done any histochemical studies in this connection as I was able to rely on the work of Dr. SCHMIDT-MATTHIESEN (Göttingen) who clearly demonstrated that histochemical changes occurred in the mesenchymal structures prior to the invasive growth of a carcinoma *in situ*.

D. F. H. Wallach: The experiments of S. J. YOUNG do show that injection of fluid produces a greater increase in hydrostatic pressure in tumours than in normal tissues, but this does not imply a chronic gradient of hydrostatic pressure between the tumour and its environment. Acute increases in pressure may be due to anomalies in vascularity and tissue architecture. Even if there is an abnormally high hydrostatic pressure in tumours it is not clear how, in an incompressible (aqueous) medium, this would affect the mobility of single cells or small cell groups.

H. Hamperl: The internal pressure of a growing mass will increase as long as its rate of new cell formation is higher than that of the surrounding tissues. It may level off temporarily or permanently if the mitotic rate decreases and stays low. But of course factors such as haemorrhages, oedema, etc. may have the same effect on the internal pressure as cell proliferation. The point about early stromal invasion is just that these other changes do not occur here.

P. Sträuli: Your statement that only the internal pressure of the tumour tissue is in active force in invasive growth is of fundamental importance. I would therefore like to aks you to what extent this statement may be applied to tumours other than carcinoma *in situ* of the human uterine cervix.

G. Barski: As regards Prof. HAMPERL'S hypothesis that invasive growth is, essentially, a function of the mechanical pressure inside the tumour: if this hypothesis is correct, the pressure would be greater inside malignant tumours than inside benign tumours. This would be easy to verify both in patients and in animal experiments.

H. Hamperl: I think Dr. BARSKI'S suggestion is a very valuable one and should be followed up.

F. Lacour: If we take the example of transplanted tumours which, despite their rapid growth, metastasize seldom if at all, it is difficult to believe that internal pressure can be a decisive factor in the diffusion of cancer cells.

It is even more difficult to explain, by reference to pressure alone, the appearance of metastases from tranplanted tumours in animals treated with cortisone or X-rays. I do not think it would be logical in these cases to disregard the possibility that immunological factors may be involved.

H. Hamperl: I cannot and will not exclude other factors besides internal pressure which may favour the formation of metastases, such as immunological disturbances. On the other hand, it should be borne in mind that cortisone and X-rays have a very definite influence on the reaction of mesenchymal tissues in the stroma surrounding a tumour; they may, as it were, open the door for a tumour to start infiltrating in the interstitial spaces. The formation of metastases seems to me more closely linked with the enhanced disjunction or lowered cohesion of tumour cells than with their infiltrating growth.

R. E. Madden: Dr. CHARLES KARPAS and myself have some evidence from our laboratory that an experimental tumour (Walker 256) growing in the lathyritic rat has an early growth advantage. In lathyrism, a disease produced by certain nitrile compounds, there is a weakness of surrounding connective tissue. If local pressure is a factor in containing the early tumour, this is the result we would expect.

Others have injected this tumour into the foot-pad of the rat, then encased the paw in a cast. At sacrifice, the tumours in the encased paws were much smaller than those of controls without casts. This is further evidence that local pressure might control the size of the tumours.

J. Leighton: There are specific clinical examples in which pressure effects are suggested. Colloid carcinoma of the breast or gastrointestinal tract appears to spread owing to the pressure exerted by the mucus produced by the tumor. A parallel might be found in infections with a pathogenic yeast, *Cryptccoccus neoformans.*

This organism synthesizes a mucoid material which help it to spread when it infects the brain.

M. Abercrombie: It is not clear to me why, in the case of an epithelial tumour growing by pressure, the direction of least resistance should be inwards into the connective tissue, and not outwards from the surface.

H. Hamperl: The superficial layers of a squamous epithelium, such as the epithelium covering the cervix, show a much greater cohesion than the epithelial cells in the more basal layers. This fact may provide an explanation as to why, when internal pressure increases precisely in these layers, the epithelium with its back to a cohesive surface "escapes" towards the stroma.

My demonstration was concerned only with the early stromal invasion of carcinoma *in situ;* this invasion provides us with a good model for assessing at least one factor influencing infiltrative growth, i.e. the basement membrane, and furthermore enables us to discuss the question of the internal pressure of a growing cell mass. I think we can rightly assume that the same factors play a role in infiltrative growth at other sites as well, in combination of course with other locally prevailing factors.

References

BAJARDI, F., and BURGHARDT, E., Ergebnisse von histologischen Serienschnittuntersuchungen beim Carcinoma colli O. *Arch. Gynäk.* **189**, 392—403 (1956).

BARSKI, G., and BELEHRADEK, J., Etude microcinématographique du mécanisme d'invasion cancéreuse en culture de tissu normal associé aux cellules malignes. *Exp. Cell Res.* **37**, 464—480 (1965).

CARTIER, R., Recherches sur les ultrastructures des épithéliomas intraépithéliaux pavimenteux cervicaux (Reconstitution topographique). *Bull. Féd. Soc. Gynéc. Obstét. franç.* **11**, 463—477 (1959).

CLAUSS, J., u. BERIC, B., Über das Mikrokarzinom am Collum uteri. *Oncologia (Basel)* **11**, 23—41 (1958).

ENTERLINE, H. T., and COMAN, D. R., The ameboid motility of human and animal neoplastic cells. *Cancer Res.* **3**, 1033—1038 (1950).

FASSKE, E., Das Verhalten der sog. Zona limitans bei Plattenepithelcarcinomen. *Z. Krebsforsch.* **61**, 240—254 (1956).

—, and THEMANN, H., Die elektronenmikroskopische Struktur menschlicher Carcinome. *Beitr. path. Anat.* **122**, 313—344 (1960).

FIDLER, H. K., and BOYES, D. A., Patterns of early invasion from intra-epithelial carcinoma of the cervix. *Cancer (Philad.)* **12**, 673—680 (1959).

GLATTHAAR, E., and VOGEL, A., Zur Ultrastruktur des Plattenepithelcarcinoms der Portio. *Gynaecologia (Basel)* **151**, 212—226 (1961).

HAMPERL, H., Definition and classification of so-called carcinoma *in situ.* Cancer of the Cervix. Ciba Foundation Study Group No 3. London: J. & A. Churchill Ltd. 1959.

LAX, H., Über Unterschiede in der Histogenese des Collumcarcinoms und daraus erkennbare Grade der Malignität. *Arch. Gynäk.* **185**, 415—440 (1955).

LIMBURG, H., *Die Frühdiagnose des Uteruscarcinoms.* Stuttgart: Georg Thieme 1956.

LUIBEL, F. J., SANDERS, E., and ASHWORTH, C. T., An electron microscopic study of carcinoma *in situ* and invasive carcinoma of the cervix uteri. *Cancer Res.* **20**, 357—361 (1960).

PAHLKE, G., Elektronenmikroskopische Untersuchungen an der Interzellularsubstanz des menschlichen Sehnengewebes. *Z. Zellforsch.* **39**, 421 (1954).

SYLVÉN, B., On the biological mechanism underlying the destructive capacity of malignant cells. *Biochim. Biol. sper.* **1**, 8—20 (1961a).

ULM, R., in T. ANTOINE (ed.), *Klinische Fortschritte „Gynäkologie".* Wien u. Innsbruck: Urban & Schwarzenberg 1954.

YOUNG, J. S., The invasive growth of malignant tumors: an experimental interpretation based on elastic-jelly models. *J. Path. Bact.* **77**, 321—339 (1959).

ZWILLENBERG, L. O., *Beiträge zur Kenntnis des geschichteten Pflasterepithels*. Basel u. New York: S. Karger 1959.

ZWILLENBERG, L. O., and BERGER, J., Einige morphologische Beobachtungen am normalen und pathologischen Pflasterepithel de Portio vaginalis uteri. *Oncologia (Basel)* **10**, 1—10 (1957).

Locomotion of Cancer Cells in vivo Compared with Normal Cells*

Sumner Wood, jr., M.D., R. Robinson Baker, M.D., Barbara Marzocchi

*Department of Pathology Johns Hopkins Hospital***
Baltimore, Maryland 21205, U.S.A.

Script by Leo L. Leveridge, M.D.

Among the various possible mechanisms by which cancer invades its host, the active motility of carcinoma cells has invited study since first observed *in vitro* with time-lapse photomicrography several decades ago-here seen accelerated 240 times.

For an understanding of the mechanisms of invasion, as they occur in the living host, methods have been developed for studying carcinoma cells *in vivo*, and for comparing them quantitatively with normal cells under similar circumstances.

To obtain tumour cells for this study, a laparotomy under aseptic conditions is performed on a rabbit, 14 to 18 days after an intraperitoneal seeding. A slightly bloody ascitic fluid has formed. It is rich in anaplastic V 2 carcinoma cells, (originally derived from a squamous cell papilloma of the rabbit skin, by Kidd and Rous) — merely one of many diverse types of cancer, but a useful model for study in the rabbit. Between 100 and 300 milliliters of ascitic fluid, containing about 10 million carcinoma cells per milliliter are harvested. A sample is removed for microscopic inspection of representative cells.

The V 2 carcinoma cell has been modified here to grow predominantly as single cells in the ascitic fluid. They have not been traumatized. Occasional large, bizarre forms are seen. These cells are inserted directly into the rabbit ear chamber by removing and replacing the coverslip.

The assembly of a rabbit ear chamber is demonstrated for the orientation of those unfamiliar with this research technic: The modified Barclay-type chamber is constructed around this one inch Tuffax plastic disc. A plastic ring is cemented with ethylene chloride to the upper surface of the perforated disc, that will be the floor of the chamber. To the under surface of the disc a cylindrical plastic plug is cemented. A skirt of wide-mesh Dacron is also cemented to the undersurface of the disc. On the upper side of the disc, a ring of Teflon $1/_2$ mil thick is laid in place to serve as a spacer that will hold the cover slip 13 microns above the floor of the chamber — the perforated disc thru which it will be vascularized.

* Grateful appreciation is expressed to Dr. George C. Gey for the *in vitro* footage employed in the introduction of this film.

** This investigation is supported in part by research funds from the USPHS (CA 5319), Susan Greenwall Foundation and the American Cancer Societyl.

This article contains the narration for a research 16 mm film, available upon request from the authors.

The fragile glass cover slip is protected by a Teflon gasket and retained by a stainless steel ring, completing the assembly of the chamber, that, after sterilization, is inserted in the long, wide ear of a Laboratory Lop rabbit. Although the insertion of the ear chamber is performed under anesthesia, the subsequent observations are made without use of anesthetics. Immediately adjacent to the central artery, a $1/4$ inch hole is punched thru the ear for insertion of the plug beneath the chamber. The skin is elevated from the cartilage to produce a pocket for the Dacron skirt. Additional skin is excised to accommodate the ring that forms the wall of the ear chamber. The plug is narrowed where it is cemented beneath the floor of the chamber, and enters the punched-out hole in the cartilage like a collar-button into a starched shirt collar. The plug prevents the skin of the back of the ear from covering the light path to the chamber. The wide-meshed Dacron skirt is inserted between skin and cartilage to prevent growth of skin under the chamber. The chamber has filled with blood.

The blood clot which formed in the chamber is replaced, through the holes in the floor of the chamber, by growth of blood vessels, lymphatics and connective tissue. The tissue matures in 2 to 4 weeks when it is ready for microscopic study and cinemicrography. Permanent film records are made that can be studied repeatedly and analyzed mathematically. When the rabbit ear chamber is placed under the microscope for inspection of the connective tissue, at low power, an arteriole is seen, and here two venules. They are connected by arterio-venous anastomoses, and capillaries. The capillaries are identified at higher power by their delicate, thin walls, lacking the muscular elements seen in the arterioles and in the anastomosing shunts. The

capillary blood flow reverses direction frequently.

These leukocytes are filmed and projected at 24 frames per second, so that what is seen here is the same as the preparation viewed directly through the microscope. When observed at the speed with which it occurs, active motility of these cells is not discernable, but with time-lapse, photographed at one frame per second, the locomotion of these cells becomes apparent, can be analysed, and rates of movement measured.

Compared to normal cinemicrography at 24 frames per second, time-lapse photography at one frame per second accelerates action 26 times. This report is based upon long continuous observations recorded by time-lapse on over 40,000 feet of 16 mm film exposed at one frame per second. To determine the rate of locomotion of a given cell, the film is projected on a Moviola screen, one frame at a time, for analysis. The initial location of a cell is marked on the screen. This granulocyte, for example, was followed frame-by-frame, as it moved within the lumen of this venous capillary or post-capillary venule, upon the endothelium. The path of the granulocyte was traced on the Moviola screen:

The path is measured, and its length converted to microns. The time interval is derived from the number of frames of film exposed while the cell migrates this distance. Division of the distance moved, by the time interval, gives the average rate of locomotion.

The same (6 to 7 microns per minute) rate of locomotion is observed with cells from rabbit skin cancer — the V 2 carcinoma. The motility of these neoplastic epidermal cells contrasts with the non-motility of normal epidermal cells.

This low power view of an autologous skin graft in a rabbit ear chamber shows that it is well-vascularized, but these normal epidermal cells remain as a firm group exhibiting strong cohesiveness. The visible keratin content confirms their epidermal character. Observed for a year, these epithelial cells continue to exhibit *no* apparent motility, even when these time-lapse photographic methods are used.

Most of the time, tissue macrophages also are virtually non motile. The nonmotility is seen again with this macrophage. During the infrequent periods when macrophages *do* migrate, a maximum of $^1/_{30}$ of a micron per minute has been calculated. The sliggishness of macrophages contrasts with the V-2 cells which move about 200 times faster. Fibroblasts move as slowly and infrequently as do macrophages.

On the other hand, granulocytes move at approximately the same average speed ($6^1/_2$ microns per minute) as the V-2 carcinoma cells. Thus, these cells move as much as the width of a red blood cell in one minute. If they moved continuously, they would travel a total distance of one centimeter in ten days.

Lymphocytes near or among the V-2 carcinoma cells move at a similar rate.

Granulocytes on the endothelium within small blood vessels were once stated to be propelled by the flow of blood. Time-lapse photomicrography however, clearly shows this granulocyte moving across stream, then against the blood flow, or with it, at approximately the same speed regardless of its direction in relation to the flow of blood. This observation was confirmed by determining the rates of locomotion with the methods demonstrated earlier.

Over 900 granulocytes in the connective tissue of rabbit ear chambers have been analysed: Their mean rate of locomotion was 6.7 microns per minute. The speediest granulocyte moved 28.2 microns per minute. Preliminary studies of a smaller

number of V-2 cancer cells gave similar results.

At low power, one month after implantation, a layer of tumour cells fills the rabbit ear chamber. At high power, this group of cells was observed first in a random arrangement. These cells then migrated into an acinar pattern which persisted for $3^1/_2$ minutes. The pattern gradually became disorganized. Finally the cells formed an epidermoid or squamous cell pattern.

The film obtained during the continuous 30 minute recordings is projected again, showing how initially undifferentiated cancer cells may form the pattern of an adenocarcinoma, then again become undifferentiated. Like granulocytes and lymphocytes (in the absence of chemotaxis) V-2 carcinoma cells exhibit non-directional motility at 6 to 7 microns per minute and lack contact inhibition. After 13 minutes, these cells changed their pattern to a squamous cell or epidermoid arrangement. From these continuous time-lapse photomicrographic records it appears that a group of the same cells is capable of forming either differentiated or undifferentiated patterns so that, what is seen in fixed and stained sections of some tumours, may be a matter of the moment in time that happened to be selected for examination. Histologic sections of this tumour growing in connective tissue outside of a chamber reveal that, while the *predominant* portion is undifferentiated, selected areas show acinar or squamous cell differentiation. They closely resemble the formations just observed in the rabbit ear chamber.

In time-lapse photography, lymphocytes, as seen near the center of the screen, are distinguished by their tails. Three small lymphocytes. Their motility attests to their viability. This lymphocyte will gradually enter the cancer cell. Meanwhile another lymphocyte has entered half-way. Now both lymphocytes are in the malignant cell ... later, the third lymphocyte starts in. A pseudopod reaches around the lymphocyte as it is engulfed by the cancer cell. All three lymphocytes now move within the cytoplasm of the cancer cell. This inter-relationship between cancer cells and the host's blood cells is shown again by repeating the film:

The engulfment of lymphocytes by other cells *in vitro* was first reported by WARREN LEWIS in 1925. The phenomenon has been rediscovered since, and eventually was termed "emperipolesis". Many have contended that it occurs only *in vitro*, but as this time-lapse photomicrography of the rabbit ear chamber first demonstrated, small lymphocytes can also enter V-2 carcinoma cells *in vivo*. An erythrocyte likewise is engulfed by another cancer cell.

The significance of this inter-reaction of normal cells with V-2 cancer cells is, so far, unknown.

The mechanisms of cellular locomotion are not fully understood either, nor the bonding of non-motile and motile cells. These time-lapse studies, however, provide evidence that the penetration of surrounding tissues by these cancer cells can be explained, at least in part, by the intrinsic motility of individual cells.

The observation and measurement of cellular locomotion *in vivo* offers a useful technic for the development and testing of methods designed to control the invasion and spread of cancer.

Discussion

Questions put to S. WOOD

D. B. Amos: 1. When lymphocytes have been observed to enter tumour cells *in vitro*, no harm appears to result to either tumour or lymphoid cell. This has been reported by several authors. Dr. WEISER has produced a film of the reactions of histiocytes and ascites tumour cells. The histiocytes can attach to the tumour cell, but damage is not observed in that system. It has been seen later in a plaque technique. Have you observed any damage in the *in vivo* system?

2. There is much interest in the conversion of lymphocytes into histiocyte-like cells. We have been following this in electron-microscope studies, and are attempting to find out whether this type of transformation precedes the damage to target cells reported by ROSENAU and MOON, ROSE, and others. Did you see any kind of conversion in your studies?

S. Wood: When lymphocytes which entered the V 2 carcinoma celle were observed and photographed *in vivo*, both the lymphocytes and the tumour cells appeared undamaged. The lymphocytes moved about within the cytoplasm of the tumour cell which continued to demonstrate activity of the nucleus and cytoplasmic membrane. In other instances, lymphocytes have been observed to intermingle with tumour cells, sometimes partially surrounding the latter. In this situation, too, the lymphocytes as well as the tumour cells appear to be unaltered.

We have not as yet detected any conversion of cell types *in vivo* in the rabbit ear chamber.

J. Leighton: Do you have any data on the movement of fibroblasts in the rabbit ear chamber? Those of us who study invasiveness of cancer in tissue cultures are frequently impressed by the motility of fibroblasts.

S. Wood: We have not observed locomotion of fibroblasts *in vivo*. The virtual absence of locomotion by macrophages during formation of the membrane of the rabbit ear chamber (wound healing) has previously been described by several authors [cf. J. Path. Bact. *48*, 79 (1939) and Quart. J. exp. Physiol. *50*, 79 (1965)]. These authors attributed any changes in position by macrophages to passive movements of the cells within the fluid milieu present at the encroaching edge of the granulation tissue. In addition, it should be pointed out that we permit our chambers to develop for 3—6 months before use to assure a mature connective tissue network with innervation of the blood vessels. At this stage in their development, movement of fibroblasts would be even less expected.

M. Feldmann: Are the spots of penetration of leucocytes through the endothelium randomly distributed, or does the spot of penetration of one leucocyte indicate a region of particular susceptibility to granulocyte penetration?

S. Wood: By *in vivo* light microscopy it has been impossible to predict in advance the precise site within the venous capillary of endothelial penetration by leucocytes. Once a leucocyte has attached to and emigrated through the endothelium, a defect may persist through which additional leucocytes [cf. Amer. J. Anat. *57*, 385—438 (1935) and J. exp. Med. *102*, 655—668 (1955)] or carcinoma cells [cf. Arch. Path. *66*, 550—568 (1958)] may pass into the perivascular connective tissue.

By electron microscopy, Marchesi and his colleagues have demonstrated that granulocytes and monocytes penetrate between endothelial cell junctions, and the lymphocyte may penetrate by entering the endothelial cell and traversing its cytoplasm [cf. Proc. roy. Soc. B *159*, 283—290 (1963/64) and Ann. N.Y. Acad. Sci. *116*, 774—788 (1964)].

E. J. Ambrose: I should like to refer to the sudden increase in the rate of movement of a group of tumour cells shown in Dr. Wood's film. In time-lapse films of tissue culture we sometimes see a cell which is firmly attached at one point to neighbouring cells. This cell is moving actively; it stretches the membrane in the region of contact. When the cell — to — cell contact breaks suddenly, the moving cell immediately increases its rate of migration. I am wondering whether a contact of this kind may be involved in the sequence shown in Dr. Wood's film.

S. Wood: I do not know what the explanation for this event may be. The ranges of locomotion of the V 2 carcinoma *in vivo* varied from a minimum of 3.1 to a maximum of 13.0 μ/min, with a mean of 6.46 μ/min, $\pm$ a standard error of 0.52.

Le Pouvoir Invasif des Cellules Transformées Étudié en Culture in vitro

GEORGES BARSKI

Laboratoire de Culture de Tissus et de Virologie, Institut Gustave-Roussy, Villejuif (Val de Marne), France

Le corollaire habituel à longue échéance de la culture *in vitro* des cellules animales est leur transformation. Les cellules que nous observons dans les cultures adaptées à la vie et à la prolifération suivie *in vitro* sont sur de nombreux points différentes de celles présentes dans les tissus lors de leur explantation *in vitro*.

Ces points de différence sont notamment:

1. l'acquisition du pouvoir de prolifération constante et apparemment illimitée;

2. des modifications de morphologie cellulaire, nucléaire et nucléolaire, aussi bien que cytoplasmique;

3. des modifications du caryotype;

4. des changements du comportement «social» des cellules transformées, vis-à-vis de leurs semblables et vis-à-vis d'autres cellules;

5. des modifications de différenciation fonctionnelle, du métabolisme et d'équipement enzymatique, dans l'ensemble mal définies;

6. l'acquisition éventuelle des propriétés invasives, attestées par le pouvoir de produire des tumeurs malignes après inoculation chez l'animal isologue.

En rapport avec cette dernière propriété qui nous intéresse tout spécialement, l'essentiel devient d'établir quels sont les rapports pouvant exister entre celle-ci et l'ensemble d'autres caracté-ristiques propres aux cellules transformées et que nous venons d'énumérer.

Il serait en effet capital de pouvoir juger et mesurer le pouvoir envahissant des cellules en dehors de l'épreuve ultime qui est l'inoculation de ces cellules à l'animal histo-compatible, c'est à-dire en greffe isologue ou autologue, et prévoir le degré de «cancérisation» de cellules d'après leur comportement en dehors de l'organisme, dans des conditions appropriées *in vitro*.

Le système des souches cellulaires, que nous avons développé dans notre laboratoire à partir du tissu pulmonaire de la souris C57BL, s'est avéré particulièrement utile dans cette étude. Au cours des expériences débutées en 1961 [1], nous avons obtenu deux souches cellulaires pulmonaires qui, au bout des premiers 6 mois de culture *in vitro*, se sont transformées dans ce sens que leur caryotype comportait régulièrement 58 à 80 chromosomes parmi lesquels ont apparu plus tard des chromosomes métacentriques inhabituels. Les cellules à caryotypes normaux, caractérisées chez la souris par 40 chromosomes télocentriques, ont finalement disparu complètement. Cette transformation s'est traduite également par un rythme de multiplication accéléré et par des modifications marquées de morphologie cellulaire.

Une de ces deux souches, la P 1, traitée au cours de passages successifs par la trypsine, produisit, lors de l'inoculation à l'animal, des tumeurs à partir du 7ème mois de culture. Cependant, la souche parallèle P 2 est restée dépourvue de tout pouvoir cancéreux pendant les premiers 20 mois de culture. Elle s'est cancérisée dans une certaine mesure par la suite.

Dans plusieurs séries d'expériences plus récentes, nous avons développé dans des conditions similaires et à partir du même tissu (poumon de la souris C57BL adulte) de nombreuses souches et clones cellulaires présentant une gamme étendue de malignité [2].

Nous avons accumulé dans l'ensemble des données concernant 9 lignées cellulaires représentant des populations primaires mixtes et 3 lignées cellulaires clonales. Dans 8 cas sur 9, les lignées primaires, essayées entre le 8ème et le 24ème mois de culture *in vitro,* produisaient, lors de leur inoculation à la souris isologue, des tumeurs à croissance progressive plus ou moins rapide. Ces lignées étant toutes d'origine identique — poumon normal de souris C57BL (femelle) — présentaient ainsi après le même délai de culture *in vitro* et le même degré d'adaptation à la prolifération illimitée en culture, une gamme étendue de malignité. Les plus malignes, comme la PTT 12 ou le clone 61, tuaient l'animal en moins de 3 mois après inoculation de 10^5 cellules; d'autres, comme la lignée P 6, ne produisaient pas de tumeurs même après inoculation de 2 à 3 millions de cellules à des souris nouveau-nées.

Ces lignées cellulaires s'ajoutaient à celles dont nous disposions antérieurement et qui provenaient des souches développées, à partir du tissu sous-cutané de la souris C3H, par K. Sanford *et coll.* [3] ainsi que des souches hybrides obtenues dans notre laboratoire [4].

En utilisant ces deux systèmes de lignées cellulaires, nous avons entrepris des expériences dont le but était de rechercher des critères «objectifs» du pouvoir invasif de ces cellules en dehors de l'animal isologue. Nous avons d'abord pu établir un parallèle entre le pouvoir cancéreux des lignées malignes, N 1 et M 1 (souche hybride) chez les souris de la souche autochtone C3H et le pouvoir invasif très prononcé de ces mêmes souches vis-à-vis du mésonéphros de poulet en cultures organotypiques préparées selon la technique de Et. et Em. Wolff [5].

Les souches de cellules pulmonaires originaires de la souris C57Bl obéissaient dans l'ensemble à la même règle. Nous pouvons citer comme exemple d'une part les souches clonales Cl 91 et Cl 92, qui, inoculées chez des souris C57Bl adultes après 18 à 21 mois *in vitro,* ne donnaient pas de tumeurs, et d'autre part, la souche PTT 12 et son clone dérivé 61 qui produisaient dans les mêmes conditions, avec des doses de l'ordre de 3×10^4 cellules, des tumeurs envahissantes à croissance très rapide et fatale. Toutes ces souches cellulaires étaient très comparables par le degré de leur adaptation à la vie *in vitro,* le rythme de multiplication et les caractéristiques caryologiques (hypotétraploidie et présence de chromosomes anormaux). Or, associées aux fragments de mésonéphros en cultures organotypiques, les cellules du clone 91 par exemple se montraient incapables d'envahir ces cultures tandis que les cellules de la souche PTT 12 les infiltraient très intensément et pouvaient être repiquées dans ces conditions de mésonéphros à mésonéphros pendant 90 jours au moins.

Par conséquent, d'après les données expérimentales dont nous disposons à l'heure actuelle, la culture en association avec le mésonéphros d'embryon de poulet semble présenter un intérêt non seulement en fournissant le moyen de reproduire *in vitro* le processus d'invasion par des cellules en provenance des tumeurs et connues comme malignes, mais en permettant aussi de reconnaître, et dans certains cas au moins, d'évaluer, la malignité des cellules, transformées en dehors de l'organisme, dont la malignité ne peut être, pour une raison ou une autre, mise à l'épreuve par greffe histocompatible.

Nous avons recherché, pour nos souches transformées *in vitro,* encore d'autres systèmes d'évaluation de malignité qui pourraient être équivalents et parallèles à l'épreuve ultime d'isogreffe. Nous avons notamment essayé avec ce matériel la technique de croissance en gélose molle de SANDERS *et coll.* [7]. Selon ces auteurs, et au moins pour certaines souches cellulaires de hamster et d'homme, il existerait un rapport entre la faculté de former des colonies en gélose et le pouvoir de former des tumeurs envahissantes chez l'animal autochtone.

D'après nos données, les cellules monodispersées de la souche maligne N 1, ensemencées en gélose selon cette technique, produisaient avec un rendement élevé des colonies repiquables. La souche hybride M 6, ayant vis-à-vis de l'animal d'origine un pouvoir cancéreux sensiblement le même, donnait également, avec un rendement comparable, des colonies facilement repiquables bien que d'aspect différent.

En revanche, les souches cellulaires non malignes, comme par exemple, le clone 91, qui chez l'animal adulte ne produisaient pas de tumeurs à croissance rapide et facilement transplantable, ne formaient pas de colonies en gélose.

Une autre technique visant l'étude directe d'interaction entre cellules cancéreuses et le tissu normal *in vitro* a été utilisée dans notre laboratoire et les résultats de ces observations partiellement publiées [8]. Cette technique fait recours à la microcinématographie au contraste de phase et au ralenti. Des cultures soumises à l'observation comportaient en premier lieu des associations de cellules hautement malignes de souris, comme celles de la lignée N 1 ou la lignée hybride M 6, avec des fibroblastes ou des cellules endotheliales isologues. Il s'est révélé que les cellules malignes envahissaient assez aisément les zones de croissance fibroblastiques lâche mais qu'elles étaient inhibées et même arrêtées totalement dans leur progression à la rencontre d'une croissance endotheliale lorsque celle-ci présentait une structuration cohérente et ordonnée.

Les conclusions générales à tirer des études d'invasion cancéreuse à l'aide de différents systèmes de culture *in vitro* peuvent se résumer ainsi:

1. Le pouvoir invasif des cellules apparaît comme une propriété héréditaire des cellules malignes, transmise au cours de générations des cellules *in vitro* comme *in vivo.*

2. Le pouvoir invasif des cellules est associé à un ensemble de différentes propriétés de ces cellules accessible à l'étude *in vitro* telles que propriétés de membranes, mobilité, cohésion mutuelle, caractéristiques de croissance en couches monocellulaires ou en gélose etc. La recherche de lien entre ces propriétés *in vitro* et le pouvoir invasif de cellules in vivo doit être poursuivie systématiquement et peut apporter des indications valables sur la malignité cellulaire.

L'observation des lignées cellulaires développées à partir de poumon de souris nous a permis de conclure dans l'ensemble qu'une lignée cellulaire de cette origin a d'autant plus de chance de se révéler maligne que ses cellules:

a) présentent un aspect fusiforme et polygonal plutôt qu'épithélioïde et pavimenteux;

b) possèdent régulièrement des ramifications cytoplasmiques s'entrecroisant facilement;

c) apparaissent réfringeantes à l'observation au contraste de phase;

d) adhèrent relativement mal au verre;

e) possèdent, lorsqu'on les observe à l'aide de la microcinématographie au ralenti, une mobilité propre intense [8];

f) sont peu inhibées dans leur mouvement par les cellules sœurs et présentent par conséquent un arrangement et une orientation intercellulaire chaotique et une tendance à l'entassement;

g) se détachent par leur mouvement propre de l'ensemble de la colonie et cheminent facilement dans la périphérie comme cellules individuelles [8].

3. La malignité des lignées cellulaires transformées est essentiellement indépendante de l'hôte. Elle peut s'exprimer *in vitro* dans un milieu tissulaire hétérologue et aussi rudimentaire que le mésonéphros de poulet en cultures organotypiques, un système tissulaire d'où toute réaction de défense spécifique et tout particulièrement immunologique est absente par définition.

4. Le phénomène d'invasion et sa contrepartie — la résistance que le tissu normal oppose dans certaines circonstances à cette invasion, peuvent être reproduits, dans une certaine mesure, et étudiés *in vitro* en utilisant l'association des cellules malignes avec une croissance cellulaire normale et un système d'observation continue à l'aide de la microcinématographie au contraste de phase.

5. Les résultats obtenus permettent d'affirmer qu'au cours du processus de transformation cellulaire *in vitro*, la cancérisation ne va pas toujours de pair avec la transformation du caryotype et l'adaptation à la croissance et à la multiplication illimitée *in vitro*. Il s'avère qu'au sein des populations transformées coexistent des variantes plus ou moins malignes ayant des propriétés invasives plus ou moins prononcées. La possibilité de faire cette distinction à l'aide de technique de culture *in vitro* apparaît à l'heure actuelle comme tout à fait réelle.

Discussion

A cinematomicrographic study of cancer invasiveness in vitro, using phase-contrast microscopy

A film produced by G. Barski and J. Belehradek jr. with the technical collaboration of M. P. Wauquier.

Investigations of the invasiveness of cells in *in vitro* cultures prompted us to study in greater detail and more directly the phenomena occurring when malignant cells are confronted with normal tissue. For this purpose, we made a continuous study of the areas of contact between malignant cells and outgrowths of cells from normal connective tissue and, in particular, from normal vascular endothelium. This study was carried out with a phase-contrast microscope and with the aid of time-lapse cinematomicrography. The methods employed have already been described in detail (Barski and Belehradek [8]).

First of all we studied tissue material from the mouse. Cells from the highly malignant line N 1, which had been transformed *in vitro,* were confronted with the outgrowth of normal fragments of mouse myocardium. This outgrowth comprised both fibroblasts and endothelial cells.

When the normal cells were present in the form of a cohesive continuous layer — as in the case of the endothelial outgrowth — the progress of the malignant cells was very clearly held up at the boundary of these layers. The cells either remained blocked or slid along the boundary. This effect was not merely a temporary one, for it was observed at the same point for several consecutive days. These *in vitro* observations may reflect a certain non-specific local resistance to tumour-cell infiltration, especially at the vascular level.

We recently carried out another series of experiments in which we confronted *in vitro* a normal outgrowth of the human kidney with human KB carcinoma cells. In this system, our observations were facilitated by the fact that the KB cells, whether isolated or in layers, were much more refringent than the kidney cells and were therefore easy to distinguish.

Under these conditions, we found that the renal cells and the KB cells, whether isolated or in colonies, did not penetrate each other without restrain. The malignant cells rarely encroached on the layers of normal cells, and did not become integrated with them. On the other hand, isolated KB cells, once they had reached the KB cell zone, readily integrated themselves in that zone.

A study of these cinematographic pictures entitled us to draw the following conclusions:

1. The phenomena of invasion and of its counterpart, resistance to invasion on the part of normal cellular structures, can be to some extent observed directly with the aid of cinematomicrography using a phase contrast microscopy.

2. As *in vivo*, the outcome of the confrontation between tumour cells and normal cells and tissues is variable. It will depend on the mobility of the malignant cells and on the nature of the normal tissue.

3. It is still too early to make generalizations; it is, for example, incorrect to say that malignant cells can invariably use the surface of normal cells as a substrate for their progression.

4. It may, however, be said that a chaotic arrangement of cells, reflecting certainly a decrease in the contact inhibition and an increase in the mobility of individual cells, was observed in particular in malignant cells.

5. On the other hand, the fact that the progress of malignant cells is arrested at the boundaries of normal tissue, particularly when the latter is composed of endothelial cells, is a typical phenomenon. It was observed also by Dr. STOKER (cf. the present colloquium), Dr. FOGH (personal communication), and other authors.

Questions put to G. BARSKI

B. Kellner: It appears that tumour cells have different speeds of movement. Sometimes they move rapidly and at other times slowly. How can the rapidly-moving type of cell be differentiated from macrophages?

M. Stoker: On the question of identifying the tumour cells, we have, as Dr. BARSKI knows made similar observations showing that polyoma-transformed cells are inhibited by contact with normal cells. Here, it is possible to mark the tumour cells with carbon, thus permitting clear identification of the immobilized tumour cells in contact with normal cells.

Furthermore, when the contact-inhibited tumour cells are removed from the normal cells and grown alone, they lose their contact-inhibition once again; in other words, it is only the phenotypic behaviour which is altered by contact with normal cells.

3*

M. Abercrombie: Are fibroblasts the only normal cells invaded *in vitro*?

G. Barski: In our material the only evidence of progressive invasion of normal tissue was obtained in areas of loose fibroblastic growth.

M. Feldman: I should like to ask both Dr. BARSKI and Dr. STOKER the following question: Tumour cells cannot apparently generate contact inhibition, but are nevertheless susceptible to contact inhibition generated by normal cells. When a tumour cell is contact-inhibited by a normal cell, does its free surface, which is not in contact with the normal cell, manifest any degree of inhibition of motion?

E. J. Ambrose: Evidence from time-lapse films indicates that only local regions of the cell membrane are involved in cell-cell adhesions. These regions are firmly adhering, while the remainder of the membrane still moves very actively. There is no general paralysis of the cell. But the areas of the membrane which are immobilized by cell-cell contact vary under different conditions. When cells transformed by polyoma virus are placed on a layer of normal fibroblasts they establish many contacts and assume the shape of normal cells. Nevertheless, the regions which have not formed stable contacts still move as actively as the isolated cells.

G. Barski: My answer to Dr. FELD-MAN's question would be rather: no. The movement of the *cytoplasm* of malignant cells in contact with normal cells in not arrested or paralyzed. The point is mainly that the surface of normal cells seems to be a rather unfavourable substrate for the malignant cells to move on.

M. Feldman: May I ask a further question along the same lines? When a tumour cell is contact-inhibited by a normal cell, will it replicate, will it continue to divide, or will the contact between a normal and a tumour cell block the replication of the tumour cell?

G. Barski: We have not observed so far cell divisions in the tumour cell area which is in direct contact with normal cells, but I have no quantitative data to affirm that there is no inhibition in the multiplication rate.

M. Abercrombie: Dr. BARSKI's film clearly demonstrated the phenomenon of contact inhibition between normal fibroblasts. Part of a film made by Dr. AMBROSE and myself with an interference microscope will serve to illustrate a failure of contact inhibition when a tumour cell encounters a normal cell *in vitro*. The tumour concerned is the mouse S 37, the normal cells are chick fibroblasts, and the culture is on a plane surface. In the series of frames reproduced from the film, A shows two white, rounded tumour cells; one (left) is resting on a darker fibroblast, and the other (above), which is the cell to observe, is approaching and being approached from the right by two fibroblasts. In C and D, the tumour cell is astride both fibroblasts. In

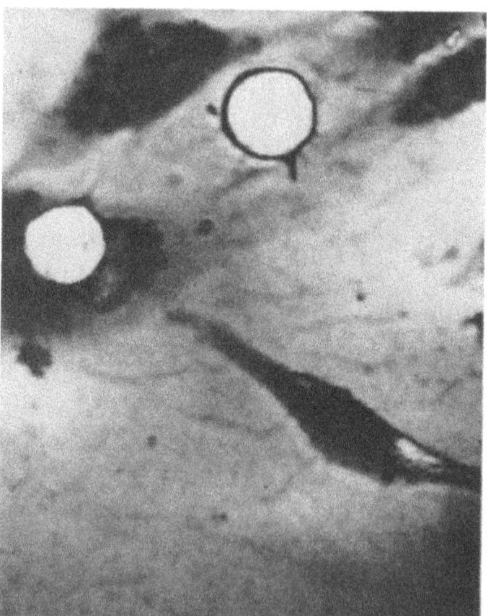

A

D, it is in the process of moving off the fibroblast surface on to the substrate again. It is rare for chick or mouse fibroblasts in culture to move across each other in this way; but it is relatively com mon for sarcoma cells to move across fibroblasts. The magnification is roughly $\times 1,000$, and the duration of the observations recorded approximately $^1/_2$ hour.

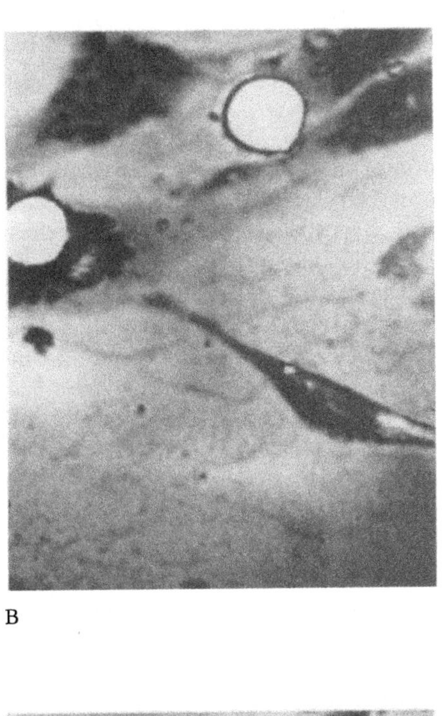

B

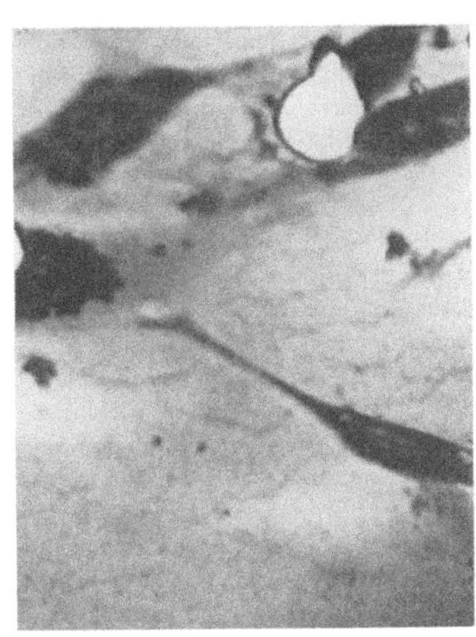

C

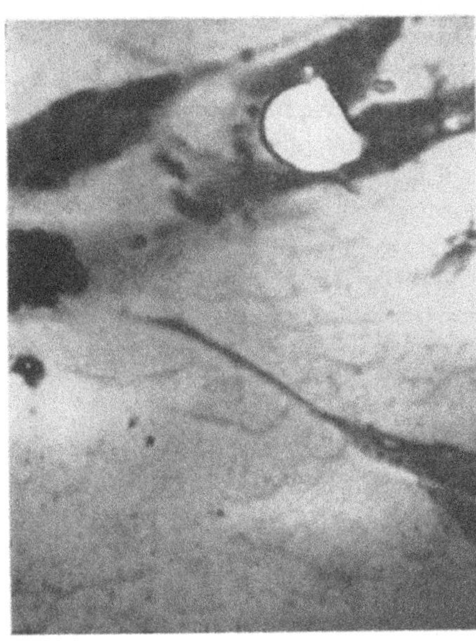

D

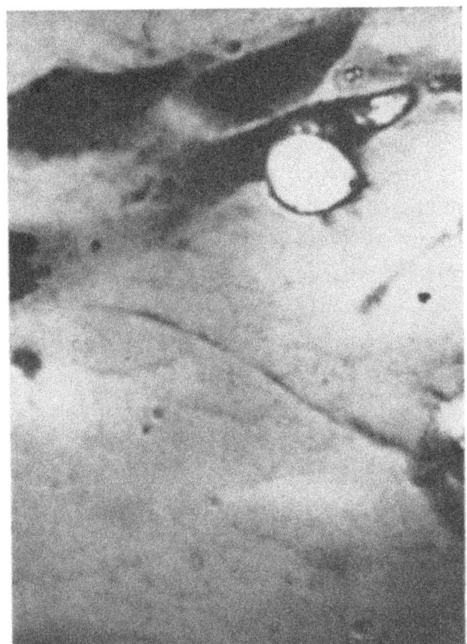

E

B. Sylvén: Could you explain in greater detail what you mean by the invasive "satellite" cells? I am puzzled by the present lack of *distinctive* data as to the cytology and cytochemistry of these cells. The other day, I raised the question about the difference between the A and B cells of solid tumours, and you have here, I believe, observations pertaining to such a cellular developmental pattern.

G. Barski: The "satellite" — or, as we call them, "sentinel" — cells are single cells characterized by energetic movement of their cytoplasmic ramifications and membranes and frequently seen at the periphery of colonies of malignant cells. We do not know whether they represent a selection of cells having particular genetically-determined properties, but we think that it would be worth while to plan experiments to test this possibility.

B. Sylvén: Such data would be pretty easy to obtain by UV microscopy and by the histochemical methods usually employed to determine, for instance, the cytoplasmic RNA content, the relative per-cell occurrence of mitochondria, etc.

G. Barski: I entirely agree with you.

I. Petrea: Dr. Barski, can you supplement your cytological criteria of malignancy, which you studied in the light microscope, with criteria of cell malignancy as established with the electron microscope?

I ask you this question because Oberling and Bernhard described a process of dedifferentiation in tumour cells. In our electron-microscope laboratory, we were able, together with Prof. Milcou, to demonstrate a similar process of cellular dedifferentiation occurring in the course of endogenous carcinogenesis in certain endocrine glands, including in particular the thyroid.

G. Barski: In collaboration with Dr. de Harven, we have successfully used electron microscopy solely with the aim of recognizing the heterogeneous nature of the cell populations in our lines which originate from the mouse lung. In this respect, we have obtained convincing results. We have not, however, tried to establish by this mean a relationship between the malignancy of a cell and its ultrastructure.

P. Sträuli: During the transformation of mouse cells two phenomena are observed at the cellular level: the appearance of new karyotypes, and the development of cytomorphological criteria of "malignancy". Does the replacement of diploid cells by polyploid or aneuploid cells facilitate the progression of the cytomorphological syndrome of "malignancy", or do these two events run parallel to each other?

G. Barski: So far as we can judge, the modifications in the karyotype and the cytological transformations go together and occur at the same period of time, but not necessarily the appearance of malignancy.

P. Vigier: Among the criteria of malignancy of his tumour cell lines Dr. Barski has mentioned infiltration of cultures of embryonic chicken mesonephros. Could you give further details about the nature of this infiltration? In particular, is it accompanied by destruction of the normal cells in the infiltrated mesonephros?

G. Barski: In the presence of very marked infiltration of the fragments of mesonephros, the latter's cells give way to invasive malignant cells, although there are no obvious signs of necrosis in the region of the invaded mesonephros.

P. Vigier: Thank you. The reason for my question was that we recently cultivated clonal cell lines of BHK 21 hamster fibroblasts transformed by two Rous viruses in association with normal chicken fibroblasts. The transformed cells were obtained in gelose by Dr. MONTAGNIER and, to judge by their appearance and behaviour in culture, they were apparently highly malignant cells. When they were cultivated with chicken embryo fibroblasts, these latter were rapidly eliminated from the cultures and only very few could still be detected after 3—4 days. This phenomenon was seen even after the transformed cells had been irradiated with 5,000 R. This suggests that the transformed cells exert a cytocidal effect on the normal cells.

G. Barski: Are any dead or necrotic normal cells to be seen in this case?

P. Vigier: No.

Bibliography

[1] BARSKI, G., et CASSINGENA, R., Malignant transformation in vitro of cells from C57BL mouse normal pulmonary tissue. *J. nat. Cancer Inst.* **30**, 865—883 (1963).

[2] — BILLARDON, CL., JULLIEN, P.-M., et CARSWELL, E., Evolution in vitro et cancérisation des cellules pulmonaires de souris. Int. J. Cancer **1**, 541—556 (1966).

[3] SANFORD, K., LIKELY, C. D., and EARIE, W. R., The development of variations in transplantability and morphology within a clone of mouse fibroblasts transformed in sarcoma-producing cells in vitro. *J. nat. Cancer Inst.* **15**, 215—237 (1954).

[4] BARSKI, G., SORIEUL, S., et CORNEFERT, F., "Hybrid" type cells in combined cultures of two different mammalian cell strains. *J. nat. Cancer Inst.* **26**, 1269—1291 (1961).

[5] WOLFF, ET., et WOLFF, EM., Le comportement, en culture in vitro, de cancers humains associés à des explants de rein embryonnaire de poulet. *C.R. Soc. Biol. (Paris)* **155**, 441—443 (1961).

[6] BARSKI, G., et WOLFF, E., Malignancy evaluation of in vitro transformation of mouse cell lines in chick mesonephros organ cultures. *J. nat. Cancer Inst.* **34**, 495—510 (1965).

[7] SANDERS, F. K., and BURFORD, B. O., Ascites tumours from BHK. 21 cells transformed in vitro by polyoma virus. *Nature (Lond.)* **201**, 786—789 (1964).

[8] BARSKI, G., et BELEHRADEK jr., Etude microcinématographique du mécanisme d'invasion cancéreuse en culture de tissu normal associé aux cellules malignes. *Exp. Cell Res.* **37**, 464—480 (1965).

Applicability of in vitro Models to a Study of the Invasiveness of Cancer

Round-Table Discussion

Leaded by G. BARSKI

G. Barski: May I open the discussion on the *applicability of in vitro models to a study of the invasiveness of cancer* by making a few remarks of a general nature?

When we approach the problem of malignant growth — a problem which can be summed up in the two key words *invasion* and *metastasis* — we are immediately aware that we are faced with a complex function, in which there are many parameters and many interdependent factors.

The essential parameters belong to two groups.

Those of the first group are connected with the intrinsic, hereditary properties of malignant cells, properties which determine their individual and social behaviour. Social behaviour, in this context, means their behaviour towards other malignant cells and towards normal cells.

The parameters belonging to the second group concern the totality of the conditions imposed by the "millieu" of the malignant growth — the passive aspect of this "millieu", the nature of its cellular and intercellular structure, and its immediate and delayed reactions to invasion, reactions which may be welcoming or defensive, specific or non-specific.

Obviously, we can simply content ourselves with saying that this is a complex situation which cannot be reproduced *in vitro*. On the other hand, we can also postulate that, precisely because the situation is complex and difficult to interpret *in vivo, in vitro* experiments will enable us to break it down into its essential elements and to find answers to certain definite, relatively simple questions.

Before we start discussing the applicability of *in vitro* models, I should like to

Table. *Elements of invasiveness*

A. Properties of tumour cells
1. Cellular proliferation and "demographic" pressure
2. Ability of individual cells to detach themselves from the body of the tumour
3. Active mobility of these cells
4. Failure to receive or perceive stopping signals
5. Positive tactism towards normal tissue
6. Ability to progress over the surface of other cells or intercellular structures
7. Ability to break down or destroy
   a) cellular barriers
   b) intercellular barriers

B. Defence reactions of the host
1. Passive, non-specific effect of the barrier provided by
   a) intercellular cohesion
   b) a liquid or solid intercellular milieu
   c) physical or chemical repulsion
2. Specific, immunological or non-immunological reactions
   a) of humoral nature
   b) of a cellular nature

C. "Suicidal" reactions of the host
1. Nutrition
2. Vascularization
3. Immunological reactions (enhancement)

draw your attention for a moment to the table in which I have attempted to list some of the essential elements of the phenomenon of invasiveness.

A glance at this table immediately shows that a considerable number of problems can be tackled by means of *in vitro* cultures.

Thus, regarding the heading A, which comprises the properties of invasive cells, it would appear that *in vitro* experiments provide favourable conditions for a study of points 1, 2, 3, 5 and 6. Even in B and C, which refer to the reactions of the host, points B 1 (a) and (c), as well as C 1 to a certain extent, appear to be perfectly accessible to *in vitro* analysis.

In vitro experiments, moreover, represent not only an additional method of investigation, but may also be the method of choice for finding answers to certain precise questions, for example those concerning tumour progression and of direct interactions between normal cells and tumour cells.

After these few general remarks, I should now like to open the discussion and to ask for your views on the applicability of *in vitro* models to a study of the invasiveness of cancer.

M. Abercrombie: I think it is impossible to discuss the applicability of *in vitro* models to the *in vivo* situation *in general*. Only particular models can be discussed profitably. Models are simplified analogies which may or may not be useful, depending on the details of the analogy proposed. One can critically discuss particular models in two ways. First, certain claims as to similarity with the organism can be refuted. For instance, YOUNG's model of invasion, mentioned this morning, claimed that tissues have the consistency of gelatin, and this is a point open to criticism. Secondly, one can investigate the correlations between behaviour *in vitro* and behaviour *in*

vivo. For example, if one can in some way influence invasion in an *in vitro* model, it should be possible to influence invasion *in vivo* in the same way. The establish ment of such correlations is the decisive test of a model. At present, for the *in vitro* models proposed, they are almost entirely lacking.

M. Feldman: Had there been a direct causal correlation between the loss of contact inhibition and the metastasizing capacity of tumours, then, from an analysis of the mechanism of contact inhibition, we could have learned the significance of points 1, 2, 3, 4, and 6 of Dr. BARSKI's scheme. However, so far, contact inhibition is a phenomenon studied *in vitro*. I was impressed this morning by Dr. WOOD's film of tumour cells which show complete loss of contact inhibition *in vivo*. Yet, you will agree, the question to be answered, before the significance of the loss of contact inhibition to cell invasiveness is appreciated, is whether *primary* tumours produced in animals manifest such a loss, and whether there is a regular correlation between such a loss and metastasizibility of these primary tumours.

J. Leighton: Can we expect any real correlation to develop between cell interactions *in vitro* and invasive behaviour in the intact animal?

M. Stoker: Those features of tumour cells cultured *in vitro* which have looked most promising for a study of *in vivo* characteristics have unfortunately not correlated too well. For example, lack of contact inhibition may be present without increased transplantability, and good contact inhibition may be present in highly malignant — i.e. highly transplantable — cells. Recently, it was hoped that growth in agar suspension would correlate well with malignancy, but again exceptions have been encountered. However, most studies on tissue culture cell lines have been correlated only with transplantability, and it is necessary to ask if this really measures invasiveness.

E. J. Ambrose: When seeking a correlation between cell contact behaviour *in vitro* and invasiveness *in vivo,* it is important to distinguish between adhesiveness to the glass surface and to neighbouring cells. Adhesiveness to glass is a comparatively non-specific reaction. I believe that intercellular contacts involve some specificity. Analysis of time-lapse films makes it possible to distinguish these two types of contact. I think that there is a definite inverse correlation between intercellular adhesiveness between tumour cells analysed from time-lapse films and invasiveness.

J. Leighton: Before we go any further, can we spend a few minutes defining what we mean by malignancy? In my experience, transplantability is not equivalent to malignancy. In the chick embryo host receiving a heterologous transplant, for example, normal adult human tissues such as skin, endometrium, and ovary are transplantable. On the other hand, although many tumours are transplantable to the embryonic chick egg, a number of highly malignant tumours of man and of laboratory animals die when transplanted to the chick embryo.

C. M. Southam: Dr. Leighton has raised the very pertinent question of what is our definition of malignancy. I should like to propose what may be regarded by many as truism: the only unequivocal criterion of neoplastic malignancy is the reproduction of the *disease* on reimplantation of the cell in question into the animal in which it originated or into an antigenically identical recipient (i.e. auto- or iso-transplantation). Reproduction of the disease implies not only the production of a cellular nodule, but local invasion or distant metastasis if

these were characteristic of the original cancer. The validity of any other test of malignancy depends upon how well it correlates with this definition. It seems to me that, of the methods now available, transplantation into a recipient animal or tissue which provides an adequate milieu for growth but has little capacity for immunologic reaction probably gives the best correlation.

J. Huppert: When I look at the excellent table prepared by Dr. Barski, I personally am convinced that questions concerning the role played by the cell in invasion can only be studied *in vitro.*

The differences in the properties of malignant cells, in their surfaces, their electrical charges, the composition of their enzymes, etc. cannot be detected in the intact organism. *In vivo,* the part played by general factors, such as immunological and hormonal reactions, predominates and masks the individual response.

E. J. Ambrose: In order to compare *in vitro* and *in vivo* effects, we need a measure of invasiveness *in vivo.* When measuring the rate of growth of an inoculum containing a known number of cells, it would be desirable to determine the extent of spread into neighbouring tissues. If such a test could be devised, it would be much easier to make *in vitro* and *in vivo* comparisons.

M. Stoker: One difficulty in deciding the important characteristics of tumour cells is lack of a proper control for comparison. Ideally, the tumour cell should be compared with the same cell before it became malignant — that is to say, with the parent cell. Clearly, this is impossible in tumours developing *in vivo.* It is here that neoplastic transformations effected *in vitro* may be useful, even if some relevance is thereby sacrificed, because they make it possible to compare normal and transformed progeny of the same single parent cell.

M. Feldman: On the subject of the morphological changes of cell surfaces and cell interactions: some years ago, it appeared that normal chick fibroblasts, when transformed by Rous virus, lose contact inhibition owing to changes in surface properties associated with the fact that the virus is completed at the cell surface. We know that other viruses, as the chicken lymphomatosis viruses or the influenza viruses, are similarly completed at the cell surface, but these do not induce a loss of contact properties of cells. Does Dr. STOKER have any comment on this?

M. Stoker: I think Dr. FELDMAN has answered this question himself. As he says, fibroblasts infected, for example, with avian myeloblastosis virus may have a new virus-like surface, but the cell behaviour is not markedly altered. On the other hand, a Rous-infected cell is dramatically changed.

The importance of the presence of Rous virus in cell behaviour is shown by recent work in our laboratory by Dr. MACPHERSON. He has transformed BHK 21 hamster cells with Rous virus leading to loss of contact inhibition and increase in transplantability, accompanied by carriage of the virus as detected by tumour production in chicken. Single transformed cells, however, may apparently segregate normal cells; these cells have regained their contact inhibition and their original low transplantibility, and have also lost the detectable Rous virus. It is believed that this reversion occurs because of loss of the virus in a rapidly multiplying cell.

D. F. H. Wallach: Is contact inhibition an all-or-none phenomenon or are there varying degrees of contact inhibition? Can contact inhibition be quantified?

M. Abercrombie: Unfortunately, one must admit that we have at present no valid way of quantifying contact inhibition. For the individual cell, contact inhibition is all or nothing: the cell either stops when it makes the contact, or goes on. But in cell populations I am confident that there are differences of degree in the proportion of collisions that result in contact inhibition.

G. Barski: The question raised by Dr. WALLACH is important. We have to realize that the accumulated data on contact inhibition are, so far scarce. They concern chiefly a limited number of experimental sarcomas confronted in most cases with normal fibroblasts. We have seen that things can change completely when the progressing malignant cells come into contact, for example, with normal endothelium. Furthermore, we know practically nothing about the contact behaviour of *carcinomatous* cells, especially when confronted with cells other than fibroblasts. On the other hand, further investigations have to be undertaken to relate the *degree* of malignancy and metastasis-forming capacity in the animal with the presence, absence, or degree of contact inhibition *in vitro*.

It would be wise therefore to refrain, for the time being, from making too far-reaching generalizations.

P. Sträuli: Coming back to your question regarding the morphological identification of cancer cells, I would like to stress one point: only in exceptional cases do we really know which normal cells are the homologous elements of a given tumour cell population. This difficulty exists even in such carefully investigated tumours as the Japanese ascites "hepatomas". Professor SATO will correct me if I am wrong.

H. Sato: Dr. STRÄULI's question about whether the tumours of the rat ascites hepatoma are homologous or not is quite difficult to answer briefly. However, I will try to consider this problem from the viewpoint of the cellular origin of the tumours. As you know, there are several kinds of cells in the liver, such as hepatic cells, bile-duct cells, reticulo-endothelial cells, etc. On the basis of the histological pictures of the original tumours, the tumours induced by giving azo-dyes are regarded as liver cancers having various of these elements in their ancestry.

The first ascites hepatoma was established in 1951 from an azo-dye-induced liver cancer of a Japanese rat. Since then, nearly sixty strains of transplantable ascites hepatomas of the rat have been established. Each strain of the tumour has its own characteristic morphology as regards its ascitic features, such as single free cell type, island-forming type, and mixed type displaying various sizes of cell complexes. On the other hand, various types of histological pattern were observed in the primary and transplanted tumours of each strain, such as hepatoma, cholangioma, mixed type, and anaplastic type.

There does not seem to be a clear-cut correlation between the histological types which would make it possible to establish the cellular origin of each strain of tumour and the ascitic features of the tumours. In some examples, of course, the island and mixed type seemed to show an epithelial structure suggestive of their epithelial origin. Even in some of the free cell type tumours, the histological structures still suggest their epithelial origin.

This series of ascites tumours cannot be said to be homologous as regards the original ancestral cells. There is no correlation between the assumed ancestral origin in the liver and the biological and pathological characteristics of each strain of tumours initiated from liver cancers

induced in the same species of animals by giving the same carcinogen, an azo dye.

M. Abercrombie: I would like to refer back to Dr. Barski's remark on the work of Dr. Halpern and others, showing that a numbers of kinds of malignant cell aggregate in suspension better than corresponding normal cells. From what Dr. Ambrose has just said, one would expect them to aggregate less. I find this puzzling, and I wonder whether Dr. Ambrose has any comment on the situation.

E. J. Ambrose: I find this ability of tumour cells to aggregate more rapidly than normal cells from a rotating flask in a fluid suspension rather surprising, and I think that the conditions must be rather special in this case. The hydrodynamics in the fluid, as well as the cell shape must be responsible to some extent, According to the other tests, tumour cells are less adhesive, as was first shown by Coman, using micro-manipulation. It is also easier to make suspensions from most tumour tissues by mechanical means. As I mentioned earlier, it is the dynamic behaviour of the contacts when the tumour cells are actively metabolizing, which gives a true measure of their intercellular adhesiveness.

J. Leighton: The architecture of carcinomas of even a single organ is so diverse in character that it may be unwise to seek a universal law based on a few laboratory tumours. Tumours from the same organ — e.g. the breast — vary widely. Some are highly organized with cells in distinct compact groups. Others are anaplastic, the tumour cells being haphazardly arranged, often without contact with one another.

J. Huppert: To answer Dr. Barski's question concering the paradox in the behaviour of malignant cells in mono-cellular layers (which have lost contact inhibition) and in suspension, I should like to mention an observation made in our laboratory. For a year now we have been cultivating hamster (BHK 21) cells transformed by polyoma virus in suspension. The cells, which are indisputably malignant, show no tendency to aggregate. If, however, the cells stop growing very suddenly for any reason (unsatisfactory milieu, for example), aggregations do appear. For us, this is a sign that the cells are damaged, and I wonder to what extent aggregation can be regarded as a specific phenomenon.

G. Barski: We have found on several occasions that among our cell lines, those which aggregate readily when the culture flasks are shaken belong to the more malignant category. But all the strains we used multiply on the surface of the glass, and do not become adapted to the culture in suspension. I believe that this latter type of culture reflects a real modification in the nature of the cells, especially as regards their surface properties. This modification would correspond to the evolution of tumour cell populations *in vivo* towards an ascitic form.

Obviously, the criteria applied to the contact behaviour of this type of cells, which are accustomed to an "aquatic" life, are completely different from those applicable to cells which can only live and multiply on a solid substrate.

R. E. Madden: Earlier in the discussion Dr. LEIGHTON spoke of the need for a generally-agreed-upon definition of malignancy as applied to *in vitro* studies. It might be pertinent to mention the idea of Prof. OTTO WARBURG, Dr. DEAN BURK, and others, that the essential lesion of malignancy is the property of aerobic glycolysis. I should like to know if any of the contributors to the present discussion have any comments to make on this point.

M. Stoker: In a study carried out with Prof. JOHN PAUL we have shown that malignant transformation by polyoma virus leads to increased acid production which is accompanied by increased glucose uptake, but not by any change in respiration. This agrees in part, but only in part, with WARBURG's original working hypothesis.

H. Hamperl: On the one hand, it will never be possible to duplicate *in vitro* the exact interrelationship between host and tumour, which is the basic problem of invasive growth — at least, as far as human tumours are concerned; the individual is as unique as his tumour. On the other hand, a pathologist has to admire the extent to which it has been possible to cumulate single factors underlying the invasive growth. In evaluating these successes, however, one should be conscious of the limitations of the method which can only provide models of parts of a most complex process. Other models, even if they do use gelatin, may prove just as good for the purpose of demonstrating a particular point.

G. Barski: This exchange of ideas clearly shows that opinions differ on many points and that in most cases we are still far from being able to draw definite, unequivocal conclusions.

Even if we can manage to reproduce invasion *in vitro*, we do not at present know how to influence this invasion, either *in vitro* or *in vivo*; hence, we lack a valuable criterion for judging whether the *in vitro* model is a true equivalent of the *in vivo* process.

On the other hand, the rule that malignant cells are invariably characterized by an absence of contact inhibition seems, as we have seen, to have numerous exceptions. It is not impossible, incidentally, that these exceptions may soon themselves constitute new rules. We, in common with other authors, have shown that malignant cells may be inhibited by contact with certain normal tissues, including in particular endothelium. The significance of various aspects of adhesion or aggregation between the cells themselves, and between the cells and the substrate, is still not very clear. In addition, attempts to establish a firm correlation between invasiveness *in vitro* and malignancy *in vivo* by means of systematic experiments are greatly handicapped by the fact that malignancy *in vivo* depends, in the last resort, on the reactions of the host irrespective of the malignancy of the cell itself.

However, despite all these uncertainties, general agreement that the cellular properties responsible for malignancy may be studied from various angles *in vitro* has emerged from our discussion. Admittedly, we are still unable to define absolute rules which would permit us to predict with certainty the behaviour of a cell *in vivo* on the basis of its behaviour *in vitro*. But it is becoming increasingly evident that various *in vitro* experimental procedures are often the most appropriate means of recognizing and classifying certain essential elements of tumour invasion.

Some Factors Relating to the Invasiveness and Destructiveness of Solid Malignant Tumours

B. Sylvén

*The Cancer Research Division of Radiumhemmet, Karolinska Institute,
Stockholm, Sweden*

I have little to add to the problem of invasiveness as such, which forms the main topic of this Conference. Other speakers will dwell upon observations and thoughts about cellular cohesion (Berwick and Coman, 1962; Coman, 1947), the role of ameboid movement (Abercrombie, 1962), contact inhibition (Abercrombie, 1962), cell aggregation (Moscona, 1962), surface characteristics pertaining to the locomotion of malignant cells (Leighton, 1963) and data from organ culture studies (Easty and Easty, 1963; Wolff, 1962). My main task will be to discuss (*a*) the composition of the fluid milieu in which tumour cells live and grow under *in vivo* conditions, and (*b*) *how the degradation of preformed macromolecular host proteins may occur* — in various ways — in connection with invasive growth of solid tumours. I am forced to present a rather over-simplified reconstruction, in terms of microscopy (Berenblum, 1958) and biochemistry, of the events we have to face. Fortunately, there are a few new approaches which may help to illuminate some of the pertinent questions. We are only at the beginning of this very complex study which requires quite advanced microtechniques for sampling and assays seldom used in solid tumour materials.

Cellular death and protein degradation *in vivo* is something which goes on all the time although the local rate may show great variations. For instance, one may notice a rapid degradation and removal of fibrous proteins in connection with infarction, certain neurogenic muscle dystrophies, necrosis due to inflammatory conditions, during the first phases of wound healing, during resorption of granulomas, involution of the post-partum uterus, etc. In the case of tumours, particularly the human ones, we have to deal with two types of concomitant growth: the expansive one and the invasive-destructive type most commonly observed in *rapidly growing sarcomas and carcinomas*. This report is limited to such solid tumours excluding lymphomas, leukemias and other special tumour types presenting a different behavior with reference to destructive activity (Ehrmann and Gey, 1956; Shelton, 1958, 1964 a.o.).

The evidence prompts us to consider both *intracellular* and *extracellular degradation reactions*. The latter take place at narrow interphases necessitating microsampling procedures for adequate biochemical study. It is clear that chemical bulk data derived from heterogeneous tumour materials and homogenates can only provide average data devoid of topical significance. During recent years we have made attempts to study the composition of the interstitial medium of solid tumours. In addition, attempts are made by combined chemical and histochemical techniques to study the localization of enzymic activity at the tumour invasion zone. Interesting cytochemical observations relating to the *release of lysosomal enzymes as well as the role of histiocytes and other phagocytic cells* have further to be considered as operative in the destructive action of tumours.

Attention will also be called to the marked frequency of *cell death* (WOLFF, 1962) at the invasion zone of tumours. We have recently obtained evidence of the occurrence of *a diffusible cytotoxic polypeptide* in tumour fluids (HOLMBERG, 1962, 1964; SYLVÉN and HOLMBERG, 1963, 1965). This seems to explain why various stromal cells become changed, paralysed and later die (cp. contributions by Dr. ABERCROMBIE) as well as certain distant alterations of host tissues forming part of the clinical syndrome of cachexia.

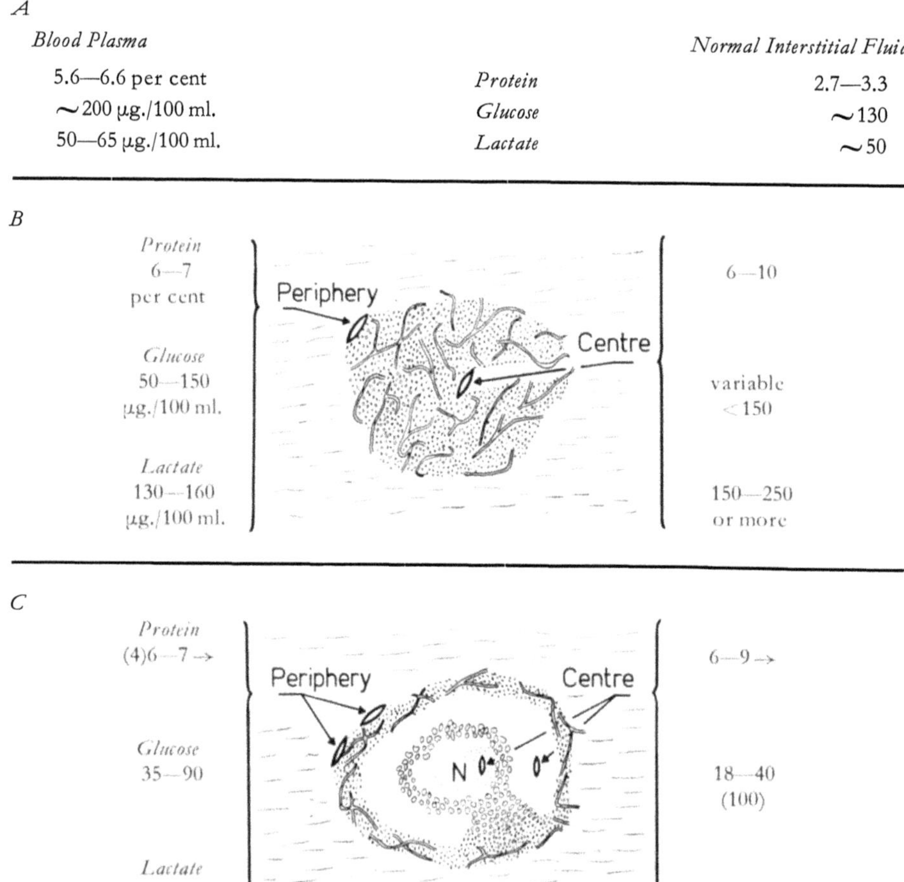

Fig. 1 A—C. Joint graphs summarizing the observed data on the content of protein, glucose and lactate in (A) mouse blood plasma and normal interstitial fluid, (B) the corresponding figures obtained on cell- and blood-free microsamples of interstitial fluid from fully vascularized young mouse tumour transplants, left part from the periphery and right part from central regions; and (C) the corresponding data on intestitial fluid from large mouse tumour transplants with necrotic tumour centers (*see* BURGESS and SYLVÉN, 1962; SYLVÉN, 1961, 1962, 1965)

I. Environmental Factors Facilitating Permeation by Tumour cells

Direct observations with a loupe or dissecting microscope on rapidly-growing and highly invasive solid mouse tumours stress the role of edema at the tumour periphery (Burgess, 1962; Sylvén, 1962). It is remarkable to see the amount of fluid filling the tissue gaps and forcing the regular host cells and fibrous structures apart. The local increase in the amount of interstitial fluid will facilitate infiltration and permeation by clusters or isolated tumour cells, which just seem to penetrate into greatly widened preformed spaces (Sylvén, 1945, 1957). Other tumour culture data seem to support this contention (Barski, 1965; Leighton, 1963; Wolff, 1962). It may provisionally be conceived that several factors are operative in the formation of edema. One is increased vascular filtration, possibly associated with release of amines from host cells (Majno, 1961), and retardation of flow (Goldacre, 1962). Another is the abnormal carbohydrate metabolism of tumour cells, leading to marked increase in the local concentration of lactate (Burgess, 1962; cp. Fig. 1). This will in turn attract water from the surrounding spaces thereby compensating for the increased molarity of tumour interstitial fluid.

For the purpose of discussion it might be added that the fluid at the tumour periphery is slowly drained away by the local lymphatics of the host (Goldacre, 1962). The driving force is the capillary pressure which is probably lower than normal due to dilatation and other changes of the capillary bed as a consequence of tumour growth. The rate of flow of the interstitial fluid can easily be measured under the microscope by means of deposited drops of suitable non-adsorbed dyes and is of the order of 300 μ per minute (Goldacre, 1962). The fluid medium of central non-vascularized tumour regions is, on the other hand, stagnant.

II. Evidence of Proteolysis

Already in the previous century the old pathologists described how solid tumours, to a different extent according to tumour types, destroy and replace fibrous host tissues including insoluble collagen, tendons, muscle and even bone. In human tumours of low and medium growth rates this degradation is mostly a slow process, but in rapidly-growing tumours the events are more easily observed. The sequence of microscopical changes of collagen fibers include (1) *denaturation* and loss of normal birefringence, (2) *swelling* into an amorphous collagenous gel often retaining some fuchsinophilia, and finally (3) *disintegration* and *digestion* of the gel. The microscopical details as described elsewhere (Sylvén, 1945, 1957, 1962) recently seem to have obtained some corroboration from electron microscopic data. In the case of muscle bundles representing a more bulky core of proteins the structural disorganization as seen under the microscope follows a similar pattern (cp. EMG data on tail regression in *Xenopus* larvae by Weber (1963, 1964).

From a number of old tumour studies including *in vitro* culture data (cp. Leighton, 1957) the impression is obtained that this destruction appears to start already at some distance from the peripheral tumour vegetations (Sylvén, 1945, 1957, 1962); most of the breakdown, however, does occur by *close contact* between the previously denatured fibrous proteins and the surrounding tumour cells and histiocytes. This is conspicuous in the case of muscle fiber degradation; remnants of non-digested tapered-off muscle fibers can be followed a few millimeters into the tumour before they disappear (Sylvén and Malmgren, 1957, Fig. 2, p. 77). On the other hand it is quite true that not all collagenous strands, especially in multifocal spontaneous tumours, are digested, although they are completely surrounded by tumour tissue.

Further interesting information relates to the topographical sites of attack in the host tissues. This seems mainly to occur at and outside the tumour periphery in close relation to the actively growing and dividing tumour cells. In this zone a considerable number of various host cells are mostly intermingling. It is not known whether any particular one of these cell types releases more enzymes or enzymic activators. Chemical data suggest, however, that the young tumour cells contain larger amounts of catheptic and peptidase activity at a per-cell level than do the mature and quiescent tumour cells (Sylvén and Malmgren, 1957; corroborated by Benz, 1959).

III. Possible Mechanisms of Fibrous Protein Degradation

The question arises how the preformed fibrous proteins of the host, such as collagen and muscle, become degraded. Some speculation seems justified until valid documentation can be provided.

The microscopical evidence favors the view that the first step is represented by *a general disorganization and denaturation*, probably involving a loosening of structural bonds keeping the orderly aggregation of polypeptide chains strictly aligned. Death of stromal cells, fibroblasts and muscle cells might initiate this autolysis. For the swelling of extracellular collagen bundles the marked

increase in lactate concentration (up to 150—350 mg/100 ml; e.g. 4—6 times the normal interstitial fluid level; Fig. 1) might also play a role (first considered by Bierich, 1927), and still more so in the case of muscle proteins where removal of metal ions (Ca^{++} or Mg^{++} or both) is deleterious. In both materials a weak solvation effect by lactate might occur at an acid pH. The electron microscopic effects of weak acid treatment on collagen fibers have been described already by Wyckoff (1949), Vanamee and Porter (1951), and Gross (1953). Similarly degraded collagen fibers were observed following collagenase digestion (Keech, 1955).

The protein gels so established would hence become susceptible to enzymatic degradation both by *extracellular enzymes* present in the medium and by phagocytic or lysosomal *endocellular hydrolases* in tumour and/or host cells. "Digestive" vacuoles have been observed in tumour cells containing foreign proteins. Still cross-banded collagen fragments appeared in fibroblasts during the post-partum uterine involution (Luse and Hutton, 1964). At which particular stage(s) catheptic and other lysosomal enzymes (de Duve, 1959, 1964) exert their action remains to be investigated. The sources and requirements of energy necessary for the hydrolysis of these proteins cannot yet be considered for lack of specific data.

IV. Evidence for the Occurrence of Extracellular Enzymes Hydrolyzing the Carbamide Bond

Data have recently been collected on the available activities of proteinases and peptidases in the cell- and blood-free extracellular medium, as it exists in its native state, in various mouse and rat tumours. The composition is highly pathological as compared with normal tissue fluid and blood plasma, suggesting that additional terms of various hydrolases are added to the tumour fluid (SYLVÉN and BOIS-SVENSSON, 1965; and Figs. 2—4). All kinds of catheptic enzymes, polypeptidases, aminoacyl-naphthylamidases (cp. SYLVÉN, 1964), aminopeptidase, regular dipeptidases as well as prolinase and prolidase show remarkably increased activities. On the other hand, despite careful search, true collagenases and proteinases active at a physiological pH range seem to be lacking or are effectively inhibited. The results suggest that the interstitial tumour fluid offers a remarkable opportunity for an enzymatic attack, in the extracellular compartment, on all kinds of denatured proteins at an acid pH and on most types of peptides at neutral and alkaline pH's.

As to the origin of these enzymes, several interesting possibilities may tentatively be considered (SYLVÉN, 1962). In independent experiments HOLMBERG (1961) has shown that living tumour cells to a very marked extent differ from the normal cells under comparison in the sense that all kinds of soluble cytoplasmic enzymes are leaking out. As an example it may be mentioned that uninjured tumour cells incubated in a perfect growth medium under *in vitro* conditions leak out proteins carrying LDH activity to an extent of approximately 1,000 units per hour per 10^7 cells (BURGESS, 1962). Another possibility is that additional lysosomal or other hydrolases might be derived from injured cells (CHAMBERS, 1964) and/or from cytolyzed stromal and tumour cells.

V. The Occurrence and Nature of a Cytotoxic Tumour Factor

Previous *in vitro* culture data have repeatedly shown that normal cells in joint culture with tumour cells mostly succumb (ref. in SYLVÉN, 1962).

4*

By means of very simple translocation experiments we have observed that cultured strain L and Chang cells became cytolyzed inside 24 hours if they were suspended in culture media to which cell-free interstitial fluid from solid mouse or rat tumours had been added (HOLMBERG, 1962; SYLVÉN, 1963). During subsequent years Dr. HOLMBERG of our group found that the effect was due to a dialysable small-sized polypeptide containing 8 different amino acids only (HOLMBERG, 1964). This polypeptide has now been isolated from many fluids from solid and ascites mouse, rat and human tumour cases (Table I). The polypeptide has nothing to do with the previous "toxohormone" of Japanese investigators (NAKAHARA and FUKUOKA, 1949). It seems to be released from tumour cells possibly during necrosis. The structure presents a unique feature, namely the constellation of — Tyrosine — Cysteine — Tyrosine — which appears to form the active group (SYLVÉN and HOLMBERG, 1965). Synchronization experiments (data to be published) suggest that this factor selectively blocks some vital synthetic process during the pre-mitotic stage of the cell cycle.

The cytotoxic activity at low concentrations is mainly effective on normal non-malignant cells. At larger concentrations, however, also the growth of some tumour cells may become impaired.

In a preliminary report, WATTS (1963) has also described the presence of a dialysable cytotoxic material in sera from carcinoma-bearing rats. The cytotoxicity was determined by addition of sera to tumour cells adhering to glass surfaces according to the method used by HOLMBERG (1962). The damaging effect of added serum increased with increasing tumour size; normal sera had no effects. Interstitial fluid from S.C.K. 1 tumours

A

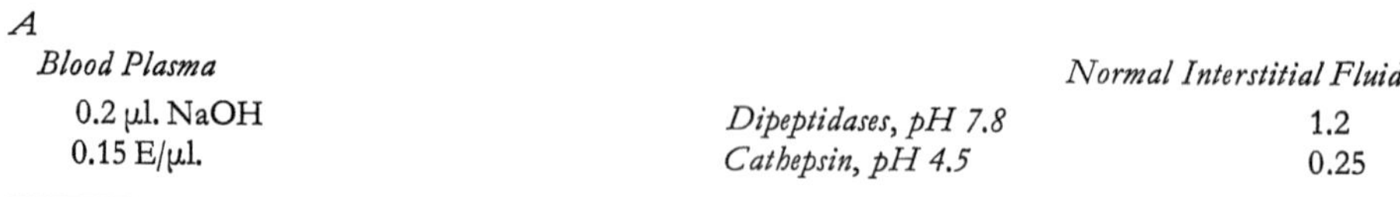

B

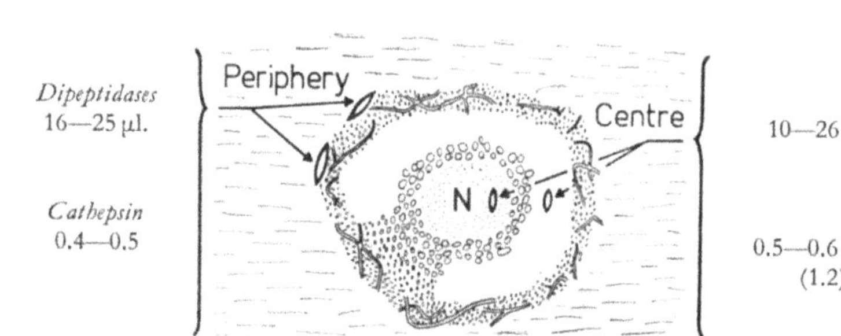

Fig. 2. Similar summarized data on the observed average activities and ranges of dipeptidase (AlaGly) and the total catheptic activity against urea-denatured hemoglobin. Section B refers to large-sized mouse tumour transplants with a necrotic center (N) (*see* SYLVÉN and BOIS-SVENSSON, 1965)

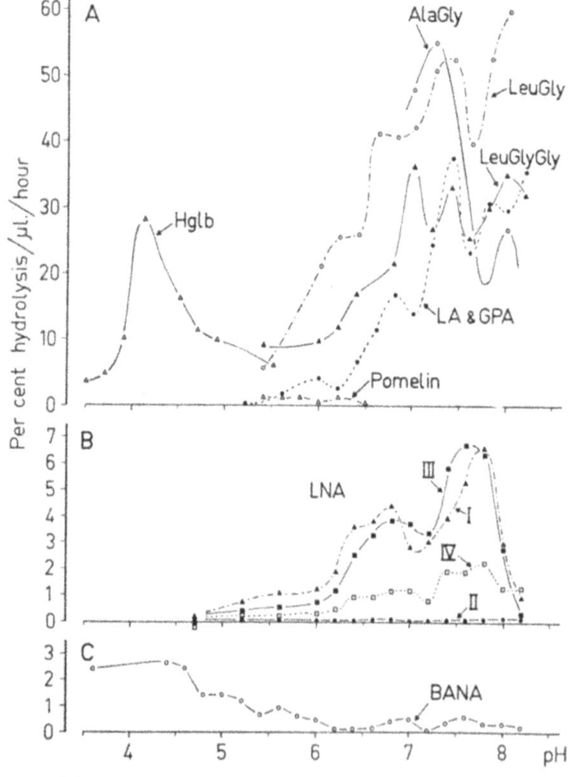

Fig. 3. Chart summarizing the pH-distribution of the catheptic and peptidase activities of central, cell-free, interstitial fluid pooled from solid Ehrlich carcinomas, representing average enzymatic levels. Common chemical abbreviations have been used for the designation of substrates. For comparison with normal interstitial fluid and detailed captions see SYLVÉN and BOIS-SVENSSON (1965). Reprinted bypermission of the Editor of *Cancer Research*

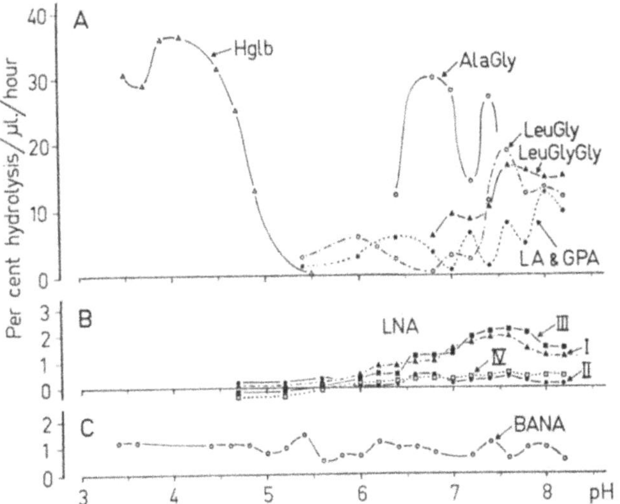

Fig. 4. Similar pH-distribution data on cell-free interstitial fluid pooled from MClM rhabdomyosarcomas. In this case the catheptic activity (mixed B and D) was greatly increased, while the average aminopeptidase, polypeptidase, dipeptidase and LNAse activities were moderately increased over those of normal interstitial fluid. For detailed captions see SYLVÉN and BOIS-SVENSSON (1965). Reprinted by permission of the Editor of *Cancer Research*

Table I. *The cytotoxic polypeptide has been isolated and analysed from ascites fluid and pleural exudates from the following tumour types (see* HOLMBERG, *1964)*

Ehrlich-Landschütz (ELD) *mouse* ascites carcinoma
Yoshida *rat* sarcoma, ascites form,
Advanced *human* cases (mostly terminal) with the following diagnoses:

Ca. abdominis	2 patients	Primary not specified
Ca. ovarii	13 patients	
Ca. corp. uteri	1 patient	
Ca. mam. gland	1 patient	Pleural effusion
Colon carcinoma	2 patients	
Hypernephroma	1 patient	
Reticulum cell sarcoma	2 patients	Retroperitoneal tumour
Carcinosis pleurae	1 patient	
Ca. bronchial.	1 patient	
Adenocarc. stomach	1 patient	

was also used, confirming our preliminary data obtained on Walker interstitial tumour fluids. The cytotoxic material was found in dialysates indicating a small molecular size. No further studies were made on the isolation or composition of the cytotoxic material, although it was assumed to be similar to that described by HOLMBERG. Cell growth inhibiting substances were also demonstrated by KATSUTA and TAKAOKA (1964). By a parabiotic cell culture technique using twin-tubes, where dialysis membranes permitted free exchange of media between the cell strains, they demonstrated that a tumour cell strain J.T.C. 1 was producing dialysable material which inhibited the growth of HeLa cells. The nature of this material was not more closely investigated.

The occurrence of this (and perhaps other?) polypeptide material and its selective action will possibly explain the marked injury and death of normal host cells as observed particularly at the invasion border of rapidly growing tumours (Sylvén and Bois-Svensson, 1964; Sylvén and Holmberg, 1965). This may further bring us to a closer understanding of the "stromal reactions" at the tumour-host interzone and also explain the increased content of hydrolases in tumour fluid, as mentioned above.

VI. Cellular Reaction as a Sequence to Autolysis

Talcum and other spontaneous granulomas are characterized by large accumulations of macrophages and histiocytes which are easily identified by their acid phosphatase reaction. It will be seen that many histiocytes die in the course of events whereby this enzyme is released to the interstitial fluid and partly adsorbed to other structures. Another group of metal-dependent aminoacyl-naphthylamidases (LNAses; Sylvén and Bois-Svensson, 1964), hydrolyzing the chromogenic substrate leucyl-β-naphthylamide (LNA) seems also to occur in autolytic vacuoles in the same cells. Following cell injury and cell death appreciable amounts of such LNAses become activated and are liberated into the extracellular compartment (Sylvén and Lippi, 1965).

Similar accumulations of histiocytes and phagocytes appear around transplanted pieces of frozen and thawed or cooked solid tumour as well as normal tissue, which then become slowly digested and removed from the periphery mainly by phagocytes. The phagocytic activity of these cells is easily demonstrated by their uptake of injected indian ink or colloidal dyes. A large number of the phagocytes die and acid phosphatase and LNAses become released into the interstitial medium (Sylvén and Lippi, 1965).

This may form an exaggeration of the reactions normally seen around rapidly growing tumours in which a smaller number of cells can be expected to die. More marked host cell reactions are found around foci of spontaneous tumour necrosis, during the homograft reaction (Chambers, 1964) as well as following necrosis by irradiation. It may be a matter of discussion to what extent such host cell reactions are due to antigenic stimuli.

VII. Stromal Reactions Around Tumours

The previous sections may help to explain the events going on at the invasion zone of the rapidly growing and highly "toxic" mouse and rat tumours. In principal, similar changes are seen in spontaneous human tumours of moderate growth rate in which, however, cell death and destructiveness generally are less marked (Sylvén, 1945, 1949).

By means of ordinary staining methods, nuclear and cytoplasmic remnants of fibroblasts, histiocytes, mast cells and possibly some tumour cells were frequently seen in the invasion zone (cp. recent electron micrographs by Barton, 1964). Phagocytosis by tumour cells of protein fragments and cytoplasmic particles as well as ingested blood cells have been described. In general, however, the phagocytic capacity of malignant cells seems rather low as compared with that of histiocytes (Easty, 1964). The histiocytes were distinguished by means of the acid phosphatase technique and marked accumulations do occur. All histiocytes as well as the growing tumour cells and injured stromal cells also showed an increased LNAse reaction confined to "lysosome-like" vacuoles (Sylvén and

Bois-Svensson, 1964; Sylvén and Lippi, 1965). Following cell death these enzymes were again released into the extracellular compartment and extensively adsorbed to denatured proteins. Only a limited number of histiocytes appeared to survive and were found in the interior of solid tumours mainly in vascularized tumour areas and around necrotic foci.

Similarly, degranulation and cytolysis of mast cells is a common feature in the invasion zone of animal and human tumours (Sylvén, 1945, 1949).

It appears that the marked activation of these enzymes as demonstrated with histochemical methods may provisionally serve as an early indicator of cell injury. This may facilitate an evaluation of the extent of cell death brought about by tumour invasion.

VIII. Concluding Remarks

The reports from this meeting bear witness to the progress made since the first informal symposium on invasiveness was held in London seven years ago (Ambrose, 1958). Since that time we have learned more of common cell physiology and our lines of thinking with respect to invasiveness and destructiveness of tumours, formation of metastases, etc. have become channelled into more fruitful areas of experimentation.

Present demands for extended knowledge concerning the surface characteristics of different cell types, their social behaviour under various circumstances and in different milieus, at different pH's (McLaren, 1959), and concerning also host cell reactions, immune responses, role of endocrine factors, cell death, phagocytosis, etc. call, however, for more crucial experimentation and more extensive use of micromethods, both for sampling and assays, preferably to be applied also to spontaneous human tumours.

As to the importance of general cytochemistry for the progress in cancer research, I should like to pay special tribute to Prof. Christian de Duve and his group. I have a feeling that his lysosomal concept (de Duve, 1959, 1964) once extended into the cancer field, will provide very useful information relating to the destructiveness of tumours and, on the whole, serve to illuminate the events at the invasion zone of tumours.

Acknowledgements

For several years this work has been supported by institutional grants from the Jubilee Fund, the Swedish Cancer Society, the Cancer Society of Stockholm, the Jane Coffin Child's Memorial Fund for Medical Research, and the Damon Runyon Memorial Fund, all of which are gratefully acknowledged.

Discussion

Questions put to B. Sylvén

B. Sylvén: Our need for more clearout definitions and crucial experimentation relating to invasiveness and formation of metastases prompts me to raise some fundamental questions. I would like to invite all of you to give your views in an attempt to arrive at a more definite standpoint, which is essential for an evaluation of the data presented at this conference.

First of all, let me remind you that all cells in a piece of solid tumour are not in the same biological state, with reference to protein synthesis, growth potential, and cell division. Long ago, as far back as 1942, Caspersson and Santesson showed by means of UV absorption measurements that the larger A-cells at the tumour periphery were the typical growing tumour cells, while the

B-cells were relatively quiescent. Now the question arises: which cells is the dangerous one, which cell produces invasion and metastases?

When we discuss experimental findings, therefore, we ought to know the biological characteristics of the material for transplantation or injection (cp. Santesson's experiments and others).

A second question that requires to be emphasized is whether metastases *in vivo* start as single cells or as clusters of tumour cells (cf. Berenblum in Sir H. Florey's text-book of pathology). This question needs much further study.

A number of additional questions not raised in this discussion concern the roles played by vascularization, interstitial fluid flow, lymphatic transport, etc. in tumour invasion, and above all the local requirements and changes associated with and/or favouring the nidation of tumour cells at other sites.

J. Leighton: Experience with the cancers of man and mouse indicates that cancer cells may spread singly, in cords, as aggregates, or as combination of these. The question you raised for discussion implies that invasive cancer cells must conform to only one of these patterns. In fact, the pattern in a single tumour nodule may be a mixed one.

B. Sylvén: Well, this may be your opinion, but I am not fully convinced as yet. I would favour the idea that generally a cluster of cells is needed.

M. Feldman: If, as suggested by Dr. Sylvén, a tumour cell population is composed of two cell types — one with a low metastatic capacity and the other with a high metastatic potency — and if the invasive properties of these two populations are stable, then when making serial transplantations of tumour cells from metastasis to normal recipients, one should select a population with an increasing capacity to form metastases.

M. Copeland: The example of bone sarcoma (osteosarcoma) was used to illustrate the A or B type of tumour cells. The test of using cochineal *in vivo* — by mouth — showed that the immature (A-type) cell without osteoid readily picked up the dye, through the phosphatase in the immature cells. The osteoid-bearing cells did not pick up any dye (B-type cells).

The metastasis usually showed little osteoid (though not always). These cells readily picked up the dye and appear to be A-type cells. This finding, obtained in bone sarcoma in the human, supports Dr. Sylvén's view that there are phases of aggressiveness in tumour cells. It is realized that histochemical tests are not entirely reliable. A positive response is significant, while a negative response is worth much less or nothing at all.

P. Sträuli: A and B cells are phenotypical adaptations of a tumour cells population to local conditions. On the other hand, the cell lines mentioned by Dr. Feldmann are genotypically fixed; they can possibly be distinguished by differences in their karyotypes. In every primary or metastatic tumour, these cell lines characterized by their genotype may be composed of A and B cells. We thus are dealing with two systems of classification: a horizontal one which comprises modifications of tumour cells (A and B cells) and a vertical one which is concerned with the tumour-cell genotypes.

M. Stoker: Although phenotypic differences may be the more probable explanation of the differences seen between cells in different parts of the tumour, we should not rule out completely the possibility that two or more genotypic variants may remain in stable association, i.e. in some sort of symbiosis.

B. Kellner: I am especially interested in the differences between necrobiotic areas, florid parts, and the vicinity of tumours. This problem has been under investigation for 30 years in my Institute and has given rise to difficulties which have not yet been solved. I should therefore like to ask some questions which are of importance in connection with our work.

1. We have not been able to make an exact differentiation between the necrotic microbiotic areas and florid tumour parts. How do you distinguish between the florid and the necrotic parts?

2. The vicinity of a tumour varies from one tumour to another, depending on the size of the tumour, reactivity of the organism, etc. How can one collect a fairly clean fluid from the stroma and connective tissue in the vicinity of a tumour?

3. Dr. BRADA mentioned Menkin's polypeptides which are produced from disorganized, dying cells during inflammation. Is there not some similarity between Menkin's factors and yours?

B. Sylvén: The answer to the first question is that fluid can be sampled from the well-vascularised tumour periphery or just outside, where no necrotic changes are seen. Fluid from central regions of unicentric tumour transplants wider than 4 mm across is always contaminated by necrotic material.

The second question has been discussed in our papers and in the present communication. The answer is that it is easy to sample a "clean" fluid owing to the peripheral edema.

With reference to all the various factors reported by my friend VALY MEN-KIN, who did pioneering work in this field, we must all realize that these factors were never sufficiently purified and chemically defined. This was not possible at Menkin's time, and hence no comparison can be made with his materials, which sometimes possibly were of a polypeptide nature.

H. Hamperl: To what extent are the peculiarities of the fluid inside and around the tumour implants characteristic of tumour cells or tumour tissue and not of a fast-growing and partially disintegrating and necrotizing cell mass in general? Could not the investigation of embryonic fast-growing cells under the same conditions provide an answer? How can one know that the pool demonstrated inside the tumour mass consists of remnants of disintegrated tissue?

The fluids surrounding the growing tumour mass may play an important role in the infiltrative growth of a tumour by weakening the cohesion of the normal tissues. But we should bear in mind that this phenomenon occurs only under special conditions and can by no means be generalized so as to provide an explanation of tumour infiltration. There are many instances in which normal and neoplastic epithelial cells lie in close contact with each other *without any interposed fluid*, and yet the normal cells show no sign of being damaged by a chemical or enzymatic action on the part of the tumour cell. The only change occurring at these sites, at which normal and tumour cells are in intimate contact with each other, is the very evident compression of the normal cells by the tumour cells, as shown diagrammatically in Fig. 1.

D. F. H. Wallach: I am curious about the mechanism of enzyme "leakage" which Dr. SYLVÉN and his associates have so beautifully shown. I believe the word "leakage" is not a properly descriptive term. For instance, remarkable losses of glycolytic enzymes occur side by side with slow, tightly regulated rates of flux of Na^+, K^+, amino acids, sugars, and inorganic phosphate, while there is no apparent loss of high-energy intermediates — at least in Ehrlich ascites

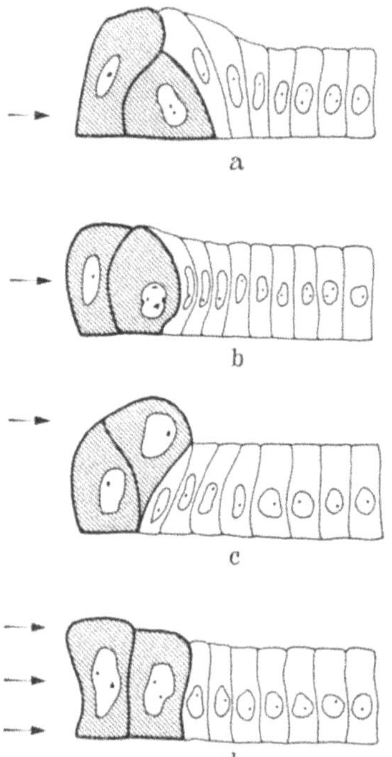

Schematic drawings based on histological sections of a carcinoma of the gall-bladder growing *in situ* and pushing aside the normal epithelium. The tumour cells (shaded) are advancing from the left and can influence the normal epithelium in different ways according to the main direction of their pressure (arrows). (From: H. Hamperl, Handbuch der allgemeinen Pathologie Bd. VI/3, 1956).

carcinoma, in which such phenomena have been extensively studied. This is all the more remarkable since the rate of pinocytosis in these cells is rather slow. It seems to me that this phenomenon must involve translocation of macromolecules across the plasma membrane. In the case of lysosomal enzymes, this would have an important bearing on the invasive process. Here, an increase in the rate of translocation of lysosomal enzymes relative to the rate of vascular perfusion could be the critical factor. It is also curious that the large loss of glycolytic enzymes occurs in cells showing a very high rate of glycolysis which can continue unabated for hours *in vitro*.

Could you give us your ideas about the mechanisms involved here? Is the "leakage" phenomenon unique to neoplasia?

B. Sylvén: We believe at present that this "leakage" or "secretion" of enzymes reflects an altered permeability of the tumour cells themselves, which in turn is due to defects or "functional pores" in their membrane structure.

Normal non-secretory cells are very tight, but all tumour cells so far investigated (except the lymphoblast strain MBIII of Dr. W. de Bruyn in Amsterdam) have been leaky.

G. Barski: You have demonstrated an increase in the products of hydrolysis and proteolysis, and at the same time an increase in enzymatic activity, in the liquid surrounding the tumours or accumulating inside them.

It is of paramount importance to know whether this increase represents a qualitative and quantitative change in the enzymatic equipment of malignant cells. If not, it could be due simply to the consequences of marked inflammatory and necrotic processes in the immediate vicinity of the tumours.

It would seem that the best way of finding an answer to this question would be to carry out parallel experiments *in vitro*. What do you think?

B. Sylvén: Cultured tumour cells and ascites tumour cells incubated under carefully controlled conditions *in vitro* in a full growth medium leak out soluble cytoplasmic enzymes, as shown by Holmberg in our Laboratory (1961) and others.

M. Feldman: Since it has to be a brief question, I will confine myself to one of the many enzymes, the increased activity of which you have described. You have demonstrated that LDH activity is elevated in the interstitial fluid of the tumour. My impression has been that the elevation of LDH in tumour-bearing animals has very little to do with the so-called destructive effects of tumour cells on normal tissues, since a similar elevation can be induced in normal animals by virus injections, without any observable "pathological" effects.

Would you care to comment on that, with regard to the general question of the relevance of the enzymes you measured to the "destructive" effects of the tumours?

B. Sylvén: The increased LDH activity has not been associated with destructiveness. As regards the role of the carbamide-bond splitting enzymes, I may refer you to my text and references.

References

ABERCROMBIE, M., and AMBROSE, E. J., The surface properties of cancer cells — a review. *Cancer Res.* **22**, 525—548 (1962).

AMBROSE, E. J., Invasiveness and surface properties of cancer cells. *Nature (Lond.)* **182**, 1419—1421 (1958).

BARSKI, G., and BELEHRADEK, J., Etude microcinématographique du mécanisme d'invasion cancéreuse en culture de tissu normal associé aux cellules malignes. *Exp. Cell Res.* **37**, 464—480 (1965).

BARTON, A. A., An electron microscope study of human breast cells in fibroadenosis and carcinoma. *Brit. J. Cancer* **18**, 682—685 (1964).

BENZ, G. VON., Die Kathepsinaktivität in normalen und malignen Geweben tumortragender Ratten (Catheptic activity in normal and malignant tissue of tumour bearing rats). *Oncologia (Basel)* **12**, 128—142 (1959).

BERENBLUM, I., *in: General pathology* (Sir H. FLOREY, ed), p. 453—456. London: Lloyd-Luke Ltd. 1958.

BERNHARD, W., Verh. Dtsch. Ges. Path. 45. Tagg, 1961, S. 7.

BERWICK, L., and COMAN, D. R., Some chemical factors in cellular adhesion and stickiness. *Cancer Res.* **22**, 982—986 (1962).

BIERICH, R., *Klin. Wschr.* **6**, 1599 (1927).

BURGESS, E. A., and SYLVÉN, B., Glucose, lactate and lactic dehydrogenase activity in normal interstitial fluid and that of solid mouse tumours. *Cancer Res.* **22**, 581—588 (1962).

CHAMBERS, V. C., and WEISER, R. S., An electron microscope study of Sarcoma I in a homologous host. II. Changes in the fine structure of the tumour cell during the homograft reaction. *Cancer Res.* **24**, 1368—1390 (1964).

COMAN, D. R., *Science* **105**, 347—348 (1947).

DE DUVE, C., *in Subcellular particles*, p. 128—159. New York: Ronald Press 1959.

— From cytases to lysosomes. *Fed. Proc.* **23**, 1045—1049 (1964).

EASTY, G. C., The uptake of fluorescent labelled proteins by normal and tumour tissues *in vivo*. *Brit. J. Cancer* **18**, 368—377 (1964).

—, and EASTY, D. M., An organ culture system for the examination of tumour invasion. *Nature (Lond.)* **199**, 1104—1105 (1963).

EHRMANN, R. L., and GEY, G. O., The growth of cells on a transparent gel of reconstituted rat-tail collagen. *J. nat. Cancer Inst.* **16**, 1375—1403 (1956).

GOLDACRE, R. J., and SYLVÉN, B., *Brit. J. Cancer* **16**, 306—322 (1962).

GROSS, J., *Ann. N.Y. Acad. Sci.* **56**, 674—683 (1953).

HINGLAIS-GUILLAUD, N., MORICARD, R., and BERNHARD, W., Ultrastructure des cancers pavimenteux invasifs du col utérin chez la femme. *Bull. Cancer* **48**, 283—316 (1961).

HOLMBERG, B., On the *in vitro* release of cytoplasmic enzymes from ascites tumour cells as compared with strain L cells. *Cancer Res.* **21**, 1386—1393 (1961).

— Inhibition of cellular adhesion and pseudopodia formation by a dialysable factor from tumour fluids. *Nature (Lond.)* **195**, 45—47 (1962).

— The isolation and composition of a cytotoxic polypeptide from tumour fluids. *Z. Krebsforsch.* **66**, 65—72 (1964).

KATSUTA, H., and TAKAOKA, T., Parabiotic cell culture. IV. Interaction between normal and ascites tumour cells of rats. *J. nat. Cancer Inst.* **32**, 963—980 (1964).

KEECH, M. K., Human skin collagen from different age groups before and after collagenase digestion — an electron microscopic study. *Ann. rheum. Dis.* **14**, 19—50 (1955).

LEIGHTON, J., Contributions of tissue culture studies to an understanding of the biology of cancer. A review. *Cancer Res.* **17**, 929—941 (1957).

— The appearance of disseminated minute tumour nodules in the chorioallantoic membrane of the chick following intravenous inoculation of ascites tumor cells. *Cancer Res.* **23**, 148—152 (1963a).

LEIGHTON, J., A method for the comparison of the fate of intravascular tumour cell emboli *in vivo* and in organ culture. *Nat. Cancer Inst. Monograph* **11**, 157—179 (1963b).

LUSE, S., and HUTTON, R., Amer. Ass. Anatomists; abstr. in *Collagen Currents* **5**, 159 (1964).

MCLAREN, A. D., and BABCOCK, K. L., *in Subcellular particles*, p. 23—60. New York: Ronald Press 1959.

MAJNO, G., and PALADE, G. E., Studies on inflammation. I. The effect of histamine and serotonin on vascular permeability: an electron microscopic study. *J. biophys. biochem. Cytol.* **11**, 571—605 (1961).

MOSCONA, A. A., Cellular interactions in experimental histogenesis. *Int. Rev. exp. Path.* **1**, 371—428 (1962).

NAKAHARA, W., and FUKUOKA, F., *Gann* **40**, 45—69 (1949).

SHELTON, E., Effect of tumour cells on pre-existing collagen and on collagen production by normal cells grown in diffusion chambers. *J. nat. Cancer Inst.* **32**, 709—722 (1964).

—, and RICE, M. E., Studies on mouse lymphomas. II. Behaviour of three lymphomas in diffusion chambers in relation to their invasive capacity in the host. *J. nat. Cancer Inst.* **21**, 137—149 (1958).

SYLVÉN, B., Ester sulphuric acids of high molecular weight and mast cells in mesenchymal tumours. Histochemical studies on tumourous growth. *Acta radiol. (Stockh.)*, Suppl. 59 (1945).

— Ester sulphuric acids in stroma connective tissue. *Acta radiol. (Stockh.)* **31**, 11—16 (1949).

— *Elfde Jaarboek van Kankeronderzoek en Kankerbestrijding in Nederland*, p. 127—133. Amsterdam: J. H. de Bussy 1961.

— *The host-tumor interzone and tumor invasion*, in: Biological interactions in normal and neoplastic growth. Henry Ford Hosp. Symp., p. 635—655 (M. J. BRENNAN and W. L. SIMPSON eds). Boston: Little, Brown & Co. 1962.

SYLVÉN, B., and BOIS-SVENSSON, I., Studies on the histochemical "leucine aminopeptidase" reaction. IV. Chemical and histochemical characterization of the intracellular and stromal LNA reactions in solid tumor transplants. *Histochemie* **4**, 135—149 (1964).

SYLVÉN, B., and BOIS-SVENSSON, I., On the chemical pathology of interstitial fluid. I. Proteolytic activities in transplanted mouse tumors. *Cancer Res.* **25**, 458—468 (1965).

—, and HOLMBERG, B., *Nord. Med.* **70**, 765—770 (1963).

— — On the structure and biological effects of a newly-discovered cytotoxic polypeptide in tumor fluid. *Europ. J. Cancer* **1**, 199—202 (1965).

—, and LIPPI, U., The suggested lysosomal localization of aminoacyl-naphthylamide splitting enzymes. *Exp. Cell Res.* **40**, 145—147 (1965).

—, and MALMGREN, H., The histological distribution of proteinase and peptidase activity in solid mouse tumor transplants. A histochemical study on the enzymic characteristics of the different tumor cell types. *Acta radiol. (Stockh.)*, Suppl. 154 (1957).

—, and SNELLMAN, O., A new metal-dependent enzyme present in cathepsin C preparations. *Biochim. biophys. Acta (Amst.)* **65**, 350—353 (1962).

VANAMEE, P., and PORTER, K. R., Observations with the electron microscope on the solvation and reconstitution of collagen. *J. exp. Med.* **94**, 255—265 (1951).

VASILIEV, J. M., The role of connective tissue proliferation in invasive growth of normal and malignant tissues: A review. *Brit. J. Cancer* **12**, 524—536 (1958).

WATTS, J., A factor in the serum of tumour-bearing rats which is deleterious to cells in tissue culture. *Nature (Lond.)* **197**, 196—197 (1963).

WEBER, R., *in: Lysosomes.* A. V. S. DE REUCK and M. P. CAMERON (eds.), p. 282—300. London: J. & A. Churchill Ltd. 1963.

WEBER, R. J., Ultrastructural changes in regressing tail muscles of *Xenopus* larvae at metamorphosis. *J. Cell Biol.* **22**, 481—487 (1964).

WOLFF, E., *in: Biological interactions in normal and neoplastic growth.* Henry Ford. Hosp. Symp. (M. J. BRENNAN and W. L. SIMPSON eds.), p. 413. Boston: Little, Brown & Co. 1962.

WYCKOFF, R. W. G., *in: Electron microscopy.* New York: Interscience Publ. 1949.

Biochemical Aspects of the Environmental Control of Tumour Growth and Spread

ZBYNĚK BRADA

Cancer Research Institute, Department of Biochemistry, Brno, Czechoslovakia

Various changes are induced in the host by the presence of tumour cells. The host's reaction may either facilitate or impede the growth and spread of tumours. Conceptions of the significance of the host's reactions are varied, and in their orthodox form they are conveyed by the term "the host's 'organic' defence". The purpose of this communication will be to review some experimental findings and to discuss, on the basis of available results, some possible hypotheses that might contribute to the understanding of these interrelations. The limits of the present communication are defined by biochemical relations, even though other factors too (above all immunological and in some cases endocrinological ones) are sure to play a most significant role.

When trying to solve these problems experimentally, investigators compare transplantable tumours with autochthonous ones. In these considerations they proceed from the assumption that between the two groups no fundamental differences usually exist and that transplantable tumours offer a number of approaches enabling a rational research to be made into these problems.

By the term "tumour growth" we mean the speed of metabolic changes connected with the division of tumour cells, while by the term "tumour spread" we mean the speed and mode of tumour infiltration. A close relationship exists between these two phenomena.

Reaction at the Tumour-Host Interphase and Formation of Tumour Stroma

In order that reactions may take place at the interzone between the tumour cells and the host, it is necessary for the tumour cells to be slightly irritant to the adjoining tissues, i.e. the existence of tumour cells means the transmission of stimuli to the host.

As yet no definite answer can be given as to the nature of these stimuli. It may, however be, presumed that a complex phenomenon is involved (Fig. 1), and that at least some of its parts are of a completely unspecific character, such as raised nutrition requirements. As a result of these stimuli and the contact of the peritumoral tissue with tumour cells there ensue angioplastic and fibroplastic reactions in the host. These reactions result in the formation of the so-called stromal bed of the tumour. It is presumed that the stromal bed is the local representative of the host and that it is here that host responses to tumour growth find their final expression (LEIGHTON, 1964).

A tumour mass can be produced in vivo by tumour cells only when the host provides a favourable environment for the growth of tumour cells. The most important condition of tumour cell growth is the supply of nutritional factors and the elimination of metabolic catabolites. This basic condition is assured because tumour cells are able to induce the production of new capillary endothelium from the host. Though this special quality is not characteristic of tumour growth, it is usually reported tissue of the stroma, then information on the constancy of hexosamine concentration would indicate the permanent ratio between the tumour cells themselves and the tumour stroma, irrespective of whether the stromal connective tissue is formed by host or tumour fibroblasts. Independently of our work this finding has been confirmed by a study of col-

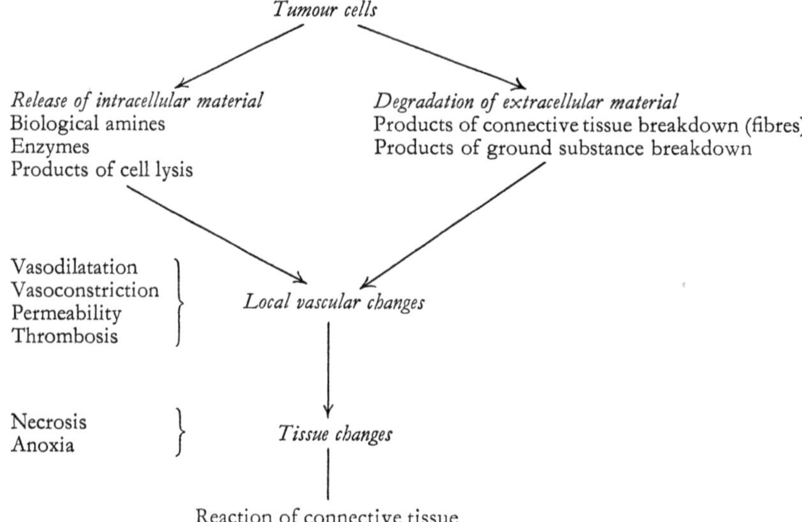

Fig. 1. Concepts of the reaction chain between tumour growth and connective tissue reactions

that proliferation of capillaries takes place three days after tumour transplantation, as contrasted with six days for normal autologous tissue. The second basic condition, which is closely connected with the first, is the formation of tumour stroma permitting diffusion of substances to and from the tumour cell. Consequently, tumour stroma formation participates functionally in the creation of the tumour's optimal architecture. In 1960 we observed (PECHAN and BRADA, 1960) that the hexosamine concentration of transplanted BS rat tumour was constant during tumour growth. If we proceed from the assumption that hexosamine contained in a solid tumour is for the greater part found in the connective lagen concentration in epithelial tumours (GULLINO and GRANTHAM, 1963; GULLINO *et al.*, 1962). These tumours are far more suitable for such studies, since it has been found that collagen is produced exclusively by host fibroblasts (SHELTON, 1964).

In spite of the fact that host fibroblasts are involved, collagen production is not regulated by the host but by the tumour cell, so that we are justified in speaking of the fibroplastic efficiency of tumour cells. Our results obtained by studying hexosamine concentration in solid Ehrlich and Krebs tumours growing on different hosts (BRADA, 1965), are in agreement with GULLINO's findings.

The Function of Peritumoral Connective Tissue from the Standpoint of Tumour Invasion

However, peritumoral connective tissue is often considered to be a barrier standing in the way of tumour cell invasion. Even though tumour cell infiltration is made possible owing to own favourable properties, it is perhaps worth considering the exact cause of infiltration. Earlier it was thought that the cause of infiltration was some pressure arising inside the tumour as a result of permanent growth (YOUNG, 1959). This view was justly criticized, because infiltration takes place even in tissue cultures where no such pressure can be manifested (EASTY and EASTY, 1963). From the biochemical standpoint it appears that the principal cause is the migration of tumour cells against the concentration gradient of the nutrients and in the direction of the falling concentration of tumour cell catabolites.

Let us now consider the possible function of the interstitial connective tissue from the standpoint of tumour infiltration. In the case of our simplified model of interstitial tissue we shall consider the function of connective tissue fibres, the half liquid amorphous intersubstance, interstitial fluid, as well as further cell components. Special biochemical data on parablastomatous connective tissue are practically unobtainable. Data on the collagen and polysaccharide content of tumours of an ectodermal origin indicate that investigations of these substance groups in solid tumours contribute more to the study of the tumour stroma than to the biochemistry of the tumour cells themselves. This is evidenced by the results of a preliminary study of hexosamine-containing substances in solid Yoshida tumours and Yoshida tumour cells (BRADA, 1964). These results have shown that isolated tumour cells contain hexos-amine predominantly in substances of a neutral type in contrast to the predominant part of hexosamine in solid tumours, where it is contained in substances of an acid character. The properties of structural components have shown that tumour cells are surrounded by substances of extremely high stability, that is not only by protein fibrils (collagen, elastin, reticulin), which are highly resistant to tension and not very elastic, but that the network of these fibrils is again stabilized and restricted in its possible movements by the influence of polysaccharide macromolecules.

As to collagen fibres visible under a light microscope, it may be stated that they most probably serve as a kind of shifting mechanism of transferred cells. This presumption has been corroborated by observations on tissue cultures. The cell movement naturally depends on the orientation of the fibres, too. On the other hand, numerous small fibrils surrounding the cell on all sides may also function as obstacles to the shifting of cells, provided they do not possess an apparatus that would enable them to loosen themselves from the hindering fibrils. In principle, some kind of enzymatic mechanism (breaking down fibrils or polysaccharides), or some influence of other chemical factors on the degradation of the connective tissue might be involved. The considerable resistance of connective tissue fibrils to proteolytic enzymes is generally known. The possibility of rapid desintegration of collagens is, however, demonstrated by the very rapid resorption of carragenin granuloma or by uterus involution following birth (WOESSNER, 1962). In carragenin granulomas and in tumour ascites fluid there are present katepsins with a pH optimum of about 4. The origin, specificity and nature of these katepsins have so far not been explained (SYLVÉN and

Bois, 1960). The question of their activation and their release is also as yet unknown. The presence of enzymes, such as collagenase, might of course explain the destruction of fibres, but so far doubt has been expressed as to the presence of such enzymes in mammal tissues. Recently, their presence has been noted in extracts from the pancreas (Houck, Jacob, 1960; Oken, Boucek, 1957) and in the skin of rats (Goldstein et al., 1964). In any case, these enzymes have not been sufficiently characterized and their presence in tumours and in various organs has not so far been verified. The same applies to elastase discovered by Baló Banga (1963) and Hall (1963). Scanty experimental data exist to throw light on the real role of the collagen fibres. It is known that lathyrogenic substances prevent soluble collagen from changing into insoluble. Experimental data on the influence of lathyrism on tumour growth do not completely agree (Karpas and Madden, 1964; McCrary et al., 1963). These substances inhibit tumour growth to a small degree, although accelerated growth has been observed at the initial stage. This fact may indicate that insoluble collagen formation might be the host's response in order to slow down tumour growth. On the other hand it is reported by Shelton that tumour cells do not possess the capacity of destroying preformed collagen (Shelton, 1964). However, the possibility cannot be excluded that even normal proteolytic enzymes can degrade fibrils after denaturation, e.g. with lactic acid. Stability against enzyme activity is most probably conditioned by the integrity of mucosaccharide-collagen complexes (Glynn, Reading, 1956). Mucopolysaccharides or mucoproteins form around individual collagen fibres an envelope consisting predominantly of hyaluronic and chondroitinsulphuric acid (Jackson, 1957). According to Chvapil and Zahradník (1960) a mere pH shift to the acid region is sufficient to split the polysaccharide material from the collagen fibres. But their views on the stabilization of collagen by polysaccharides are not generally accepted (Glynn, 1957). Sometimes, it is explained by the special structure of the collagen alone. Another variant of these considerations in the view that collagen fibres do not locally disintegrate into their fundamental structural elements, but that they dissociate into their subunits, which then associate again, thereby enabling the cell to move. Acid polysaccharides, which morphologically represent the ground substance of connective tissue, could be eliminated by mucolytic enzymes. According to Grossfeld's data, hyaluronidase is produced by tumour cells of epithelial origin, and sarcomata do not contain any hyaluronidase. The molecular weight of hyaluronic acid isolated from Rous chicken sarcoma is about one third lower than that of hyaluronic acid from healthy tissues (Caputo and Marcante, 1960). This finding may be connected with the possible regulation of the intrinsic viscosity of hyaluronic acid during its synthesis.

Acid polysaccharides can be also degraded in another way than by the action of mucolytic enzymes. Various substances and systems that have the power to induce radical formation (e.g. ascorbic acid) bring about degradation of hyaluronic acid (Pigman, 1963; Pigman, Rizvi, 1959; Ropes et al., 1947). Proteins carrying free SH-groups are able to degrade hyaluronic acid, which can also be demonstrated during the incubation of serum with hyaluronic acid (Robert, Robert, 1963).

If connective tissue or its components are really degraded by the action of the tumour, the products of degradation could be of specific significance to tumour-host relationship, about which there are reported data in the literature (HANO, 1960; LINDNER et al., 1960; RUBIN et al., 1954; SCHWEINITZ et al., 1960; VOSS et al., 1963). These data concern the cytotoxic effect of glucosamine, the inhibition of mucolytic processes and the inhibition of cell mobility (LEHMAN). It has been stressed above that the stromal connective tissue is very important for substance exchange between the tumour cell and the host. The very existence of the tumour stroma suggests that the destruction of the connective tissue must at least be of a limited character, because it would be very hard to explain why it is stromal connective tissue, as contrasted with peritumoral connective tissue, that should resist the degradation effect of infiltrating tumour cells.

The flow of interstitial fluid as also influenced by the viscosity of the ground substance (its permeability). In the case of ascitic tumours, we have interpreted the retarded outflow in a different way since we assume that the lymphatics become less passable as a result of connective tissue proliferation and thrombus formation.

In this case, the reason why interstitial connective tissue inside the tumour remains intact might be: 1. the limited diffusion of substances, so that from the standpoint of nutrition of tumour cells the interstitial fluid would not represent a field with a concentration gradient of nutrients; 2. the presence of some katabolites that would reduce invasion; 3. a change in the chemical character of connective tissue. When studying hexosamine concentration in necrotic and living tissue, no differences were found. But considerable difference in the content of hydroxyproline containing material were observed. Necrotic tumour

tissue contains less hydroxyproline than living tissue. When determining hydroxyproline concentration in slices obtained from cryostat we found no difference in collagen content between the peritumoral and tumour tissue. But considerable differences between the peritumoral connective tissue, living tumour tissue and necrotic tumour tissue were found when hydroxyproline determinations were performed in extracts at pH 9 and pH 3. These results are shown in Fig. 2. A more extensive degradation

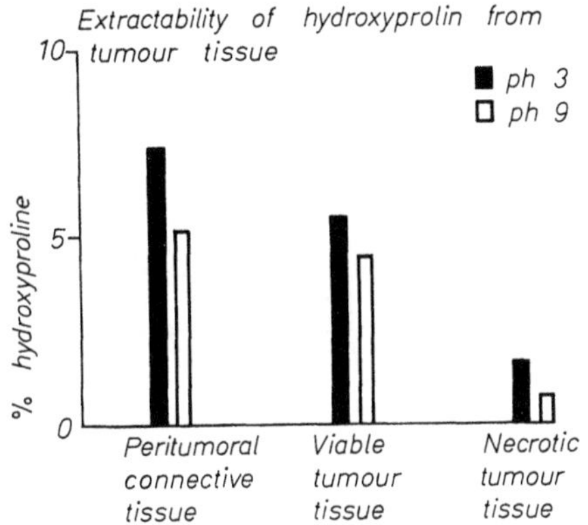

Fig. 2. Extractability of hydroxyproline from Jensen tumour homogenate expressed in percentage of total hydroxyproline

of collagen and of related proteins could be accompanied by raised concentrations of the material containing hydroxyprolin in the serum. Although such a substance has been proved to exist in the serum, no information is so far available on its behaviour in tumour-bearing animals (LEROY et al., 1964). During the growth of Jensen tumour of rats there were observed almost no changes in the hydroxyproline excretion in urine. But in the terminal stage there appeared a high maximum, in which the ration free (total hydroxyproline showed a marked increase) (Fig. 3). Histological examination has revealed that this stage corresponds to the degradation of spinal bone collagen caused by direct infiltration of cells from the near by primary tumour (Vermousek *et al.*, 1967). Excretion of hexosamine containing low-molecular substances in different patients with disseminated cancer was compared with the situation in healthy persons (Pechan, 1964). It was found that, with the exception of a group of patients with cancer of the stomach, where decreased excretion was observed, no differences existed between the control groups of the same age. Moreover, no marked

substances in tumour-bearing animals cannot be brought into play. By eliminating liver function in animals with tumours as a result of intoxication induced with tetrachlormethan, it is possible largely to lower the concentration of these substances in the serum, but to a smaller degree than was observed in animals with sterile abscesses. Under these conditions the concentration of glycoproteins and mucoproteins is closely related to the relative size of the tumour (Tobiška *et al.*, 1964). This rela-

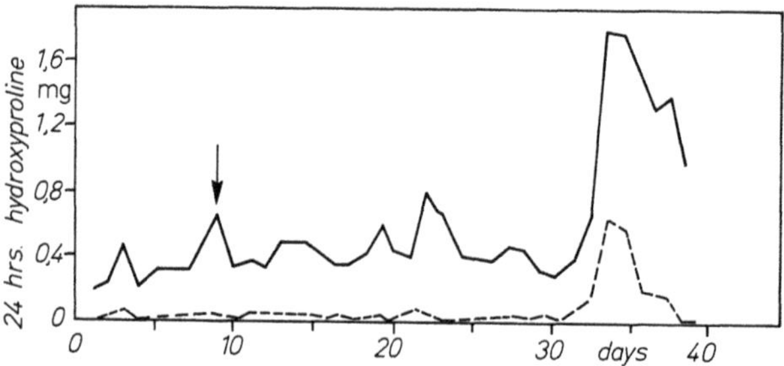

Fig. 3. Excretion of total (———) and free (------) urine hydroxyproline in Jensen tumour bearing rats. Arrow indicate the time of tumour transplantation

differences have been ascertained in the content of hexosamine containing low molecular substances between normal human serum and tumorous ascitic fluid (Kolářová *et al.*, in preparation for press). The concentration of these substances is very low, being somewhere below 1 mg-%. The concentration of hexosamine containing high molecular substances (glycoproteins, mucoproteins) is raised in the serum of human beings and of animals with tumours. Although according to one of the hypotheses they arise as a result of depolymerisation of the ground substance (Catchpole, 1950; Pirani, Catchpole, 1951), most of these substances originate in the liver (Miller and Bale, 1954; Tobiška *et al.*, 1964; Werner, 1949). This does not of course mean that extrahepatic synthesis or the release from extrahepatic tissues of these

tion need not, however, be only the consequence of the extrahepatic or directly peritumoral origin of these substances, but may express a close correlation between the biosynthetic activity of the functionally intact remaining part of the liver and the metabolic requirements of the tumour, although we cannot exclude the possibility that even a part of these substances may be released in the course of infiltration from the peritumoral connective tissue. It has been observed that substances of this type are released from Jensen tumours (Irwine *et al.*, 1961) during cell cultivation.

An essentially better criterion of connective tissue degradation would be the determination of acid polysaccharides in the serum. However, no information is available in this respect, apparently owing to their very low level of concentration (lower than 1 mg-%).

Concentration changes of substances present in the blood and consequently also in the tumorous interstitial fluid may be considered from another angle too, irrespective of the site of their origin, that is from the viewpoint of their functional role in the course of tumour growth. In these considerations we shall not only discuss metabolic processes taking place at the interface between tumour and host, but we shall extend the problems from the standpoint of the nutrition requirements of the tumour cell and in particular to regulation relationships between tumour and host.

The Influence of Biochemical Changes in the Host on the Creation of Tumour-Host Relationship

When considering the role played by substances of a high-molecular character in the growth and spread of cancers, we cannot limit our considerations to their direct inhibitory or growth-promoting effect. Consequently, it is not necessary for all these growth-promoting or inhibitory factors to be chemical entities in all cases. By regulating the permeability of the blood capillaries, by influencing the permeability of the connective tissue, by the presence of substances capable of transporting physiologically active factors, etc., it is possible indirectly to influence proliferation of tumour cells and the spread of tumour cells both in the growth-promoting and in the inhibitory direction. Also the very changes in the concentration of some components in the tumour cell environment can have an influence on the mitotic activity of tumour cells, in accordance with observations made by Glinos (1960) on a model of a liver following partial hepatectomy. On the other hand, the concentration of these substances may be influenced directly both by their utilization by the

tumour cell and its formation in the tumour cell, or indirectly by influencing their synthesis in the host. Consequently, we can imagine, to a certain degree, that mitotic activity in the tumour cell is directed by feedback regulation, but with the tumour progress the importance of the feedback control keeps gradually decreasing, and finally the bond is broken either at tumour cell or host level. One of the possible approaches to the study of these problems is analysis of the interstitial tumour fluid. Attempts have been made to obtain this fluid by various methods (Gullino *et al.*, 1964; Mauer, 1938; Sylvén, Bois, 1960; Vozejl, Zajicek, 1962). The first more detailed information on this fluid was obtained by Sylvén and Holmberg (1963), and later by Gullino *et al.* (1964).

Tumour interstitial fluid is surrounded on one side by a tumour cell membrane, on the other by the endothelium of blood capillaries. Consequently, it is a fluid that rinses tumour cells and contains metabolic products of tumour cell activity, products of tumour and non-tumour cell cytolysis, products of ground substance and connective tissue fibril disaggregation, and especially substances passing from the vascular bed through the network of capillary endothelium. Interstitial fluid is then transported through lymphatic pathways as far as the blood. A model of ascites tumours can also be used for similar purposes. Here too, one of the boundaries is formed by the tumour cell walls and the other by the endothelium of blood capillaries, because the barrier of peritoneal mesothelium is broken and the interstitial fluid flows directly from the peritoneal wall into the abdominal cavity (Fig. 4).

It may be presumed that, just as in the case of solid tumours, the origin of ascites tumours is closely connected with the host's response to tumour stimulus

(WHEATLEY, 1964; WHEATLEY *et al.*, 1963). In subcutaneous application, ascites tumour cells possess a greater ability to induce a fibroplastic reaction than solid tumour cells. Following infiltration even retrograde lymph flow, which is evidenced by a higher concentration of some immunoglobulins, much higher in the ascites fluid than in the serum (ANACKER and MUNOZ, 1961).

The mechanism of ascites tumour formation

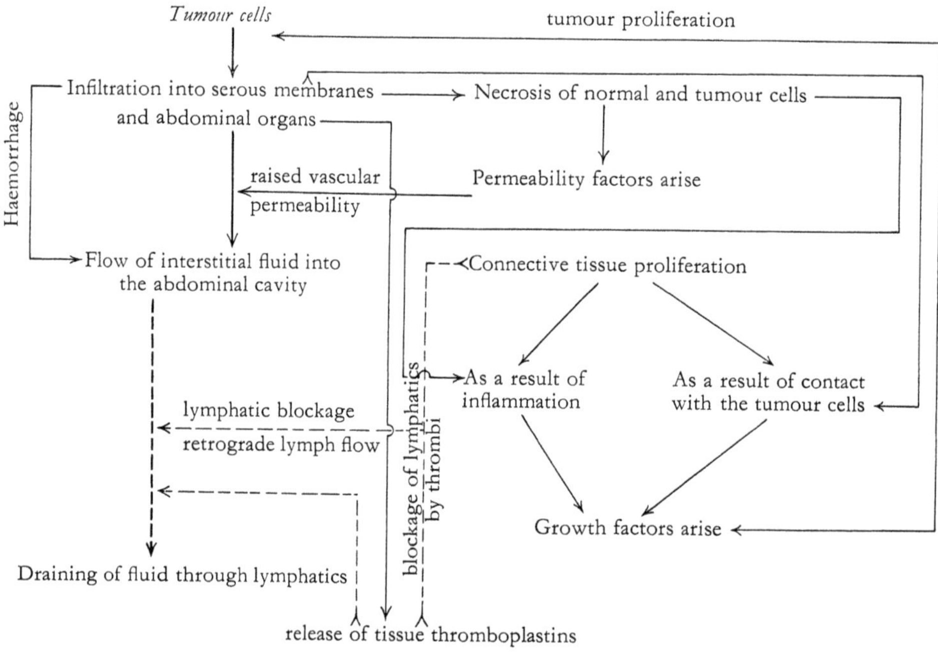

Fig. 4. Mechanism of ascitic tumour formation from the standpoint of tumour-host relationship. The broken line represents inhibition effects

into serous membranes and abdominal organs, connective tissue proliferation takes place (MENKIN, 1960) this being the result of contact with the tumour cell and of inflammation induced by necrosis of normal and of tumour cells. Simultaneously, growth factors arise which again have an effect on tumour cell proliferation. As a result of inflammation various permeability factors are brought into play and increase vascular permeability in the peritoneum.

In consequence of connective tissue proliferation and perhaps as a result of thrombus formation there results not only lymphatic blockade but probably

High-Molecular Substances in Ascitic Fluid

The concentration of total proteins is constantly lower both in the interstitial tumour fluid (GULLINO *et al.*, 1964) and in the cell-free ascites fluid (DOLEŽA-LOVÁ *et al.*, 1964) than in the blood serum. Although no correlation exists between total protein concentration in the blood serum and total protein concentration in defibrinated cell-free ascites fluid, a very close correlation exists between a number of protein components. This may be observed for example, with mucoproteins and sialoproteins. The concentration of total proteins and of protein-bound hexoses correlates significantly with ascites tumour size. It may be concluded that ascites fluid composition is in close correlation with changes in the composition of the corresponding blood serum; consequently, the changes induced by tumour growth in blood protein anabolism and katabolism are directly reflected in the composition of the fluid rinsing tumour cells. Semiquantitative investigation of the passage of individual serum proteins into the ascites fluid (DOLEŽALOVÁ and BRADA, 1964), has revealed that it is serum components alpha$_1$ A, alpha$_1$ B, alpha$_1$ D, alpha$_2$ F, alpha$_2$ B and alpha$_2$ C that pass into the ascites fluid in the greatest amounts. As to mucoproteins (protein soluble in sulphosalicylic acid), it has been found that a number of substances take part in the increase of these substances in the blood and ascites serum, in particular the fractions containing alpha$_2$B-globulin (haptoglobin), alpha$_2$C-globulin, beta-A-globulin (haemopexin). Acid polysaccharides containing fractions are much less responsible for this increase (DOLEŽALOVÁ and BRADA, 1964). The concentration of protein groups classified according to their molecular weight varies in the course of tumour growth (CAPUTO and MARCANTE, 1962; DOLEŽALOVÁ and BRADA, 1966). Most marked is the increase in the macroglobulin fraction.

Relation of the Biosynthesis of Glycoproteins and Mucoproteins to the Processes at the Tumour-Host Interphase and their Functional Significance

On the basis of these experimental results no further information can be obtained on the functional significance of changes in the concentration of some proteins. However, these results create conditions for further study of these problems along the lines suggested.

The greatest changes in serum and ascites protein concentrations take place in the group of glycoproteins and mucoproteins. The possibility cannot be excluded that the synthesis of these substances in the host is stimulated by some degradation products arising at the tumour-host interface. It appears, however, that bacterial toxins released from the tumour, or the activation of latent infection in the host (PATTERSON et al., 1963) are also very important factors. JAYLE, BOUSSIER (1955), and ROBERT, ROBERT (1963) have expressed the opinion that glycoproteins and mucoproteins are very important to connective tissue synthesis. Their importance as growth-promoting factors has been also demonstrated by a number of other observations (GLINOS, 1962; KENT and GEY, 1957; KENT and GEY, 1960; LEADERS et al., 1962; LIEBERMANN and OVE, 1958; MARR et al., 1962; TOBIŠKA and BRADA, 1963). Furthermore, some of their other functions are also known. We assume that the tumour stimuli discussed in the present communication do not induce any specific metabolic reactions in the host but are part of the general adaptation syndrome.

In consequence of this, the otherwise adequate adaptation reactions of the organism, the purpose of which is to get the noxious factors under control, do not always terminate favourably for the organism in the case of malignant tumours, because in the first stage these reactions appear to promote cell dedifferentiation and proliferation (STICH, 1960). It is true than reactions of the second stage of the regenerative proces soon come into play, but owing to the fact that the tumour stimulus continues to be active throughout tumour growth until the organism dies, both these reactions occur simultaneously. As to the equilibrium or changes in the equilibrium of these two reactions, only working hypotheses can as yet be expressed.

References

ANACKER, R. L., and MUNOZ, J., Characterization and properties of antibody in mouse peritoneal fluid. *J. Immunol.* **87**, 426 (1961).

BANGA, I., Signification biologique des enzymes élastolytiques. *Exp. Ann. Biochim. Méd.* **24**, 151 (1963).

BRADA, Z., Mucoproteins and mucopolysaccharides in tumour cell. *Acta Un. int. Cancer* **20**, 945 (1964).

— Host-tumour relationship. XX. The hexosamine content of the tumour as an marker of relations between the tumour stroma and tumour cells. *Neoplasma (Bratisl.)* **12**, 373 (1965).

BURGESS, E. A., and SYLVÉN, B., Glucose lactate and lactic dehydrogenase activity in normal interstitial fluid and that of solid mouse tumours. *Cancer Res.* **22**, 581 (1962).

CAPUTO, A., and MARCANTE, M. L., On the structure of hyaluronic acid-protein complex isolated from Rous chicken sarcoma. *Clin. chim. Acta* **5**, 477 (1960).

— — Protein changes occuring in blood serum and ascitic fluid in rats with Yoshida ascites tumours. *Acta Un. int. Cancr.* **18**, 99 (1962).

CATCHPOLE, H. R., Serum and tissue glycoproteins in mice bearing transplantable tumours. *Proc. Soc. exp. Biol. (N.Y.)* **75**, 221 (1950).

CHVAPIL, M., and ZAHRADNÍK, R., A study of the chemical shrinkage and relaxation of collagen fibres. *Biochim. biophys. Acta (Amst.)* **40**, 329 (1960).

DOLEŽALOVÁ, V., and BRADA, Z., Host-tumour relationship. XVII. Quantitative changes in some fractions of sulphosalicylic acid soluble substances in the serum and ascites fluid of Yoshida ascites tumour bearing rats. *Neoplasma (Bratisl.)* **11**, 459 (1964).

— — Host-tumour relationship. XXI. Proteins distribution according to molecular size between the serum and ascites fluid in the course of development of Yoshida ascites tumours in rats. *Neoplasma (Bratisl.)* **13**, 35 (1966).

— —, and KOČENT, A., Host-tumour relationship. XIII. Proteins, mucoproteins and their saccharide components in the serum and ascitic fluid of rats in the course of growth of Yoshida ascitic sarcoma. *Neoplasma (Bratisl.)* **11**, 257 (1964).

— — —, and HEKELOVA, J., Host-tumour relationship. XV. Comparison of proteins in the blood and ascites serum of rats with Yoshida ascites tumour. *Neoplasma (Bratisl.)* **11**, 361 (1964).

EASTY, G. C., and EASTY, D. M., An organ culture system for the examination of tumor invasion. *Nature (Lond.)* **199**, 1104 (1963).

GLINOS, A. D., Environmental feedback control of cell division. *Ann. N.Y. Acad. Sci.* **90**, 592 (1960).

— On relationship between the D_2 serum globulins and normal and neoplastic cell growth. VIII. Int. Cancer Congr. Abstr. 476, Moskva 1962.

GLYNN, L. E., *Int. Symposium on diseases of collagen*, Milano 1957.

—, u. READING, C. A., *7. Colloquium d. Ges. f. Physiol. Chem.* Mosbach 1956. Berlin-Göttingen-Heidelberg: Springer 1957.

GOLDSTEIN, E. R., PATEL, Y. M., and HOUCK, J. C., Collagenolytic activity of intact and necrotic connective tissue. *Science* **146**, 942 (1964).

GULLINO, P. M., CLARK, S. H., and GRANTHAM, F. H., The interstitial fluid of solid tumours. *Cancer Res.* **24**, 780 (1964).

—, and GRANTHAM, F. H., The influence of the host and the neoplastic cell population on the collagen content of a tumour mass. *Cancer Res.* **23**, 648 (1963).

— —, and CLARK, S. H., The collagen content of transplanted tumors. *Cancer Res.* **22**, 1031 (1962).

HALL, D. A., Elastase and its inhibitors. *Exp. Ann. Biochim. Méd.* **24**, 165 (1963).

HANO, K., Studies on the cancerostatic activities of aminosugars and mucopolysaccharides in vitro. *J. Osaka Med. Coll.* **20**, 86 (1960).

HOUCK, I. C., and JACOB, R. A., Systemic response of collagen to local inflammation. *Fed. Proc. A* **19**, 149 (1960).

IRWINE, E. S., WHITTLE, W., SHIRLEY, B., CONWAY, E., and McCoY, T. A., Production of extracellular material by Jensen sarcoma cells in vitro. *Proc. Soc. exp. Biol. (N.Y.)* **108**, 629 (1961).

JACKSON, S. F., *Connective tissue.* Oxford: Blackwell Sci. Publ. 1957.

JAYLE, M. F., et BOUSSIER, G., Les séromucoides du sang. Leurs relations avec les mucoprotéines de la substance foudamentale du tissu conjonctif. *Exp. Ann. Biochim. Méd.* **17**, 157 (1955).

KARPAS, CH. M., and MADDEN, R. E., Lathyrism in an experimental model modifying host response to transplantable tumors. *Proc. Amer. Ass. Cancer Res.* **5**, 34 (1964).

KENT, H. N., and GEY, G. O., Changes in serum proteins during growth of malignant cells in vitro *Proc. Soc. exp. Biol. (N.Y.)* **94**, 205 (1957)

— — Selective uptake of serum globulins and glycoproteins by cells growing in vitro. *Science* **131**, 667 (1960).

KOLÁŘOVÁ, M., BRADA, Z., and VERMOUSEK, I., *in preparation for press.*

LEADERS, F. E., DIXON, R. L., OSBORNE, J. W., and LONG, J. P., Erythropoietic stimulating factor (ESF) as a stimulant of tumour growth. *Proc. Soc. exp. Biol. (N.Y.)* **110**, 436 (1962).

LEIGHTON, J., Invasion and metastasis of heterologous tumors in the chick embryo. In: HOMBURGER, F., *Progress in tumor research*, vol. 4, p. 198. Basel: S. Karger 1964.

LIEBERMANN, I., and OVE, P., A protein growth factor for mammalian cells in culture. *J. biol. Chem.* **233**, 637 (1958).

LINDNER, J., SCHWEINITZ, H. A., u. BECHER, K., Über die geschwulsthemmende Wirkung von Grundsubstanzbestandteilen. II. Mitt. Stoffwechseluntersuchungen. *Klin. Wschr.* **38**, 763 (1960).

MARR, A. G. M., OWEN, J. A., and WILSON, G. S., Studies on the growth-promoting glycoprotein fraction of foetal calf serum. *Biochim. biophys. Acta (Amst.)* **63**, 276 (1962).

MAUER, F. W., Isolation and analysis of extracellular muscle fluid from the frog. *Amer. J. Physiol.* **124**, 547 (1938).

McCRARY, C., AKAMATSU, J., and ORBISON, J. L., Lathyrism effect on tumour-host relationships in the rat. *Arch. Path.* **76**, 95 (1963).

MENKIN, V., Biologic cocarcinogens. In: HOMBURGER, F., *Progress in experimental tumor research*, vol. 1, p. 279. Basel: S. Karger 1960.

MILLER, L. L., and BALE, W. F., Synthesis of all plasma protein fractions except gammaglobulins by the liver. The use of zone electrophoresis and lysin-C^{14} to define the plasma proteins synthetized by isolated perfused liver. *J. exp. Med.* **99**, 125 (1954).

OKEN, D. E., and BOUCEK, R. J., Enzymatic proteolysis of rat sponge biopsy collagen tissue. *Proc. Soc. exp. Biol. (N.Y.)* **96**, 367 (1957).

PATTERSON jr., M. K., MAXWELL, M. D., and McCOY, T. A., Influence of secondary infection on tumour host serumbound carbohydrates. *Proc. Soc. exp. Biol. (N.Y.)* **113**, 689 (1963).

PECHAN, Z., Hexosamine containing substances in cancer. III. Excretion of dialyzable hexosamine in urine. The influence of age and malignant tumour disease. *Neoplasma (Bratisl.)* **11**, 37 (1964).

PECHAN, Z., and BRADA, Z., Host-tumour relationship. V. Hexosamine distribution in rat organs in dependence on growth of the BS tumour. *Neoplasma (Bratisl.)* **7**, 366 (1960).

PIGMAN, W., Acide hyaluronique et facteurs de perméabilité tissulaire. *Bull. Soc. Chim. biol. (Paris)* **45**, 185 (1963).

—, and RIZVI, S., Hyaluronic acid. *Biochem. biophys. Res. Commun.* **1**, 39 (1959).

PIRANI, C. L., and CATCHPOLE, H. R., Serum glycoproteins in experimental scurvy. *Arch. Path.* **51**, 597 (1951).

ROBERT, L., and ROBERT, B., Mécanismes enzymatiques de la dégradation du tissu conjonctif a l'état normal et pathologique. *Exp. Ann. Biochim. Méd.* **24**, 269 (1963).

ROPES, M. W., VAN ROBERTSON, W. B., ROSSMEISEL, E. C., PEABODY, R. B., and BAUER, W., Synovial fluid mucin. *Acta med. scand.* **128**, Suppl. 700 (1947).

ROY, E. C. LE, KAPLAN, A., UDENFRIEND, S., and SJOERDSMA, A., A hydroxyprolin-containing, collagen-like protein in plasma and a procedure for its assay. *J. biol. Chem.* **239**, 3350 (1964).

RUBIN, A., SPRINGER, G. F., and HOGUE, M. J., The effect of D-glucosamine hydrochloride and related compounds on tissue cultures of the solid form of mouse sarcom 37. *Cancer Res.* **14**, 456 (1954).

SCHWEINITZ, H. A., LINDNER, J., u. VOSS, H., Über die geschwulsthemmende Wirkung von Grundsubstanzbestandteilen. III. Mitt. Die Beziehung zwischen Überlebensratten, Stoffwechseluntersuchungen und cytologischen Befunden. *Frankfurt. Z. Path.* **70**, 150 (1960).

SHELTON, E., Effect of tumor cells on preexisting collagen and on collagen production by normal cells grown in diffusion chambers. *J. nat. Cancer Inst.* **32**, 703 (1964).

STICH, M. F., Regulation of mitotic rate in mammalian organisms. *Ann. N.Y. Acad. Sci.* **90**, 603 (1960).

SYLVÉN, B., and BOIS, I., Protein content and enzymatic assays of interstitial fluid from some normal tissues and transplanted mouse tumors. *Cancer Res.* **20**, 831 (1960).

—, and HOLMBERG, B., Current approaches in the study of the destructive capacity of malignant tissues. *Yearbook of Swedish Cancer Soc.* **3**, 202 (1963).

TOBIŠKA, J., and BRADA, Z., Host-tumour relationship. IX. The erythropoietic activity of rat plasma in the course of the growth of the Jensen tumour as studied by means of ^{53}Fe. *Neoplasma (Bratisl.)* **10**, 597 (1963).

Tobiška, J., Brada, Z., Kočent, A., and Pechan, Z., Hosttumour relationship. X. The role of the liverin serum glycoprotein synthesis during the course of experimental inflammation. *Neoplasma (Bratisl.)* **11**, 3 (1964).

— — — — Host-tumour relationship. XI. The role of the liver in the synthesis of serum glycoproteins during the course of growth of Jensen's sarcoma. *Neoplasma (Bratisl.)* **11**, 13 (1964).

Vasiljev, J. M., The role of connective tissue proliferation in invasive growth of normal and malignant tissues. A review. *Brit. J. Cancer* **12**, 524—536 (1958).

Vermousek, I., Brada, Z., and Tobiška, J., Host-tumour relationship. XXII. Hydroxyproline excretion in the course of tumour growth and sterile abscess in rats. *Neoplasma (Bratisl.)* **14**, 59 (1967).

Vozejl, J. M., and Zajicek, J., Quantitative determination of enzymic activities in cells and in extracellular fluid aspirated from human tumors by needle biopsy. *Experientia (Basel)* **18**, 143 (1962).

Voss, H., Becher, K., u. Lindner, J., Über die geschwulsthemmende Wirkung von Grundsubstanzbestandteilen. VI. Vergleichende Untersuchungen über den Einfluß des Glucosamins auf den Stoffwechsel des Yoshida-Ratten und Ehrlich-Mäuse-Ascites-Tumores. *Z. Krebsforsch.* **65**, 228 (1963).

Werner, S., On the regeneration of serum polysaccharide and serum proteins in normal and intoxicated rabbits. *Acta physiol. scand.* **19**, 27 (1949).

Wheatley, D. N., Influence of various substances on production of ascites tumour. *Nature (Lond.)* **202**, 1348 (1964).

— Ambrose, E. J., and Easty, G. C., Infiltration of intra-abdominal organs by ascites tumours. *Nature (Lond.)* **199**, 188 (1963).

Woessner jr., J. F., Catabolism of collagen and non-collagen protein in the rat uterus during post-partum involution. *Biochem. J.* **83**, 304 (1962).

Young, T. S., The invasive growth of malignant tumors: an experimental interpretation based on elastic-jelly models. *J. Path. Bact.* **77**, 321 (1959).

Studies on Metastasis of Spontaneous and Transplantable Tumours at High Altitude

Pablo Mori-Chavez

Laboratorio de Investigación de Cancer, Instituto de Investigaciones de la Altura, Universidad Peruana "Cayetano Heredia", Lima, Peru

Studies on the effects of high altitude on neoplastic growth were started in Peru in 1954 taking advantage of a unique geographic situation which permitted the establishment of a high-altitude laboratory in Morococha, a mining town 14,900 feet above sea level with a barometric pressure of 446 mm Hg, and with 13 per cent atmospheric oxygen. The travel time from the sea-level laboratory in Lima is less than four hours by automobile.

An animal colony of several inbred strains of mice was established. These were strain C3H mice for mammary tumours, strain C58 for leukemia, and strain A for pulmonary tumours. Since the animals did not breed at high altitude, they were bred at sea level and at the time of weaning were similarly distributed between the two locations by litter and sex. The environmental conditions in regard to temperature, humidity, food and water supply were kept as nearly alike as possible.

The first observations established that spontaneous or induced tumours of several strains of mice can grow at a natural high altitude of about 15,000 feet. This environment affected the various tumours which we studied in different ways. The incidence of spontaneous leukemia in strain C58 mice was significantly lower at high altitude than at sea level (Mori-Chavez, 1958), while that of spontaneous pulmonary tumours in strain A mice was higher at high altitude than at sea level (Mori-Chavez, 1962a). Urethan proved to be more carcinogenic in the induction of lung tumours at high altitude than at sea level (Mori-Chavez, 1962b).

The results obtained to date on the effect of natural high altitude on the occurrence of metastasis may open a way to explore the mechanisms of metastasis, "one of the most important fields in cancer research, too long underemphasized and neglected" (Tannenbaum, 1964).

In this paper, I will present and discuss observations of metastasis from spontaneous mammary carcinomas and other tumours of mice transplanted subcutaneously or intravenously.

Metastasis from Spontaneous Mammary tumours in C3H Mice

Observations on the incidence of spontaneous mammary tumours and their metastases are summarized in Table I.

The overall incidence of mammary tumours was equal at both locations, though tumours occurred 10 weeks earlier at high altitude than at sea level. Pulmonary metastasis was twice as frequent in mice at high altitude as at sea level. The size of mammary tumours and the period of morbidity were equal in the two locations (Mori-Chavez unpublished data).

Metastasis Following the Subcutaneous Transplantation of a Hemangioendothelioma of BALB/c Mice

This tumour was kindly provided by Dr. Richard L. Swarm of the National Cancer Institute, National Institutes of Health, Bethesda, Maryland. Sixty-two BALB/c mice were subcutaneously transplanted at the age of 16 weeks, and were shipped by air to Lima. They were equally distributed between the high-altitude and sea-level locations.

All mice at both levels developed the tumour. No differences were found in the rate of growth or in the life span after transplantation which averaged 11 weeks.

Metastatic spread was greater at high altitude than at sea level (Table II). The differences in the incidence of metastasis

to the lung, spleen, subcutis and muscle were, respectively, 21.6 ± 7.19, 51.6 ± 10.87, 25.8 ± 11.40, and 18.7 ± 8.96 per cent. The frequency of peritoneal implants was 12.9 ± 12.25 per cent greater at sea level than at high altitude, not a significant difference.

Transplantation experiments from BALB/c to (BALB/c $\times$ A) F1 hybrids were successful in 100 per cent of mice at both locations with 66.7 per cent metastasis at high altitude and 38.9 per cent at sea level, mostly limited to the lungs. Transplantation experiments to and from (BALB/c $\times$ A) F1 hybrids were also 100 per cent successful. The percentage of metastasis to the lungs was 19.5 at high altitude and 9.1 at sea level. Tumour transplants from F1 hybrids back to the BALB/c mice were 100 per cent successful but the metastasizing ability practically disappeared (Mori-Chavez, 1964).

Table I. *Metastasis of spontaneous mammary tumours in C3H mice at high altitude*

Experimental groups		Tumour incidence		Average age (weeks)		Morbidity (weeks)	Metastasis to lung	
Location	No. of mice	No.	Per cent	Tumour appeared	At death		No.	Per cent
High altitude Morococha (14,900 feet)	261	175	67.0	62.3 ± 1.78	70.7 ± 1.73	8.4 ± 0.33	53	29.7 ± 2.82
Sea level Lima	273	184	67.0	72.1 ± 1.70	80.7 ± 1.73	8.6 ± 0.28	26	14.1 ± 2.2
Differences			$- 0.4$	$- 9.8 \pm 2.46$	-10.0 ± 2.45	-0.2 ± 0.43		$+15.6 \pm 3.56$

Table II. *Metastasis of hemangioendothelioma subcutaneously transplanted in BALB/c mice at high altitude*

Exper. groups		Lung		Spleen		Peritoneum		Subcutis		Muscle		Erythropoiesis	
Location	No. of mice	No.	Per cent	No.	Per cent	No.	Per cent	No.	Per cent	No.	Per cent	No.	Per cent
High altitude Morococha	31	30	96.8 ± 3.16	23	74.2 ± 7.86	10	32.2 ± 8.39	14	45.1 ± 8.93	8	25.2 ± 7.80	27	87.1 ± 6.02
Sea level Lima	31	23	74.2 ± 7.86	7	22.6 ± 7.51	14	45.1 ± 8.93	6	19.3 ± 7.08	2	6.5 ± 4.43	17	54.8 ± 8.94
Differences		$+7$	21.6 ± 7.19	$+16$	51.6 ± 10.87	-4	12.9 ± 12.25	$+8$	25.8 ± 11.40	$+6$	18.7 ± 8.96	$+10$	33.3 ± 10.77

Metastasis Following Subcutaneous Transplantation of 678-Ascites Carcinoma in C 3 H Mice

Groups of mice of the C3H strain kept at the high altitude and sea level locations were subcutaneously transplanted with 678-ascites carcinoma (Mori-Chavez, 1962c). The ascites fluid harvested from the donor mice was diluted with sterile isotonic saline to a concentration of 4×10^5 tumour cells per 0.1 ml, the amount of the inoculum. Three different groups of inoculated mice were established at each location for killing at 30, 25, and 20 days after transplantation.

The results are summarized in Table III. The percentages of distribution of metastasis by site are referred to the number of mice bearing metastases at any or all sites indicated. At all three intervals after transplantation metastasis was more frequent at high altitude than at sea level. The percentage difference was most significant in the 20-day groups, 24.6 ± 9.5 greater at high altitude than at sea level.

Metastasis to the lung was significantly greater in mice kept at high altitude than at sea level. The percentage differences in the 30-day, 25-day, and 20-day groups were, respectively, 11.4 ± 3.78, 19.0 ± 6.38, and 35.7 ± 14.14 greater at high altitude than at sea level. The metastatic growths in the heart were also greater at high altitude than at sea level. The differences for the above groups were, 14.9, 8.1, and 3.6 per cent, respectively. The extent of metastatic growth in the lung and heart was also much greater at high altitude than at sea level. This difference could not be evaluated by counting and measuring tumour nodules, because infiltration was often so extensive and diffuse that individual nodules were not seen.

Metastasis to lymph nodes was next in frequency to lung metastasis at both levels. It was increased at high altitude in the 30-day group, equal at both levels in the 25-day group, and greater at sea level than at high altitude in the 20-day group.

"Artificial Metastasis" Following the Intravenous Injection of 678-Ascites Crcinoma in to C 3 H Mice.

An experiment was designed to ascertain whether *"metastasis"* at high

Table III. *Metastasis of 678-ascites carcinoma subcutaneously transplanted into C3H mice at high altitude*

Experimental groups			Frequency of metast.		Distribution of metastasis (per cent $\pm$ S.E.)		
Days	Location	No. of mice	No.	Per cent $\pm$ S.E.	Lung	Lymph nodes	Heart
30	High altitude	152	144	94.7 ± 1.82	95.1 ± 1.79	69.4 ± 3.84	22.2 ± 3.46
	Sea level	147	123	83.7 ± 3.05	83.7 ± 3.33	56.1 ± 4.47	7.3 ± 2.36
	Differences			$+11.0 \pm 3.54$	$+11.4 \pm 37.8$	$+13.3 \pm 5.89$	$+14.9 \pm 4.41$
25	High altitude	75	63	84.0 ± 4.20	92.1 ± 3.39	77.8 ± 5.23	11.1 ± 3.95
	Sea level	87	67	77.0 ± 4.51	73.1 ± 5.41	77.6 ± 5.09	3.0 ± 2.08
	Differences			7.0 ± 6.16	$+19.0 \pm 6.38$	$+ 0.2 \pm 7.29$	$+ 8.1 \pm 4.46$
20	High altitude	50	28	56.0 ± 7.02	85.7 ± 6.61	17.8 ± 7.22	3.6 ± 3.52
	Sea level	51	16	31.4 ± 6.49	50.0 ± 12.50	50.0 ± 12.50	—
	Differences			$+24.6 \pm 9.55$	$+35.7 \pm 14.14$	-32.2 ± 14.43	—

P. Mori-Chavez

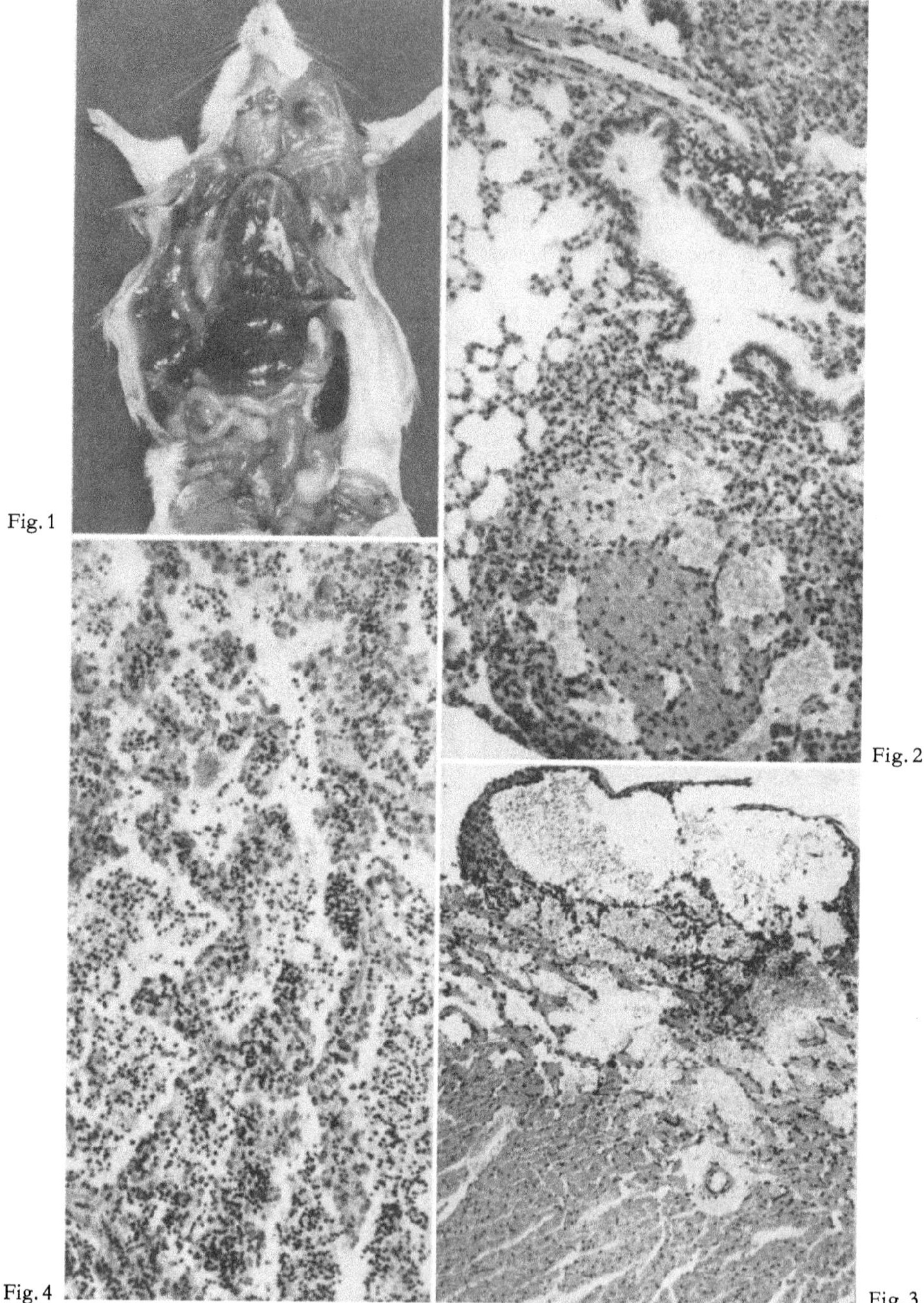

Fig. 1

Fig. 2

Fig. 4

Fig. 3

Fig. 1. BALB/c mouse at high altitude, transplanted with hemangioendothelioma. Widespread metastasis to lung, chest wall, subcutis and spleen

Fig. 2. Section of lung of BALB/c mouse at high altitude showing metastasis of hemangioendothelioma. Hematoxylin and eosin. $\times 120$

altitude would differ from that at sea level when equal numbers of tumour cells were *artificially* introduced into the circulation.

At the age of 10 weeks the acclimatized high-altitude mice were taken to sea level at Lima on the morning scheduled for transplantation and were returned to Morococha the same day. Individual mice of the two altitude groups were injected alternately with 678-ascites carcinoma. Each mouse received a suspension of tumour cells in sterile isotonic saline at a concentration of 5×10^4 viable tumour cells per 0.1 ml. The injected mice from each altitude level were divided in four groups: (1) allowed to die spontaneously; (2), (3), and (4) killed at 15, 10, and 6 days after injection (MORI-CHAVEZ, 1965).

Mice dying spontaneously or killed 15 days after tumour injection often had the paratracheal lymph nodes and mediastinum infiltrated with tumour. Usually hemorrhagic effusion containing many free tumour cells accompanied the infiltration. Tumour nodules in the lungs were most numerous and largest, irrespective of altitude, in the groups of mice that survived longest after tumour injection. Metastatic infiltration of the heart was a common finding at both altitude levels, especially noted in those mice of the group allowed to die spontaneously which survived for relatively long periods. Table IV summarizes the results of these experiments.

In group No.1 of mice that died spontaneously, the mean survival time after intravenous transplantation was much shorter at high altitude than at sea level, 18.6 days compared to 26.1 days. The overall incidence of metastasis in the groups of mice killed at shorter intervals after tumour injection was greater at high altitude than at sea level. In all four groups there were larger average numbers of pulmonary nodules at high altitude than at sea level. Tumour infiltration of the heart was less at high altitude than at sea level in the group of mice that died spontaneously. Differences at the two levels were not significant in the other two groups. Metastasis to the mediastinal lymph nodes was noted only in the group of mice that died spontaneously and in the group killed at 15 days after tumour injection. In the latter group the difference was more than twice as great at high altitude as at sea level.

Mice killed 6 days after tumour injection had grossly and microscopically apparent tumour nodules only in the lung. The difference in incidence was significantly greater at high altitude than at sea level by 24.0 ± 7.7 per cent. A total of 149 tumour nodules were found in the lungs of 54 mice at high altitude, averaging 2.76 nodules per mouse. At sea level, 70 nodules were counted in 33 mice, averaging 2.12 per mouse. The percentage of measurable or grossly visible nodules (0.25 mm) was greater at high altitude than at sea level.

Summary and Discussion

Experiments on tumourigenesis at natural high altitude and at sea level have shown interesting differences that vary somewhat with the tumours used and the inbred strains of mice. An important

Fig. 3. Section of spleen of a BALB/c mouse at high altitude, showing area of metastasis of hemangioendothelioma. Branching sheets of neoplastic cells are limiting spaces partly filled with cells in active erythropoiesis. Hematoxylin and eosin. $\times 350$

Fig. 4. Section of heart of a BALB/c mouse showing metastatic growth of hemangioendothelioma below the epicardium. $\times 80$

Table IV. "*Metastasis*" *following i.v. injection of* 5×10^4 *tumour cells of 678-ascites carcinoma in C 3 H mice*

Experimental groups				Frequency of metastasis		Distribution					
No.	Days after i.v. tumour cells	Location	No. of mice	No. of "takes"	Per cent ± S.E.	Lung				Heart	Lymph nodes
						%	Aver. No. nod/mouse	Aver. size mm		%	%
1	18.6	High altitude	76	66	86.8±3.88	100.0	20.2	1.50		57.6	69.7
	26.1	Sea level	76	62	81.6±4.44	98.4	7.4	1.94		72.6	64.5
	(Spontaneous death)	Difference			+5.2±5.89	+1.6	+12.8	−0.44		−15.0	+ 5.2
2	14.6	High altitude	73	73	100.0±0	100.0	24.58	1.48		15.0	52.05
	14.9	Sea level	69	61	88.4±3.85	98.36	11.15	1.61		14.7	19.67
		Difference			+11.6±3.85	+1.64	+13.43	−0.13		− 0.3	+32.38
3	10.0	High altitude	76	74	97.4±1.82	100	12.97	1.12		8.1	0
	10.0	Sea level	69	53	76.3±5.11	100	6.46	0.85		9.2	0
		Difference			21.1±5.42		+ 6.51	+0.27		− 1.1	
4	6.0	High altitude	73	54/149 *	74.0±5.13	100	2.76	≧0.25=44%		0	0
	6.0	Sea level	66	33/70	50.0±6.15	100	2.12	− =35		0	0
		Difference			+24.0±7.7		+ 0.64	+9			

* Number of mice with "metastasis"/total number of tumour nodules.

observation is the greater frequency at high altitude of metastasis of spontaneous mammary tumours in C3H mice and of certain transplantable tumours.

A hemangioendothelioma transplanted subcutaneously in BALB/c mice and in (BALB/c × A) F1 hybrids showed a greater metastatic spread in mice kept at high altitude than in those at sea level.

Mice transplanted subcutaneously with 678-ascites carcinoma and killed thereafter at various intervals showed a greater frequency of metastasis, especially to the lung, at high altitude than at sea level. The percentage difference in metastasis was relatively more significant in the groups of mice killed at the shorter intervals after transplantation. This suggests that the tumour cells may have been released earlier into the bloodstream and/or have established their growth sooner at high altitude than at sea level.

Interesting results were obtained also in the experiments on tumour spread following the artificial introduction of viable tumour cells into the circulation. In all four groups of mice, the "artificial metastasis", especially to the lung, was significantly more frequent at high altitude than at sea level. The percentage differences in the overall incidence of tumour growths at the two levels was greater in the groups of mice killed in the shorter intervals after tumour injection. Since equal numbers of tumour cells were injected into mice maintained at both altitude levels, the differences observed would indicate that mechanical

factors contribute at least some of those high-altitude conditions which favor the lodgement and growth of tumour emboli. These are hemoconcentration due to the polycythemia of high altitude, and dilatation and increase of the capillary bed, an adaptive response to the environment (Mori-Chavez, 1935; Valdivia, 1956), which contribute at least some of the high-altitude conditions that favor the lodgment and growth of tumour emboli. If metastasis had been equal at both levels, the differences observed in the spread of tumours transplanted subcutaneously could be considered as residing entirely in the tumour cells.

The possible role of humoral or endocrine factors, especially the adrenal gland response to the hypoxia of high altitude, might be considered in studying the mechanism of the above differences in metastasis. It is known that cortisone treatment enhances metastasis of transplantable tumours (Agosin et al., 1952; Baserga and Shubic, 1954; Wood et al., 1956), but it is not known whether this hormone acts upon the reticuloendothelial system to prevent a tissue-specific immune reaction (Pomeroy, 1954), or whether it favors embolic arrest by increasing the stickiness of capillary endothelium (Zeidman, 1962). It has been demonstrated that a mucopolysaccharide coat on tumour cells establishes their metastasis by fostering adhesion to the vascular endothelium (Gasic and Gasic, 1962). Roentgen irradiation increases the frequency of pulmonary

Fig. 5. Five pairs of lungs of C3H mice at high altitude showing metastatic nodules of 678-ascites carcinoma subcutaneously transplanted. Three hearts on left side also show metastasis.

Fig. 6. Section of the heart of a C3H mouse killed 4 weeks after subcutaneous transplantation with 678-ascites carcinoma. The ventricle is filled with a tumour mass. Hematoxylin and eosin. ×65

Fig. 7. A diffuse spread of metastatic growth is shown in this section of lung of a mouse killed 30 days after subcutaneous transplant of 678-ascites carcinoma at high altitude. Hematoxylin and eosin. ×35

 P. Mori-Chavez

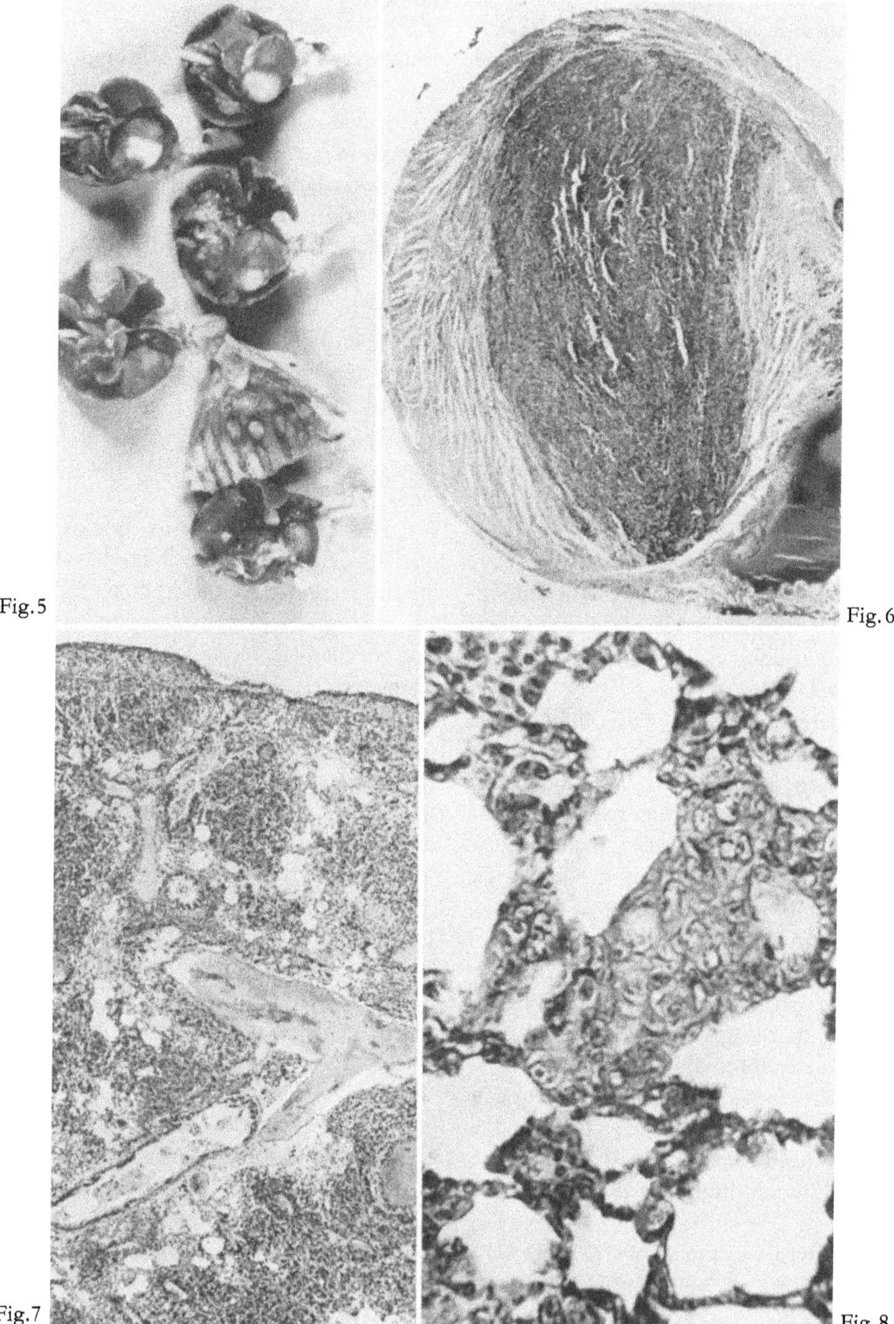

Fig.5

Fig.6

Fig.7

Fig.8

Fig. 8. Section of a lung of a C3H mouse killed 10 days after the intravenous injection of 678-ascites tumour cells. A small tumour nodule deep in the parenchyme, and the capillaries next to it infiltrated by tumour cells. Hematoxylin and eosin. ×430

metastasis by interfering with defense mechanisms of the host (KAPLAN and MURPHY, 1949; ESSEN and KAPLAN, 1952). Such effects may be mediated through the adrenal gland. Investigators have observed changes in the adrenal glands of the rabbit (ARMSTRONG and HEIM, 1938) and rat (DARROW and SARASON, 1944; DALTON *et al.*, 1944; ALTLAND, 1948) following exposure to decreased barometric pressure. The mechanism of increased metastatic spread of experimental tumours at high altitude in comparison to sea level may be dependent on some of these factors. The possibility might also be considered that there are differences in local or general immune reaction to the lodgement and growth of tumour emboli at the two altitude levels.

Acknowledgements

This investigation was supported by Grants DRG-321 and 726 from the Damon Runyon Memorial Fund for Cancer Research, Inc., and by research grant CA-06597 from the National Cancer Institute, National Institutes of Health, U.S. Public Health Service.

Grateful recognition is given to the Cerro de Pasco Corporation for facilities to establish the High Altitude Laboratory in Morococha, Peru. We also acknowledge the help of Mr. GEBHARD GSELL in the preparation of the photomicrographs.

Discussion

Questions put to P. MORI-CHAVEZ

H. Hamperl: Is it possible to duplicate the effect of high altitude on tumour growth and number of metastases by keeping the animals in low-pressure chambers? Does the keeping of animals in high-pressure chambers have an effect opposite to that of high altitude?

P. Mori-Chavez: Natural high-altitude conditions cannot be reproduced by keeping animals in low-pressure tanks. Some studies on tumour growth in such artificial conditions have been done in the past-mostly short-term experiments with transplantable tumours. The results indicated a lower rate of growth or a regressive effect.

G. Barski: It should be possible to dissociate the essential factors peculiar to high altitude — i.e. low barometric pressure, low O_2 tension, and increased cosmic radiation — by breeding animals at a high altitude in tanks with barometric pressure and oxygen content adjusted to normal values.

P. Mori-Chavez: These experiments could indeed be performed. The well-known physiological changes observed at high altitudes as a result of an adaptation mechanism are mainly due to the low oxygen tension. We are inclined to believe that hypoxia is also perhaps the main factor related to the differences observed in the incidence of tumours in mice and their rate of growth and of invasiveness. With regard to the cosmic radiation you mentioned, it was measured both in Morococha, at a high altitude, and in Lima at sea level. At Morococha, the amount of cosmic radiation is only 3 stars per 1 c.c. of photographic emulsion, after 1 day exposure, which is probably too low to induce any effect on tumour growth. Even so, this amount is 30 times greater than the cosmic radiation at Lima at sea level.

E. J. Ambrose: I am wondering whether the degree of vascularization of the tissues could play a role in the dependence of various types of tumour growth on high-altitude conditions.

P. Mori-Chavez: The various mechanisms of adaptation to high altitude include at the tissue level a dilatation and a real increase of the capillary bed. These vascular changes are probably more difficult to evaluate comparatively when dealing with tumour growth, in which great variation occurs even in animals maintained in equal conditions.

O. Mühlbock: In Amsterdam, O. Kluft has performed experiments with transplanted mammary tumours in mice kept in tanks with hyperbaric oxygen up to 3 atm. The growth of the transplanted tumours did not differ from that observed in animals kept under normal conditions, but the formation of metastases did show differences. The number of metastases in the animals under hyperbaric oxygen was significantly lower than in animals under normal oxygen pressure. Taking into consideration the results of Dr. Mori-Chavez, one could say that more oxygen means less metastases or, vice versa, less oxygen means more metastases. The results with hyperbaric oxygen indicate that the role of oxygen — and not of other factors, e.g. cosmic rays — is of primary importance in experiments at high altitude.

Another interesting finding of Dr. Mori-Chavez is the acceleration in the appearance of primary mammary tumours in mice at high altitudes. In the development of this tumour, hormones, especially from the ovary and the hypophysis, play an important role. It would be worth while to study the changes in the endocrine system at high altitudes; perhaps in this way an indication can be found as to the pathway by which the high-altitude factors act.

P. Mori-Chavez: I appreciate Dr. Mühlbock's reference to O. Kluft's experiments with mammary tumours in mice kept in tanks at pressures of up to 3 atmospheres, in which he observed the opposite effect upon tumour metastasis, e.g. a significantly lower frequency than

in animals kept under normal oxygen conditions. I entirely agree with Dr. Mühlbock about the importance of the role played by the endocrine system in adaptation to high-altitude environment, as well as in some of the differences observed in tumour incidence, rate of growth of various tumours, and increase in metastasis formation at high altitudes.

J. Leighton: Dr. Mori-Chavez's experiments on the effect of high-altitude on the formation of metastases have provided an added stimulus to studies in our laboratory on the influence of a number of environmental variables on metastasis.

We use the embryonated egg inoculated with a suspension of ascites tumour cells as our model system. We are studying the effects of differing environmental temperature, $p O_2$, and $p CO_2$, on the formation of metastases in the chorio-allantois, the respiratory organ of the chick.

One technical problem, that of obtaining an adequate sample of the chorio-allantois in a single histological specimen, has been solved.

One week after intravenous inoculation of the 11-day-old chick embryo with Walker ascites tumour cells and incubation at 37.8^0 C, random histological sections of the chorio-allantois show many foci of metastatic growth in an alveolar pattern. Recent developments in technique permit us to survey the entire chorio-allantoic membrane of the chick in a single histological section. Metastases are found to be evenly disseminated throughout the chorio-allantois.

The procedure is as follows:

The chorio-allantoic membranes are prepared by opening the shell at the air space. The embryo and residual yolk sac are removed, leaving intact the shell, shell membrane, and chorio-allantoic membrane as a single cup-shaped struc-

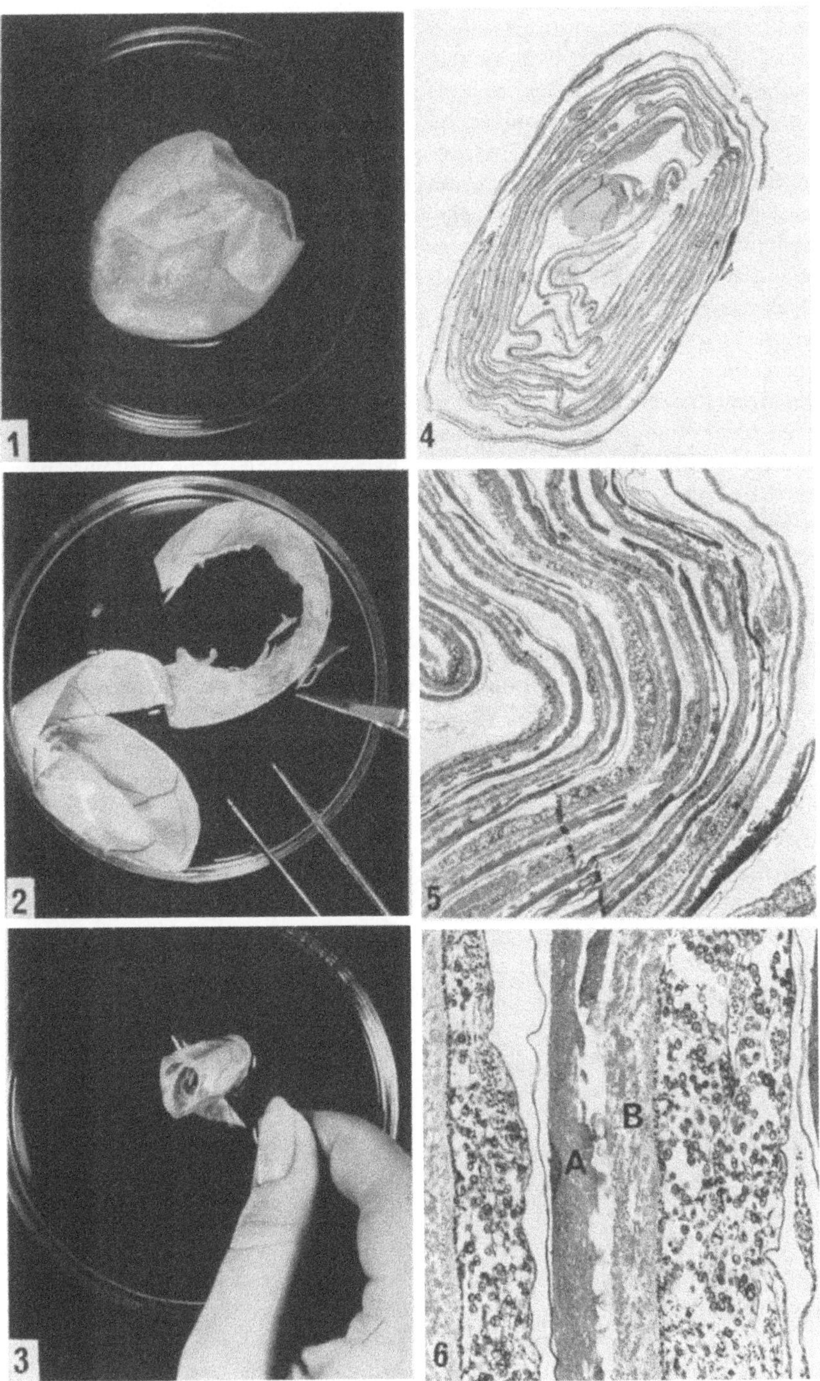

Fig. 1

ture. The shell and the two membranes encased in it are immersed in a solution of Bouin's fixative. After two days in this solution, the entire calcareous component of the shell has been dissolved by the acetic acid in the fixative. The specimen, consisting by this time of a sac made up of shell membrane and chorio-allantoic membrane, is washed briefly in water and stored in 80% ethyl alcohol. Fig. 1 shows such a sac after decalcification.

This sac is cut with scissors in a spiral pattern from the open air space to the apex as a continuous ribbon between 1.5 and 2 cm in width. In Fig. 2 about half of the membrane has been cut. The larger vessels of the chorio-allantois can be seen in the ribbon, as well as in the remaining part of the specimen. The entire membrane is cut in this fashion to complete the formation of the ribbon. We now prepare the membrane for embedding by grasping the end where the incision began with blunt forceps and then rolling the ribbon into a small scroll. The scroll is kept together with an insect pin, as illustrated in Fig. 3, during the process of dehydration, clearing, and infiltration with paraffin. The pin is removed just before the last embedding. After the paraffin has hardened, the scroll is removed from the mold and is cut in half along the length of the ribbon, making two scrolls. Each scroll is re-embedded with the cut surface down for better infiltration of the paraffin. The width of the ribbon finally examined is less than 1 cm. The length of the average ribbon before it is rolled into a scroll is between 20 and 25 cm. A representative microscopic section of a complete scroll is seen with very low magnification in Fig. 4. The pattern of metastatic involvement with cancer, which is seen throughout the length of the chorio-allantois, is illustrated with

increasingly higher magnification in Figs. 5 and 6. In Fig. 6, at approx. X 150, the residual matrix of the decalcified shell is labelled A, and the shell membrane B; the thick cellular tissue is the chorio-allantois itself.

Knowing that we can study the intravascular dissemination of cancer cells throughout the chorio-allantois, we have begun to study the effects of alteration of gas exchange on the development of metastases in the chorio-allantois. Our present technique is a simple one. We block the exchange of gas through half of the surface of the cell by coating half of the shell with paraffin. This research is in its early stages.

D. F. H. Wallach: Exposure of animals to a low p O_2 would result in very different effects in different tissues as far as p O_2 is concerned. Adaptive changes in blood flow and hemoglobin concentration would tend to maintain the p O_2 at the mitochondrial surface rather close to normal levels in those tissues which are normally above their "critical oxygen tension" (e.g. brain).

On the other hand, the lung would experience a very large change in its oxygen environment. Might this make the lung particularly susceptible to metastasis? What is the role of alveolar macrophages with their high aerobic metabolism?

P. Mori-Chavez: Polycythaemia, together with an increase in haemoglobin and in the total blood volume, is the immediate response to oxygen deficiency.

At the tissue level there is an increase in myohaemoglobin, and probably metabolic changes to adjust to the hypoxic condition. It is indeed quite possible that the continuing influence of oxygen deficiency at high altitudes may give neoplastic cells in the lung and other tissues a competitive advantage over neoplastic cells at sea level.

I. Petrea: 1. Are there any statistical data available in Peru concerning the geographical distribution of cancer and the process of metastasization at sea level and at high altitudes? Can any parallel be drawn between the clinical data and the results of your experiments?

In my opinion, the very interesting experimental conditions you used are not entirely applicable to clinical cases of cancer since patients living, for example, at high altitudes already possess their regulating mechanisms which permit them to adjust to such conditions.

2. With regard to mechanisms, it seems to me that altitude may represent a stress, a process in which the diencephalo-pituitary-adrenal system is often involved.

P. Mori-Chavez: We have no statistical information on the geographical pathology of cancer at high altitudes. The scattered populations living in the high plateaux of the Andes are mostly Indians. A ten-year survey of the records of a small hospital in Oroya, Peru, at 13,000 feet above sea level, revealed a very high incidence of cancer of the uterine cervix in women; the most common types of cancer in men were those of the stomach and intestine, i.e. the same as at lower altitudes in Peru.

C. Southam: Is there not, at high altitudes, an increased respiratory effort and increased pulmonary blood flow to compensate for the low atmospheric p O_2 tension? Might not these purely mechanical factors affect the dissemination of tumour cells and increase the frequency of implantation in the lungs? Perhaps such factors could be reproduced at normal barometric pressure by production of pulmonary fibrosis or by pneumonectomy?

P. Mori-Chavez: Pulmonary hyperventilation and increased blood flow at high altitudes may contribute, as mechanical factors, to the increased frequency of tumour implantation in the lung. Your suggestion of reproducing such factors at sea level is certainly appreciated.

References

AGOSIN, M., CHRISTEN, R., BADINEZ, O., GASIC, G., NEGHME, A., PIZARRO, O., and JARPA, A., Cortisone-induced metastases of adenocarcinoma in mice. *Proc. Soc. exp. Biol. (N.Y.)* **80**, 128—131 (1952).

ALTLAND, P. D., Acclimatization response of the adrenal glands of rats during discontinuous exposures to high altitude. *Proc. Soc. Penn. Acad. Sci.* **22**, 35—43 (1948).

ARMSTRONG, H. G., and HEIM, J. W., The effect of repeated daily exposures to anoxemia. *J. Aviat. Med.* **9**, 92—96 (1938).

BASERGA, R., and SHUBIC, P., The action of cortisone on transplanted and induced tumors in mice. *Cancer Res.* **14**, 12—16 (1954).

DALTON, A. J., MITCHELL, E. R., JONES, B. F., and PETERS, V. B., Changes in the adronal glands of rats following exposure to lowered oxygen tension. *J. nat. Cancer Inst.* **4**, 527—536 (1944).

DARROW, D. C., and SARASON, E. L., Some effects of low atmospheric pressure in rats. *J. clin. Invest.* **23**, 11—23 (1944).

ESSEN, C. F. VON, and KAPLAN, H. S., Further studies on metastasis of a transplantable mouse mammary carcinoma after roentgen irradiation. *J. nat. Cancer Inst.* **12**, 883—892 (1952).

GASIC, G., and GASIC, T., Removal of sialic acid from cell coat in tumor cells and vascular endothelium and its effects on metastasis. *Proc. nat. Acad. Sci. (Wash.)*, **48**, 1172—1177 (1962).

KAPLAN, H. S., and MURPHY, E. D., The effect of local roentgen irradiation on the biological behaviour of a transplantable mouse carcinoma. I. Increased frequency of pulmonary metastasis. *J. nat. Cancer Inst.* **9**, 407—413 (1949).

MORI-CHAVEZ, P., Manifestaciones pulmonares del cuy en el "soroche" agudo. Thesis. *An. Fac. Cienc. Méd. (Lima)* **18**, 126—172 (1935).

— Spontaneous leukemia at high altitude in C 58 mice. *J. nat. Cancer Inst.* **21**, 985—997 (1958).

— A carcinoma of the forestomach of a C3H mouse. Its conversion to the ascites form by intraperitoneal passage. *Proc. Amer. Ass. Cancer Res.* **3**, 346 (1962).

— Development of spontaneous pulmonary tumors at high altitude in strain A mice. *J. nat. Cancer Inst.* **28**, 55—73 (1962).

— Lung tumors induced at high altitude by urethan (ethyl carbamate) in strain A mice. *J. nat. Cancer Inst.* **29**, 945—961 (1962).

— Study of metastasis after the intravenous injection of ascites carcinoma 678 into C3H mice at high altitude. *J. nat. Cancer Inst.* **35** (in press) (1965).

POMMEROY, T. C., Studies on the mechanisms of cortisone-induced metastases of transplantable mouse tumors. *Cancer Res.* **14**, 201—204 (1954).

TANNENBAUM, A., Statement in discussing P. Mori-Chavez' paper. *Nat. Cancer Inst. Monogr.* **14**, 335 (1964).

VALDIVIA, E., Mechanisms of natural acclimatization. Capillary studies at high altitude. Rept. 55-101. School of Aviation Med. USAF, Randolph Field, Texas 1956.

WOOD, S. S., HOLYOKE, E. D., and YARDLEY, J. H., An experimental study of the influence of adrenal steroids, growth hormone and anticoagulants on pulmonary metastases formation in mice. *Proc. Amer. Ass. Cancer Res.* **2**, 157—158 (1956).

ZEIDMAN, I., The fate of circulating tumor cells. II. A mechanism of cortisone action in increasing metastases. *Cancer Res.* **22**, 501—503 (1962).

The Tumour Cell and Vascular Bed Size Relationship in Experimental Metastases*

Robert E. Madden

Department of Surgery, New York Medical College, New York, N.Y., U.S.A.

An involved discussion of the soil-versus-seed theory of metastases might seem academic if not solely historical today. There are presently available for review many investigations in which varying conditions have been applied experimentally to manipulate the patterns of metastases. Of most general interest has been the manner in which intravascular spread of tumour could be controlled. To quote some examples: local injury, either chemical or physical (Alexander, 1964; Robinson, 1962) general anesthesia (Agostino, 1964) cortisone (Baserga, 1954; Zeidman, 1962) surgical "stress" (Kallenbach, 1962; Buinauskas, 1958) growth hormone (Wood, 1956) reticuloendothelial blockade (Fisher, 1961) proferrin (Fisher, 1962) pancreatic inhibitor (Cagliani, 1962) orotic acid (Chu, 1964) pituitary homogenates (Fisher, 1961) epsilon amnio caproic acid (Cliffton, 1964) and host irradiation (Driessens, 1963) have been observed to increase incidence of metastases; heparin (Agostino, 1962; Gallinotto, 1964) fibrinolysin (Grossi, 1960) chymotrypsin (Cagliani, 1962) neuraminidase (Gasic, 1962) coumadin (Agostino, 1963) surgery (Ketcham, 1961) and x-irradiation of donor (Hoye, 1961) have been observed to reduce incidence of metastases. Increased survival time and numbers of tumour cells in the blood have been noted to accompany heparin-induced decreased metastases when these parameters have been studied (Koike, 1964). Thus if the cell does not arrest it continues to circulate. The capillary-tumour cell size relationship as well as the plasticity of the tumour cell itself have also been studied under direct vision (Zeidman, 1961). In short, a considerable body of evidence suggests that if a sufficient number — and this is probably quite small — of tumour cells can arrest, or be made to arrest, in the vascular bed a metastasis will eventuate.

Most investigators in the field will agree that the vast number of circulating tumour cells fail to establish themselves and die. Some studies have shown, however, that intravenously inoculated tumour cells distribute widely throughout the viscera in numbers sufficient to induce metastases when blood or organ brei are grafted into secondary recipients. Yet metastases do not occur in these organs in the primary recipient (Greene, 1964). Although the dormant cancer cell now is an experimentally established fact

* This work was supported by Grant # U-1121 from the Health Research Council of the City of New York, and by Grant # CA 07587. National Institutes of Health, U.S. Department of Health, Education and Welfare. A portion of this work was presented in partial fulfillment of the requirements for degree of Master of Arts in the Hunter College of the City University of New York.

(FISHER, 1959; SFORZA, 1962) it must until demonstrated otherwise remain a special case with limited occurence.

It would seem to us that certain organs have greater resistance to the support of metastases even when tumour cell dosages can be standardized. This supposition finds support in clinical studies. Some organs or tissues such as muscle and G.I. tract exhibit near immunity to vascular metastases. Yet if we accept published series on clinical material in which tumour cells are demonstrated in peripheral blood then we must accept that all organs and tissues have been subjected to malignant cytemia. Two factors must be considered before postulating the presence of a specific organ immunity or a local soil factor. The first of these is the percentage of total blood born tumour cells to which a given vascular bed is exposed. This would vary with the proportion of cardiac output that a given organ receives. The second factor is the percentage of these tumour cells which is successfully arrested. Only the absolute numbers of viable tumour cells which lodge in the vascular bed can be considered as potentially metastasizable. A favorable size relationship between tumour cell and vascular channel may allow easy transvascular passage reducing the effective cell dose in the organ. A specific biologic interaction between tumour cell and vascular bed is of course possible and may result in lodgement and death for some blood born tumour cells. The relative number of tumour cells arrested however would seem to be of equal if not more importance. It would be informative therefore to carry out two types of studies:

1. Determination of the limiting vascular diameters in various organs;

2. Correlation of the ability of an organ to retain cancer cells (biological filtration) with its vulnerability to metastasis formation.

One method of assaying the ability to retain cancer cells is to measure the opposite effect, i.e. the tendency to transvascular passage. This is done by relating several organs to the same secondary tumour cell filter, the lung.

Materials and Methods

Vascular Sizing. Female Wistar rats weighing between 200 and 250 gm were used in all experiments. Known numbers of plastic microspheres of a specific gravity of 1.056 were injected as a dilute suspension in EARLE's salt solution intravascularly into nembutal anesthetized animals. These microspheres were of two size ranges, a "small" 10—30 micra, and a "large" 28—37 micra in diameter. The stated size ranges include roughly two standard deviations on either side of the mean. The spheres were injected during a one minute period in a volume of 0.5 cc through a PE 10 catheter placed in the appropriate vessel. Blood from the organ or tissue injected was with-drawn simultaneously and during the succeeding minute into a heparinized syringe from a catheter placed in the efferent blood vessel (the aorta in the case of lung). Aliquots of the injected samples and of the effluent blood were examined microscopically in thin cover glass smears with the aid of an ocular micrometer scale. Seven smears were made and examined for each blood aliquot.

The various studies were carried out according to the following protocol:

1. *Muscle*: Injection into femoral artery; withdrawal from femoral vein.

2. *Kidneys* (including adrenals and ovaries): Injection via catheter placed in left carotid artery and inserted down to a ligature-isolated segment of abdominal aorta opposite renal arteries; withdrawal from catheter at a similar level in inferior

vena cava placed from left jugular vein.

3. *Liver*: Injection into hepatic portal vein; withdrawal from catheter placed at level of hepatic veins in inferior vena cava.

4. *Lungs*: Injection with catheter placed in right atrium; withdrawal from catheter placed in ascending aorta.

In most cases 100,000 microspheres were injected, but in some cases 50,000 or 25,000 were injected. One animal was used in each experiment.

Analytical Method for Vascular Sizing. The method of probit analysis was used to treat these data (FINNEY, 1947). Between 190 and 200 microspheres were counted in each smear. These were enumerated according to size in five micron increments. Size-frequency distribution diagrams (usually bell shaped) were constructed for each experiment, and from these the cumulative size-frequency curves (usually sigmoidal) were derived. When the cumulative frequencies are transformed to the probit scale and replotted against size an easily interpreted straight line function results. Occasionally because of skewing to the right of the bell shaped curve it is necessary to plot the probit scale against the logarithm of the microsphere size to produce a straight line. Such skewing to the right may indicate the presence of arteriovenous shunts and will be discussed below.

According to the theory of probit analysis the point on the probit line which has the value of 0.5 on the ordinate scale has a value on the abscissal scale which corresponds to the mean microsphere size. Thus the mean size of the injected sample of microspheres or of the microspheres in the effluent blood may be read off the graph. Probit values between 0.4 and 0.6 correspond on the abscissa to a range of two standard deviations.

Mean effective vascular channel size can be calculated from the mean size of the injected sample and that of the microspheres in the effluent blood. This is illustrated in Fig. 1. The original sample M has been distributed in part to the effluent sample M' and in part to the vascular bed C (where a proportion of the microspheres have become trapped). Let us construct a graph with three probit lines, one each for M and M' which have been experimentally determined, and one for C which lies midway between. The probit curves are straight line functions of the form $Y = kX + b$ where Y is the probit value and X the size of the microspheres. Thus we might say that for any given particle size, say

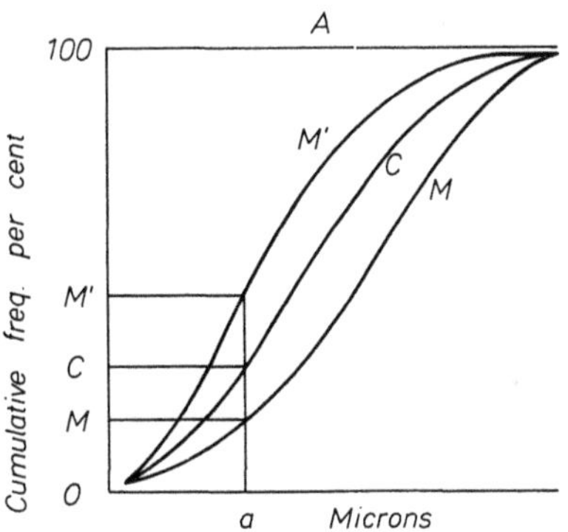

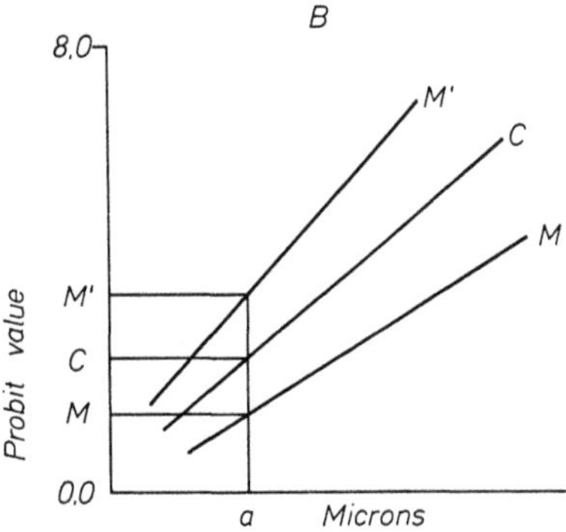

Fig. 1. Cumulative frequency and probit curves for determining mean effective vascular channel size

(a) $Y_M = Y_C - (Y_{M'} - Y_C)$ where Y_M represents a given injected sample probit value, Y_C represents that for the proportion of the sample of size (a) or less trapped in the vascular bed, and $(Y_{M'} - Y_C)$ represents that for the proportion of the original sample of size (a) or less which has transversed the vascular bed to reach the effluent blood. By transposition:

$$Y_C = \frac{Y_M + Y_{M'}}{2}.$$

The channel size X, which corresponds to the probit value, is the mean effective limiting diameter. These calculations have been carried through for each experiment.

Biological Filtration Studies. Groups of Wistar rats were injected with 10^6 Walker 256 ascites tumour cells in a volume of one cc. EARLE's solution. Intravascular injections into the target organ made over one minute were as described in the microsphere studies. In addition an aortic shower group was injected via the aortic arch. With muscle and kidney additional groups included occlusion of venous outflow during and for one minute following injection. In the preconditioned groups 5 mg cortisone was injected subcutaneously daily for four days prior to tumour cell injection. In another muscle group 40 micrograms of acetylcholine was added to tumour cells immediately before injection.

Finally in two groups of animals tumour cell injections were made directly into muscle tissue of the leg or into subcutaneous tissue of the flank. A subcutaneous viability control was provided for each animal in all groups (except the subcutaneous group itself). The number of animals surviving for assay in each group varied from 17 to 51 but in most groups was between 20 and 30. The site, method and conditions of injection are summarized in Table I.

Animals were sacrificed at 26 to 30 days or sooner if moribund. A standard autopsy search was made for tumours. Liver, spleen and kidneys were cut into one mm slices. Positive or suspicious areas in these organs or elsewhere were submitted for histologic confirmation and were recorded as positive only if so confirmed. The lungs in addition to gross examination were submitted to a standard search for tumours. They were inflated with carbon black saline solution through the trachea, fixed in formalin overnite, and cut into one mm cubes. Areas not filling with carbon black either on the surface or on cubing were regarded as grossly positive for tumour, if microscopically confirmed. Five or more sections of lungs of each animal, grossly positive or not, were submitted for microscopic examination.

Cholinesterase activity of tumour cell suspension was assayed using the guinea

Table I. *Types of experiments performed*

Type of experiment	Muscle	Direct muscle	Kidney	Liver	Lung	Aorta	Sub-cutaneous
Vein not occluded	+	+	+	+	+	+	+
Vein occluded	+		+				
Cortisone, v. not occluded	+		+	+	+	+	
Cortisone, v. occluded			+				
Acetylcholine	+						

pig ilium technique. Tumour cells and acetylcholine solution were mixed and immediately added to the bath. It was found that under the conditions used, i.e. 10^6 tumour cells in one cc volume and 40 micrograms of acetylcholine, there was no detectable loss of acetylcholine activity within two minutes, the time necessary to mix and inject tumour cells with the ester.

Rationale of Assay for Primary Take and Transvascular Tumour Cell Passage

For the purposes of this study the following categories of tumour take and their criteria were set up:

I. a) Total number of injected animals surviving 26 to 30 days or those dying sooner with tumour in primary target organ = total for primary count.

b) Number of these with tumours in primary target organ = proportion for primary take.

II. a) Total number of injected animals surviving 26 to 30 days or those dying sooner with tumour in distal primary organ = total for distal primary count.

b) Number of these with tumours in distal primary organ = proportion for distal primary take.

III. a) Total number of injected animals with negative lung cubes surviving 26 days = total for distal secondary count.

b) Number of these with negative lung cubes but positive histologically for tumour surviving 26 days = proportion for distal secondary take (applies only to injections other than lung).

Twenty six to thirty days was chosen as the maximal survival time at this tumour cell inoculum without excessive mortality. Tumours in animals in categories I were regarded as having resulted from the original injections, either via blood stream or directly into tissue. Tumours in animals in categories II were regarded as having resulted from immediate transvascular passage of tumour cells at the time of original injections. The site of distal primary implant was the lung in all cases except the lung itself, in which it was any systemic organ. In both categories I and II the tumours would have been grossly positive by the 26 day sacrifice time or at least microscopically evident if sacrificed earlier. Hence the standard microscopic search for tumours. Tumours in animals in categories III were regarded as having resulted from tumour cells exfoliated from an established primary. They would therefore be much smaller and assumed to be only microscopic at the 26 to 30 day sacrifice time. Very few such distal secondary tumours occurred. This separation into distal primary and distal secondary is admittedly artificial but is based on the fact that the primary tumour must be established and therefore be several days old before exfoliating its own cells. There is evidence that this exfoliation does not begin until about the seventh day (ROMSDAHL, 1961) from a grossly transplanted tumour. The time is probably even later with the tumours in this experiment since they originated from a much smaller tumour inoculum (only 10^6 cells).

Analysis of Biological Filtration Data. The proportion of animals in each group developing tumours gave a fraction used for statistical analysis. Pairs of proportions were tested for significance of difference using the chi square method at the five percent level. Groups were compared in two ways: 1, The proportions of primary, of distal primary, and of distal secondary take were compared separately among all of the seven target organs. Note that a distal primary group does not exist for direct muscle and subcutaneous target organs since blood vessels were not injected. Note also that the lung does not possess a distal secondary group since the target organ itself, lung, would be the site of secondary deposit, indistinguishable from the primary. 2, The proportions of primary, of distal primary, and of distal secondary take were compared separately for each experiment type within each organ where multiple types of experiments were carried out (see Table I). This gave rise to a total of 110 individual chi square tests.

Results

Vascular Bed. In Table II the results of vascular bed sizing experiments are given.

between the organs however allows them to be ranked as indicated.

Biological Filtration Studies. These data are summarized in Figs. 2 and 3. In Fig. 2 the ability of each target organgroup to support the Walker 256 tumour as a primary is shown and ranked. Statistically significant difference exists beyond the length of bars. Clearly there is a difference among the organ groups at the extremes but a broad overlap when the five organs injected intravascularly are compared. Direct injection has provided a slightly better condition for tumour take.

Table II. *Limiting vascular diameters of various organs as determined by the method of microspheres*

Organ	Number of determinations	Mean effective diameter (microns)	Range (microns)
Liver	4	17.7	10.0—21.8
Muscle	5	20.6	15.6—25.5
Lung	5	21.2	19.1—23.7
Kidney	5	23.0	20.6—24.8

These sizes are limiting vascular diameters as determined by microsphere passage and are not to be construed as those of capillaries. The relative size

In Fig. 3 the data for transvascular passage studies is depicted. Take in the distal primary site is ranked as a measure of transvascular tumour cell passage.

Primary take

Proportion of take	Injection site	Interorgan comparisons Occurrence of no difference in primary take						
23/23 Direct muscle		Direct muscle	Subcutaneous					
49/51 Subcutaneous								
27/30 Muscle				Muscle				
12/17 Aortic shower								
15/22 Lung					Aortic shower	Lung		
18/28 Kidney							Kidney	
12/21 Liver								Liver

Fig. 2. Comparison between organ categories in the support of a standard tumour inoculum (10^6 cells)

Muscle, kidney, and the total systemic capillary bed (aortic shower) are not significantly different in their tendency to allow tumour cells to pass. Lung, and liver, however, whilst similar to each other differ significantly from the others.

The intra organ comparisons, those between type of experiment within a given organ, showed almost uniform non significance of difference either in the primary or the distal primary categories. The two exceptions were in the distal primary category:

Discussion

The relative sizes of tumour cell and capillary loop have been studied directly using microcinematography (WOOD, 1958). It has appeared that a size disproportion as well as lack of cell plasticity favored tumour cell arrest (ZEIDMAN, 1961). Adhesiveness of the cell endothelial interface, possibly augmented by cortisone (ZEIDMAN, 1962) or lessened by neuraminidase (GASIC, 1962), is also thought to effect cell arrest. The present studies are of a statistical nature applied

Distal primary take

Proportion of take	Injection site	Interorgan comparisons Occurrence of no difference in distal primary take		
13/18 Aortic shower		Aortic shower	Kidney	Muscle
14/23 Kidney		Aortic shower	Kidney	Muscle
12/25 Muscle		Aortic shower	Kidney	Muscle
2/16 Lung			Lung	Liver
1/19 Liver			Lung	Liver

Fig. 3. Comparison between organs in transvascular passage of tumour cells

1. In the kidney experiment without cortisone preconditioning there was a lower incidence of distal primaries when the vena cava was occluded during injection than when it was not.

2. In the liver experiment there was a higher incidence of distal primaries after cortisone preconditioning.

Distal secondary take comparisons among the seven primary groups or among the different types of experiments in the same organ failed to show significance of difference in any case. The proportions of take in these groups were all quite small and indicate that, at the sacrifice time chosen, 26—30 days, primaries in any site failed to give rise to a significant number of gross metastases.

to the entire population of vascular channels of specific organs. Examination of Table II indicates that among the organs studied a ranking according to limiting vascular diameter can be given. It must be stressed that this mean size as determined by rigid microspheres cannot be interpreted as the resting diameter of the capillary loop or precapillary arteriole. SAUNDERS and KNISELY (SAUNDERS, 1954) have observed the precapillary sphincters of rat mesentery using vital microscopy and reported an average diameter in this structure of 5.95 micra. ZEIDMAN (ZEIDMAN, 1962) reported capillary diameters of 11.3 and 10.4 micra in the same tissue. The values reported here do not reflect capillary size but rather that of larger available vascular passages. This is a more pertinent parameter since cells exfoliated from solid tumours are larger than normal formed elements of the blood and sometimes occur as clumps. They could be arrested or passed through at this level rather than at the capillary level. This would provide an explanation for both the clinical and experimental observation of transvascular passage of tumour cells. The values of limiting vascular diameters reported here do however indicate a relative relationship among the various visceral organs and muscle. In a few of the vascular sizing experiments there was a skewing to the right of the bell shaped size distribution curve. This indicates a relatively high proportion of channels for these organs with greater than average diameters. Alternatively the presence of arteriovenous shunts as demonstrated by others (PRINZMETAL, 1948) provides a ready explanation of this phenomenon.

If the mechanical lodgement of tumour cells were the decisive factor in metastasis formation the average vascular channel size of an organ or tissue should relate to its metastatic liability. If, on the other hand, local biologic factors were of decisive importance, the cell-vascular channel size relationship would have little bearing on metastasis formation. A comparison of Table II with Fig. 3 indicates that the latter could be the case. The ascending ranking according to vascular size is stepwise from liver to kidney. But transvascular passage studies clearly separate two groups. Most striking is the position of the lung. Here the limiting vascular channel size was found to lie between that of muscle and kidney, yet the facility for transvascular passage was significantly less than either. The evidence against mechanical arrest is not uniform however since it is seen that the organ with least transcapillary passage, liver, also has the smallest vascular channels. These data on vascular channel size must be interpreted keeping in mind that the injected blood supply of both liver and lung, the portal vein and pulmonary artery respectively are under considerably less blood pressure than the injected arterial supply of the other organs. If tumour cells are able to deform in passing through vascular channels the blood pressure could be an important factor.

It was felt that venous outflow occlusion with its attendant venous stasis and congestion might favor tumour cell lodgement and increase primary take. This was not demonstrated in the case of either muscle or kidney, but the incidence of transvascular passage through the kidney did drop significantly as judged from distal primaries. In the muscle series venous occlusion produced no effect on transcapillary passage.

Cortisone has been reported to increase vascular metastases (ZEIDMAN, 1962; KOIKE, 1963). In the present studies in which muscle, kidney, and liver were directly challenged with standard doses of intravascular tumour cells in preconditioned animals this was not demonstrated. If the effect of cortisone is to increase adhesiveness a decrease of distal primaries might be expected. This likewise did not occur. In fact with the case of liver the incidence of distal primaries was actually increased.

Acetylcholine is a powerful vasodilator and is rapidly destroyed, probably with passage through one organ. Injection of acetylcholine with tumour cells would produce maximal vasodilation in the target organ but little in the organ of distal primary deposit, the lung. Such an alteration of vascular size might reduce retention of tumour cells and increase transvascular passage. Injection of acetylcholine with tumour cells into the femoral artery however had no effect on either primary or distal primary take.

The above lines of evidence are not conclusive but certainly suggest that the tumour cell vascular channel size relationship is not of decisive importance in metastasis formation. The explanation could lie in the fact that the limiting diameters, as demonstrated by microspheres, are larger than most tumour cells. Under a normal systemic blood pressure they would be swept through an organ and be unavailable for metastasis formation. The smallest channels, capillaries, are frequently non perfusing and hence not exposed to tumour cells. In the cases of lung and liver, blood supplies are under lower pressure, increasing the probability of tumour cell lodgement, even in larger channels. This concept of a vascular bypass is offered as a possible explanation for lowered metastatic incidence of some organ sites. It cannot however be concluded that organ specific antibodies do not exist or that local organ environment may be hostile to the tumour cell. Organ specific antibodies have been reported by others (MAISKII, 1963).

The choice of Walker 256 as a tumour system deserves some comment. This is an old tumour of uncertain genetic make up, unsuitable for many types of studies. In the present investigations it has been shown to be capable of near 100% take with no tumour regression and thus does not invoke a major immunologic response. It is therefore a good tumour in which to study a mechanical problem involving relatively few cells; or in which more

subtle organ reactive differences to tumour are involved.

Summary

A series of experiments has been carried out to test the importance of the size relationship between tumour cell and vascular channel in metastasis formation. The mean effective limiting vascular diameters of several visceral organs and of muscle was determined using microspheres. These same organs were individually challenged with standard doses of tumour cells intravascularly and the incidence of primary take and of transvascular tumour cell passage was assayed. In some animals venous occlusion, cortisone preconditioning and acetylcholine were adjunctively used. These in general did not alter the results. Analysis of data suggests that the tumour cell vascular channel size relationship is not decisive in determining metastasis formation. The normal limiting vascular diameter is larger than most tumour cells and the latter may bypass vascular beds imparting an apparent immunity to metastases. An individual organ specific factor is not excluded.

A review of the literature relating to the control of experimental metastases has been given.

Acknowledgements

The author wishes to recognize the assistance of Dr. CHARLES KARPAS, who has read all of the histological sections and Dr. MELVIN SCHWARTZ who has aided in the statistical analysis. Valuable technical aid has also been rendered by Mr. NORMAN SILVERSMITH, Mr. ANTHONY PAPARO, Mrs. JENNY WU, Mrs. BEVERLY JOYCE, Mr. EDWIN LOVE and Mrs. JACQUELINE BUCKLEY.

Discussion

Questions put to R. E. Madden

S. Wood: These experiments re-emphasize the following observations already recorded by vital microscopy in several laboratories: the microcirculation does not serve as a simple mechanical filter of embolic cancer cells since the extraordinary adhesive properties of carcinoma cells enable them to remain securely attached to vascular endothelium (most particularly in the venous capillaries or capillary veins) without regard to blood flow rate or luminal size [cf. Arch. Path. **66**, 550—568 (1958) and Canad. Cancer Conf. **4**, 167—223 (1961)]. They fail, however, to take into consideration the plasticity of embolic cells [cf. Cancer Res. **21**, 38—39 (1961) and Bull. Swiss. Acad. Med. Sci. **20**, 92—121 (1964)].

Experimental data suggest that the mean effective vascular sizes in microns in the rat are: kidney 23.0, lung 21.2, muscle 20.6, and liver 17.7. Plastic microspheres of the size designated may well pass through the microcirculation, but probably not through the *true capillaries*. The mathematical calculations are unclear and doubtful. The most important facts yielded by vital microscopy, however, are: 1. The *smallest* diameters of the microvascular system are generally to be found in the terminal arterioles (approx. 5—7 microns); 2. these values are far removed from the actual vascular diameters within these organs studied in the rat. They are at least double those recorded in the literature.

I believe that a very considerable number of the plastic spheres may pass through the various arteriovenous anastomoses rather than through the capillary system. Furthermore, the experimental data indicating that the smallest particles (or vessel diameters) occurred within the liver suggest that this organ had the fewest shunts, as is generally believed.

Dr. Madden's data on the effect of cortisone on hepatic metastases are at variance with those previously recorded for the Walker tumour [cf. Cancer Res. **20**, 492—496 (1960)].

R. E. Madden: Dr. Wood and I have had previous discussions on the size of capillaries as determined by microspheres. Microspheres are rigid and do not mold and deform as do tumour cells. They would force themselves under the existing blood pressure through the pre-capillary arteriole and capillary itself. There are perhaps three immediate reasons, then, why our data differ from data on capillary or pre-capillary arteriole size as determined by vital microscopy:

1. The rigidity of microspheres,

2. The fact that our experiments were carried out *in situ*, i.e. without the manipulation and disturbed physiology inevitable in vital microscopy.

3. We are not measuring true capillaries but rather larger limiting vascular channels.

With regard to the mathematics let me expand a bit. Microspheres with a broad and normal distribution are injected but, in nearly every case, their mean size is in excess of effective vascular size (as calculated subsequently). At any rate, this is not essential since the total range goes from 1 to over 100 microns. Spheres enter the vascular beds and some are retained. Those which pass through are normally distributed, i.e. give a bell-shaped distribution curve. These reflect, but do not equal, the size of the channels. Since they are of vascular channel size and smaller, their mean must lie below that of the trapped spheres, which represent the true channel size. In order to calculate channel size, we refer back to the text and the use of probits:

$$Y_C = \frac{Y_M + Y_{M^1}}{2}.$$

Curves M and M^1 are derived from the experimental data (see Fig. 1). In the example YM is the probit for any size of injected microspheres (A) we wish to select and YM^1 the probit for the proportion of microspheres passing the capillary bed. YC is the probit for the trapped spheres. Please note that all of these sizes are normally distributed, and that they do not represent a single size. The expression $YM^1 - YC$ in the original equation represents the proportion of the original sample of size (A) *or less* reaching effluent blood. YM and YM^1 vary inversely, which means that the line C lies midway between.

Let me illustrate: if a large-size sample M, with a mean, say, of 35 microns, were injected and the mean vascular size were 20 microns, the proportion of spheres in the outputs of the original sample or less would be small. Conversely, if a small-size sample, with a mean, say, of 18 microns, were injected, this proportion would be larger. Referring this to the figure, lines M and M^1 vary outwards or inwards from line C equally in opposite directions. The position of C is therefore independent of the size of the injected spheres. This was indeed exactly borne out by the experimental data. The mean size determined, using either the large range or the small range microspheres, was the same within experimental error.

Referring to Dr. Wood's statement that the liver has few if any shunts, we agree, as we saw no skewing to the right here. But we do not agree that this is the reason why we found the smallest vascular size in this organ. Rather do we suggest that the small size determined was due to the fact that these spheres were under the lowest pressure (portal vein pressure), and hence did not stretch the available pore size as much. Thus, we made the qualification that effective vascular size may depend on the blood pressure of the vascular supply injected (see text).

L. B. Thomas: Some patients with acute leukaemia die because of multiple haemorrhagic leukaemic nodules in the white matter of the brain. These intra-cerebral haemorrhagic leukaemic nodules occur most often in patients with "blastic crises" — that is to ray, in patients with a rapidly rising leukaemic cell count in the peripheral blood. At the National Institutes of Health we have studied a number of patients with these intra-cerebral leukaemic nodules. The nodules do not develop in the smallest capillaries, which would be the expected site of localisation if the only factor was simply stasis of the blood with plugging of capillaries by the leukaemic cells. In fact, the leukaemic nodules all develop first within venules and small veins. I present this information because I believe it is a good example in the human of the principle that many tumour cells actually localise in venules and form metastases there rather than in capillaries.

R. E. Madden: I thank Dr. Thomas for his remarks and I have no specific reply to offer.

D. F. H. Wallach: Are the microspheres polystyrene? If so, are they stabilised with anionic detergents as is commonly done with latexes? If so, they may be expected to have a very high negative potential, much greater than that of mammalian cells. This might produce capillary expansion secondary to electrostatic repulsion between the microspheres and the negatively charged endothelium.

R. E. Madden: The spheres are polystyrene and were obtained from the

Minnesota Mining and Manufacturing Company. I have no way of knowing their surface charge but they were suspended in EARLE's salt solution, in which they were well dispersed.

S. Wood: Commenting on the remarks of Dr. THOMAS, it would be worth noting that leucocytic sticking and emigration, as well as the adhesion and endothelial penetration of V 2 carcinoma cells in the rabbit ear chamber, first occur in the venous capillary or capillary venule.

D. Schwartz: I should like to ask Dr. MADDEN a question about statistical methodology. As a rule, the method of probits is employed for variables which cannot be measured directly (such as the minimum lethal dose for an animal). Now, it seems that in this particular case the diameter of the spheres was measured directly. I do not therefore understand why the probit method was used instead of simply calculating the mean and the variance.

R. E. Madden: The method of probit analysis was chosen by my statistical colleague, Dr. MELVIN SCHWARTZ. This is a method by which sigmoidal curves, those of cumulative frequency, are converted into straight lines. Straight line functions are more easily dealt with.

P. Lazar: May I make a comment of a purely technical nature. I did not quite understand Dr. MADDEN's calculation in connection with determining of capillary size. It seems to me that the distribution of sphere sizes in the outputs may well provide an *indication* as to the diameter of the vascular channels, but I do not see how one can *evaluate* their mean diameter as simply as Dr. MADDEN suggests.

In particular, why is the probit line for fraction C of the spheres remaining in the capillaries *exactly midway between* the other two? Besides, one would rather expect to find the M line (relating

to the spheres entering the capillaries) between the two others, the large spheres being separated from the smaller ones by their inability to pass through the vascular channels.

R. E. Madden: The spheres represented by line C are those trapped in the vascular bed, i.e. those which are precisely of the critical size required to plug a channel. Those which pass through before-hand without plugging the channel are of course smaller, represented by M^1. It is true that after a channel is plugged, spheres of that particular size and larger are trapped and denied access to effluent blood. I quite understand why you may think therefore that C, i.e. the trapped spheres, should be larger than M since some, the smaller spheres, of M have already passed through. Dr. WOOD has also raised this question. Let me point out, however, that after plugging not only that size and larger but also that size and smaller of injected spheres are denied access to effluent blood. Thus, the filtering at this point is not selective but total. C does not represent those spheres backed up in the microcirculation, but only those spheres which first occlude the capillary or precapillary arteriole. C, therefore, does in fact reflect capillary size.

This effect of plugging may introduce an error if the total dose or mass of injected spheres is great compared to the total capacity of the circulation. Spheres would then back up in arterioles and successively occlude larger vessels, giving a false high figure for C. We believe we have solved this problem by injecting the spheres in four doses varying from 25,000 to 100,000 particles. There was no change in the size distribution of effluent spheres, M^1. Hence, this error is small and not detectable within the limits of our experimental accuracy.

B. Halpern: First: What percentage of neoplastic cells is trapped by Kupffer cells following injection into the portal vein? Can this phenomenon account for the fact that primary tumours "take" poorly in the liver?

Second as regards acetylcholine, it tends to act rather on the arterioles than on the capillaries, and its effect is transitory.

In order to draw valid conclusions from the effects of pharmacological agents, other vaso-active substances exerting a prolonged action on the terminal vascular network would have to be employed, such as Priscol.

R. E. Madden: In reply to your first question this is precisely what we are attempting to show. The biological activity towards neoplastic cells, whether due to Kupffer activity, specific organ immunity, or some other cause, is more important than the simple mechanical relationship of cell-capillary size.

Thank you in your second comment. We realize that this is a weak point since we have not directly measured the vasodilator effect of acetylcholine. We reasoned that this is a powerful vasodilator capable of producing a marked fall in blood pressure. Peripheral vascular resistance is controlled largely at the pre-capillary arteriole level. Acetylcholine is also very rapidly hydrolysed. By injection it selectively into one organ (muscle) with tumour cells we could produce maximal vasodilation locally but few of the generalized depressant effects that may promote tumour cell arrest. At any rate, no effect one way or the other on primary take or on transcapillary passage occurred.

I may add that venous congestion produced by causing venous obstruction simultaneously with tumour cell injection likewise had no effect.

References

AGOSTINO, D., and CLIFFTON, E. E., Anticoagulants and the development of pulmonary metastases. Anticoagulant effect on the Walker 256 carcinosarcoma in rats. *Arch. Surg.* **84**, 449 (1962).

— — The coagulation factor in the production of metastases. Effects of fibrinolysin and heparin. *Osped. Ital.-Chir.* **9**, 393 (1963).

— — Anesthetic effect on pulmonary metastases in rats. Development of metastases of Walker 256 carcinosarcoma. *Arch. Surg.* **88**, 735 (1964).

ALEXANDER, J. W., and ALTMEIER, W. A., Susceptibility of injured tissues to hematogenous metastases: An experimental study. *Ann. Surg.* **159**, 933 (1964).

BASERGA, R. and SHUBIK, P., The action of cortisone on transplanted and induced tumors in mice. *Cancer Res.* **14**, 12 (1954).

BUINAUSKAS, P., McDONALD, G. O., and COLE, W. H., Role of operative stress on the resistance of the experimental animal to inoculated cancer cells. *Ann. Surg.* **148**, 643 (1958).

CAGLIANI, P., MARINO, V., and SFORZA, M., Administration of fibrinolysin activators and of antifibrinolysins and the hematogenic distribution of metastases of Walker carcinosarcoma. *Biol. lat. (Milano)* **15**, 171 (1962).

CHU, E. W., and MALMGREN, R. A., Effect of orotic acid on the metastasis of mammary tumors in mice. *Cancer Res.* **24**, 671 (1964).

CLIFFTON, E. E., and AGOSTINO, D., Effect of inhibitors of fibrinolytic enzymes on development of pulmonary metastases. *J. nat. Cancer Inst.* **33**, 753 (1964).

DRIESSENS, J., CLAY, A., VANLERENBERGHE, J., GIAUX, G., ADENIS, L., and QUANDALLE, P., Intravenous injection of Guerin epithelioma homogenates. I. In the rat after X-irradiation. *C.R. Soc. Biol. (Paris)* **157**, 1981 (1963).

FINNEY, D. J., *Probit analysis.* London: Cambridge University Press 1947.

FISHER, B., and FISHER, E. R., Experimental evidence in support of the Dorman tumor cell. *Science* **130**, 918 (1959).

FISHER, E. R., and FISHER, B., Experimental studies of factors influencing hepatic metastases. VII. Effect of reticulo-endothelial interference. *Cancer Res.* **21**, 275 (1961).

— — Experimental studies of factors influencing hepatic metastases. IX. Pituitary gland. *Ann. Surg.* **154**, 347 (1961).

FISHER, E. R., and FISHER, B., Experimental studies of factors influencing hepatic metastases. X. Effect of reticuloendothelial stimulation. *Cancer Res.* **22**, 478 (1962).

GALLINOTTO, G., and ZAMPOGNA, S., The influence of heparin upon the metastatic spread of malignant tumors. Experimental studies. *Minerva chir.* **19**, 347 (1964).

GASIC, G., and GASIC, T., Removal of sialic acid from the cell coat in tumor cells and vascular endothelium, and its effect on metastases. *Proc. nat. Acad. Sci. (Wash.)* **48**, 1172 (1962).

GREENE, H. S. N., and HARVEY, E. K., The relationship between the dissemination of tumor cells and the distribution of metastases. *Cancer Res.* **24**, 799 (1964).

GROSSI, C. E., AGOSTINO, D., and CLIFFTON, E. E., The effect of human fibrinolysin on pulmonary metastases of Walker 256 carcinosarcoma. *Cancer Res.* **20**, 605 (1960).

HOYE, R. C., and SMITH, R. R., The effectiveness of small amounts of pre-operative irradiation in preventing the growth of tumor cells disseminated at surgery. *Cancer (Philad.)* **14**, 284 (1961).

KALLENBACH, H., Über die Veränderung der Metastasenhäufigkeit nach operativen Eingriffen im tierexperimentellen Modellversuch. *Chirurg* **33**, 340 (1962).

KETCHAM, A. S., WEXLER, H., and MANTEL, N., Studies on the effects of surgery on transplanted animal tumors and their metastases. *J. nat. Cancer Inst.* **27**, 1311 (1961).

KOIKE, A., Mechanism of blood born metastases. I. Some factors affecting lodgement and growth of tumor cells in the lungs. *Cancer (Philad.)* **17**, 450 (1964).

— NAKAZATO, H., and MOORE, G. E., The fate of Ehrlich cells injected into the portal system. *Cancer (Philad.)* **16**, 716 (1963).

MAISKII, I. N., Effect of organ specific sera on the localization of metastases from the Brown-Pearce tumor. *Byull. éksp. Biol. Med.* **54**, 784 (1963).

PRINZMETAL, M., ORNITZ jr., E. M., SIMKIN, B., and BERGMAN, H. C., Arteriovenous anastamoses in liver, spleen, and lungs. *Amer. J. Physiol.* **152**, 48 (1948).

ROBINSON, K. P., and HOPPE, E., The development of blood born metastases. *Arch. Surg.* **85**, 720 (1962).

ROMSDAHL, M. M., CHU, E. W., HUME, R., and SMITH, R. R., The time of metastasis and release of circulating tumor cells as determined in an experimental system. *Cancer (Philad.)* **14**, 883 (1961).

SAUNDERS, E. A., and KNISELY, M. H., Living mesenteric terminal arterioles before and immediately after embolism. *Arch. Path.* **58**, 309—344 (1954).

SFORZA, M., and COGLIANI, P., Surgical operations and metastatic manifestations of latent tumor cells. Experimental studies. *Biol. lat. (Milano)* **15**, 183 (1962).

WOOD jr., S., Pathogenesis of metastasis formation observed *in vivo* in the rabbit ear chamber. *Arch. Path.* **66**, 550 (1958).

— HOLYOKE, E. D., and YARDLEY, J. H., An experimental study of the influence of adrenal steroid, growth hormone, and anticoagulants on pulmonary metastasis forma tion in mice. *Proc. Amer. Ass. Cancer Res.* **2**, 157 (1956).

ZEIDMAN, I., The fate of circulating tumor cells. I. Passage of cells through capillaries. *Cancer Res.* **21**, 38 (1961).

— The fate of circulating tumor cells. II. A mechanism of cortisone action in increasing metastases. *Cancer Res.* **22**, 501 (1962).

Morphogenesis of Lung Metastases in a Transplantable Reticulum-Cell Sarcoma of the Golden Hamster (HaTu No. 25)*

PETER STRÄULI and GISELA HAEMMERLI

*Department of Cancer Research and Experimental Pathology, Institute of Pathology, University of Zurich, Zurich, Switzerland***

A spontaneous reticulum-cell sarcoma of the golden hamster, made transplantable in the solid and the ascitic form, has been maintained in our laboratory for the past 5 years. Transplantation behavior and cytogenetic characteristics of this tumour have been described recently (HAEMMERLI, ZWEIDLER, and STRÄULI, 1966). In the majority of its hosts, the tumour displays a leukemia-like mode of dissemination which, irrespective of site of transplantation, results in the death of the animals between the 6th and 7th day. In the present communication, one facet of the spread of the tumour, the formation of lung metastases, will be analysed.

Material and Method

150 adult golden hamsters of both sexes, obtained from the Centraal Proefdierenbedrijf T.N.O. (Zeist, Netherlands), were subcutaneously implanted with 50×10^6 ascites tumour cells. The animals were randomly distributed in groups of 20 and sacrificed on 7 consecutive days, beginning with the first day after transplantation. The remaining animals lived up to the 10th day, and were killed when they had attained a moribund state. Tumour and thoracic organs were fixed partly in Susa for staining with hematoxilin/eosin and elastin/van Gieson, partly with 4% formalin for the demonstration of fibrin by means of the Pikro-Mallory method (LENDRUM et al., 1962). The lungs were cut in steps, in some cases in serial sections.

Microscopic Anatomy of the Pulmonary Vessels of the Golden Hamster

Knowledge of the pulmonary vasculature is indispensable for the study of lung metastases. Therefore, a short description of the different types of blood vessels in the hamster lung is inserted. Useful hints may be drawn from investigations on the vascular architecture of the lung in other small mammals (KARRER, 1959; WEIBEL, 1960; BEST, 1961; WAAGENVORDT, 1964).

Pulmonary Arteries. Major branches are of elastic, smaller branches of muscular type. The media is bounded by two very distinct elastic membranes. The outer layers of the adventitia form a sheath filled with very loose connective tissue; lymphatics may be distinguished within this space.

* This study was supported by grant No. 2877 from the Swiss National Foundation for Scientific Research and by a grant from the Swiss League against Cancer.

** Reproduction of figures 4 and 5 authorized by F. K. Schattauer-Verlag, Stuttgart.

Bronchial Arteries. These are systemic arteries supplying the bronchi and the walls of the pulmonary arteries and veins (vasa vasorum). In relation to the diameter of the lumen, the media is much

Capillaries. No special description is required.

Venules. These vessels are devoid of musculature. They use to join the pulmonary veins rather abruptly and often

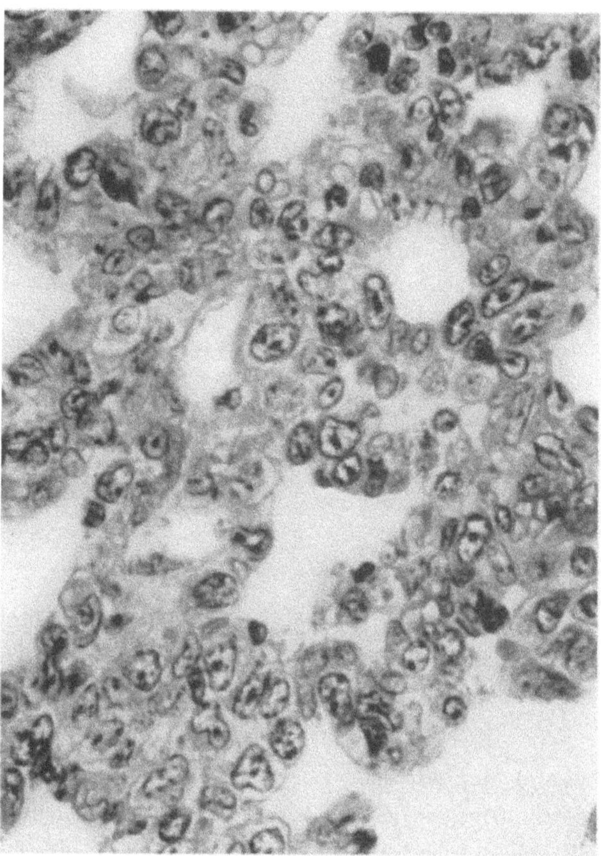

Figs. 1 to 4. Spontaneous reticulum-cell sarcoma of the golden hamster (HaTu 25) on the 8th day after subcutaneous implantation of 50×10^6 tumour cells. — Fig. 1. Pulmonary capillaries packed with tumour cells. $\times 360$

thicker than in pulmonary arteries. An internal elastic lamina is well developed whereas an external elastic lamina is incomplete or absent. Despite their functional significance, the bronchial arteries of the hamster are small vessels, and we could only find them in the vicinity of the hilus.

Arterioles. This term is used for arterial branches with a muscular media at their origin and none in their remaining portion.

at a right angle. Without connexion to a vein, the venules cannot be distinguished from the non-muscular portions of arterioles.

Pulmonary Veins. Their most characteristic feature is a layer of cardiac muscle fibers within the adventitia. The media consists of a thin layer of smooth muscle bordered by an external and a less distinct internal elastic membrane. Apart from the cardiac muscle coat, the adventitia corresponds to that of the pulmonary arteries.

Bronchial Veins. These inconspicuous vessels consist mainly of a thin layer of fibroelastic tissue.

veins. Small numbers of tumour cells were seen in the adventitia of the larger pulmonary vessels.

On the 3rd and 4th day, sporadic sarcoma cells were found to be attached to

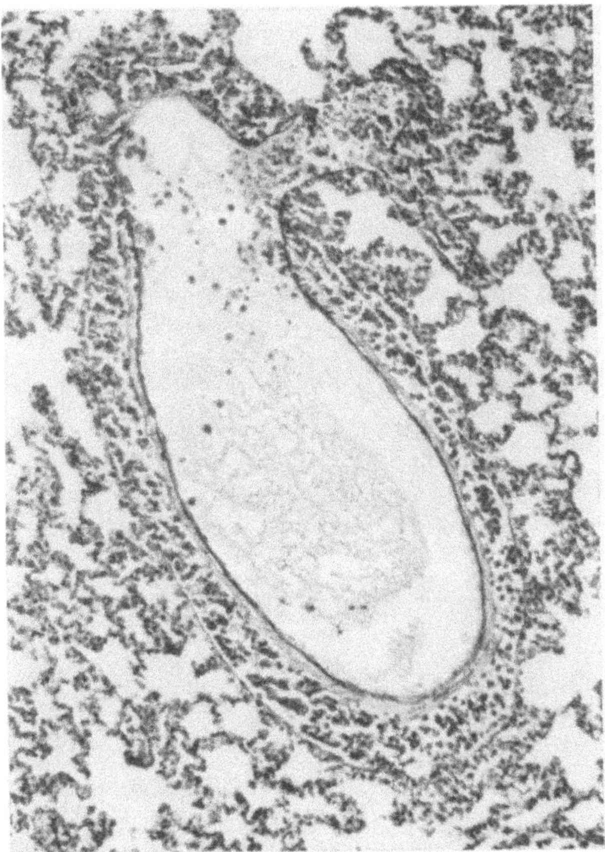

Fig. 2. Tumour cell aggregate in the adventitial space of a medium-sized pulmonary vein. At upper right entry of a venule containing tumour cells and thrombotic material. ×110

Histologic Findings in the Lungs of Tumour-Bearing Golden Hamsters

Twenty-four hours after subcutaneous implantation of 50×10^6 sarcoma cells the lung vessels were free of tumour elements.

On the 2nd day, sarcoma cells in considerable numbers were detected in pulmonary arteries and, less conspicuously, in arterioles, capillaries, venules and

the endothelial lining of small arteries and arterioles, some of them even undergoing mitosis. In the capillaries, the number of tumour cells had increased; the cells, often elongated and distorted, formed single-file columns in many loops. In the adventitial sheaths, loose aggregates of tumour cells could be seen.

By the 8th day, most arterial branches were filled with dense suspensions of tumour cells. Columns of sarcoma cells had obstructed numerous segments of the capillary system, and within ill-defined masses of tumour tissue, remains of capillary walls could be detected (Fig. 1). The

additional features could be observed. In the lumina of medium-sized pulmonary veins, mushroom-like masses, consisting of tumour cells, erythrocytes, fibrin, and cellular debris, were seen. Serial sections

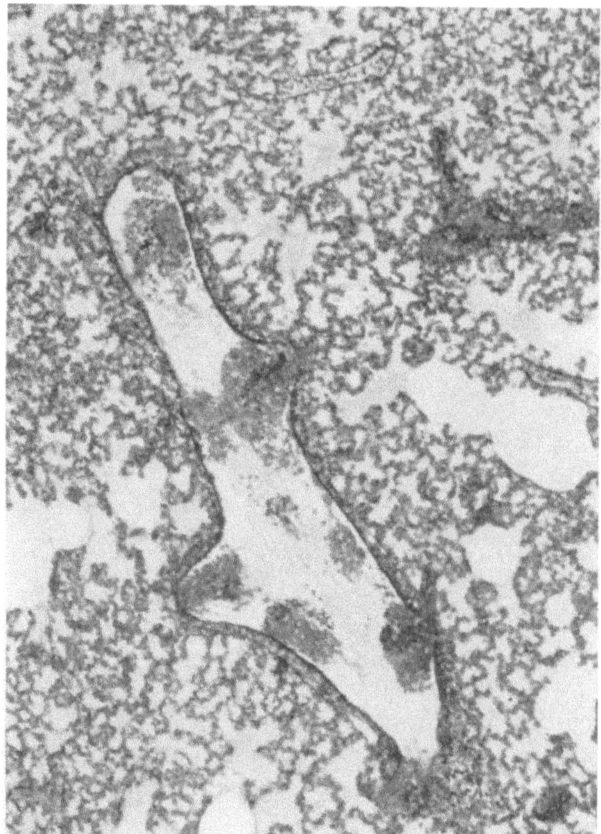

Fig. 3. Tumour thrombi in a medium-sized pulmonary vein. The mushroom-like masses are located at sites of entry of venules. ×90

tumour cell aggregates in the adventitial sheaths of pulmonary arteries and veins had increased and formed cuff-like, perivascular foci (Fig. 2). Within these infiltrates, the heart muscle layer of the veins was destroyed; the media of arteries and the elastic membranes of both arteries and veins generally had remained intact. Adventitial lymphatics also often contained sarcoma cells. In the lungs of animals sacrificed in a moribund state,

revealed these aggregates to be located at the sites of entry of venules (Figs. 3 and 4). Many veins were completely filled with compact masses of tumour cells and fibrin.

Discussion

According to the histologic findings, the development of lung metastases takes place in three vascular compartments of the lung: in the capillary system, in the adventitial sheaths of arteries and veins, and within the veins.

1. Capillary Metastases. Their origin is easily understood. Due to the increasing number of transported tumour cells,

(1965). In most cases an initial adhesion of tumour cells to the endothelium of pulmonary vessels, especially arterioles, and a subsequent migration of these elements to an extravascular "interstitial"

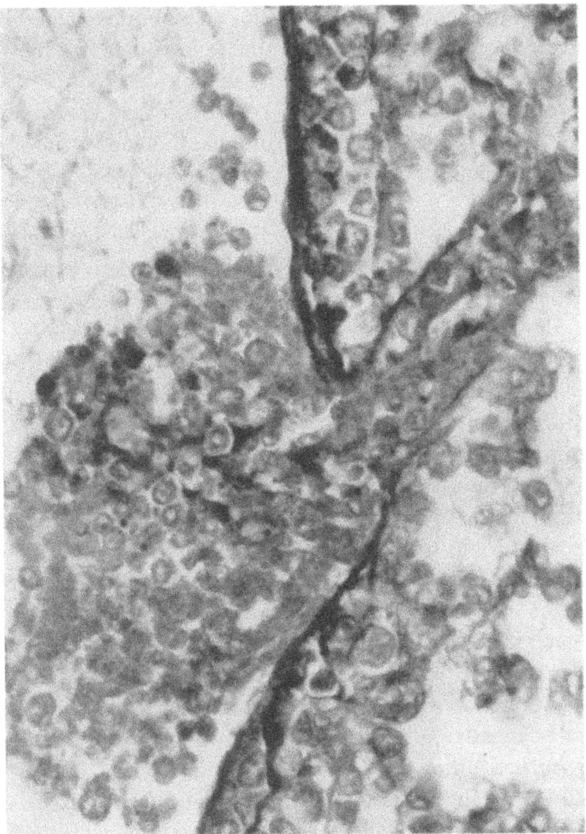

Fig. 4. Higher magnification of tumour thrombus shown at lower right of Fig. 3. ×360

the local circulation breaks down. The resulting stasis encroaches on the precapillary arterioles. The capillary walls are destroyed, and the tumour cells proliferating inside and outside the vessels form ill-defined aggregates.

2. Adventitial Metastases. The early appearance of tumour cells in extravascular positions is a well-known fact. Pertinent observations have been discussed in the monographs of COLE *et al.* (1961), and of GRIFFITHS and SALSBURY

tissue space have been described. This mechanism, however, seems of little importance in the present tumour-host system where the adventitial metastases originate in large and medium-sized arteries and veins. Adhesion of tumour cells to the endothelium of these vessels is an exceptional finding, and no observations sustaining the possibility of penetration through the unimpaired vessel wall are available. So we have to look for other explanations.

It can be assumed that tumour cells attain the adventitia by way of the vasa vasorum. A certain number of tumour cells, after passage through the pulmonary circulation, could be expected to re-enter the lungs via the systemic circulation, i.e. the bronchial arteries. However, we were not able to detect tumour cells in bronchial arteries or even in the vasa vasorum.

Another assumption is the transport of tumour cells by means of the perivascular lymph system. Obviously, a lymph circulation does occur, either through the whole adventitial space, or through lymphatics within the adventitial sheath. Yet, the relation of lymphogenous dissemination of tumour cells to the appearance of tumour infiltrates in the adventitia still has to be clarified.

3. Intravenous Metastases. These are the most conspicuous features in the present tumour-host system. It may be conceived that the mushroom-like masses, encountered in medium-sized pulmonary veins, emerge from fibrin-mediated tumour cell aggregates in venules (Sträuli, 1966). Microcoagulation within the slowly advancing tumour cell suspension begins in the venules already. When these aggregates are pushed into the large lumen of the veins, they unfold in a fanlike fashion, the firmness of the whole structure being guaranteed by fibrin. Experiments are under way to investigate whether a special coagulative capacity of the sarcoma cells concurs with this phenomenon.

Summary

In a transplantable reticulum-cell sarcoma of the golden hamster (HaTu No. 25), three morphogenetic mechanisms for the development of lung metastases can be distinguished:

1. Capillary metastases. Due to tumour cell columns in the capillary loops, the circulation breaks down and the vessel walls are destroyed. The tumour cells, proliferating inside and outside the vessels, form ill-defined aggregates.

2. Adventitial metastases. Infiltration of the adventitial sheaths of pulmonary arteries and veins leads to the formation of cuff-like perivascular tumour foci. The mode of entry of the tumour cells to the adventitia has not been clarified. An eventual significance of the vasa vasorum and of the perivascular lymphatic system is discussed.

3. Intravenous metastases. In advanced stages of tumour spread, the lumina of the medium-sized pulmonary veins contain tumour masses attached to the sites of entry of venules. It is assumed that a hypercoagulable state in the venules leads to the formation of tumour-fibrin aggregates which are pushed into the large lumen of the veins. Here the tumour thrombi form mushroom-like masses and gradually merge to compact intravenous metastases.

References

Best, P. V., and Heath, D., Interpretation of the appearances of the small pulmonary blood vessels in animals. *Circulat. Res.* **9**, 288—294 (1961).

Cole, W. H., McDonald, G. O., Roberts, S. S., and Southwick, H. W., *Dissemination of cancer. Prevention and therapy.* New York: Appleton-Century-Crofts 1961.

Griffiths, J. D., and Salsbury, A. J., *Circulating cancer cells.* Springfield (Ill.): Ch. C. Thomas 1965.

Haemmerli, G., Zweidler, A., and Sträuli, P., Transplantation behavior and cytogenetic characteristics of a spontaneous reticulum cell sarcoma in the golden hamster. *Int. J. Cancer* **1**, 599—612 (1966).

KARRER, H. E., The striated musculature of blood vessels. I. General cell morphology. *J. biophys. biochem. Cytol.* **6**, 383—390 (1959).
— II. Cell interconnections and cell surface. *J. biophys. biochem. Cytol.* **8**, 135—150 (1960).
LENDRUM, A. C., FRASER, D. S., SLIDDERS, W., and HENDERSON, R., Studies on the character and staining of fibrin. *J. clin. Path.* **15**, 401—413 (1962).

STRÄULI, P., Intravascular clotting and cancer localization. *Diffuse intravascular clotting. Thrombos. Diathes. haemorrh. (Stuttg.)*, Suppl. **20**, 147—160 (1966).
WAAGENVORDT, C. A., HEATH, D., and EDWARDS, J. E., *The pathology of the pulmonary vasculature.* Springfield (Ill.): Ch. C. Thomas 1964.
WEIBEL, E. R., Early stages in the development of collateral circulation to the lung in the rat. *Circulat. Res.* **8**, 353—376 (1960).

Studies of Circulating Cancer Cells in Cancer Patients

R. A. Malmgren

*Pathologic Anatomy Branch, National Cancer Institute, National Institutes of Health,
Public Health Service, US Department of Health, Education and Welfare,
Bethesda 14, Md., USA*

In human cancer, metastasis poses one of the most critical problems associated with the treatment of the disease and control of this phenomenon is essential to acheving a favorable prognosis. Unfortunately, despite our long awareness of metastasis as a clinical entity, the mechanism of the metastatic process remains obscure.

In current thinking on the mechanism of cancer invasion the problem is generally considered in terms of (1) the factors that cause or permit the malignant cells to leave the primary tumour, (2) the factors that influence their transportation to other tissues and (3) the factors that determine their ability to lodge and grow in their new location.

Dissemination from the site of origin to the metastatic site via the circulatory or lymphatic systems is, *a priori*, basic to the metastatic process and, in the study of factors which influence metastasis in humans, the demonstration of cancer cells in transit from the primary tumour represents an important aspect of the inquiry for several reasons. First, if the demonstration of cancer cells in the blood can always be directly related to the development of metastasis, then the factors associated with cancer cells gaining access to the blood-stream are of primary importance. If, on the other hand, finding cancer cells in the blood is not invariably associated with metastasis development then the factors related to the lodgement, survival and growth of the cells assume added significance in explaining the metastatic process.

The first reported attempt to study metastasis by looking for cancer cells in the blood was carried out by Ashworth (1869). Following Ashworth's observation there were several other reports of the demonstration of cancer cells in the blood of patients with cancer, but prior to 1934 no systematic search was made for malignant cells in the circulatory system. At that time Poole and Dunlop (1934) studied 40 cancer patients and found cells which they thought to be cancer cells in the blood of 17 of them. After this report another 20 years passed before this aspect of the metastasis problem was again examined. In 1955, Fisher and Thurnbull reported a careful study of the local blood from 25 colo-rectal carcinoma specimens and Engell (1955) reported his findings on the local and peripheral blood of 107 cancer cases. Since 1955 many reports have appeared in the literature in which patients with a variety of types of cancer in different stages of their disease have been studied for the presence of cancer cells in both local and peripheral blood.

Much of the impetus for these studies undoubtedly came from acceptance of the idea that individual cancer cells were recognizable by morphologic criteria.

This idea was, of course, a direct outgrowth of the exfoliative cytology techniques developed by Papanicolaou which were felt to be equally suitable for identifying cancer cells in the blood.

Methods

For the cytologic examination of blood, it is necessary to separate the cancer cells, which may be few in number, from the other cellular elements of the blood without cell loss and morphologic distortion and to mount the specimens in a way that assures easy microscopic detection. In the course of studies designed to develop suitable techniques, eleven methods and modifications of these methods have been described (Engell, 1955; Fawcett and Valle, 1952; Sandberg and Moore, 1957; Malmgren et al., 1958; Roberts et al., 1958; Long et al., 1959; Seal, 1959; Pimenta de Mello, 1960; Spriggs and Alexander, 1960; Kuper et al., 1961; Nedelkoff et al., 1961; Eriksson, 1962; Stein et al., 1962; Foss et al., 1963; Seal, 1964; West et al., 1964). Although each of the methods and modifications reported had certain advantages and disadvantages, each was reportedly successful for the recovery of cancer cells from the blood of cancer patients making it possible to study the factors which influence metastasis by observing cells in transit.

In our laboratory we developed and used the streptolysin 0 and the millipore filter technique (Malmgren et al., 1958) for the isolation of cancer cells in the blood, because this method, which permitted the quantitative recovery of the cancer cells provided, at the same time, a satisfactory preparation for cytologic examination.

Initially, many studies were made establishing base-line information on how frequently cancer cells could be found in the blood of patients with a particular type of cancer at a particular stage of the disease. These studies involved many different techniques, many different types of cancer in various stages of the disease, and the results were expressed in different ways. As a consequence, the range for finding cancer cells in the peripheral blood has varied widely, and it would be impossible to reduce these highly varied reports to a single norm or even to correlate the variables which might account for these differences. Despite this wide variation there is general agreement on many points.

Factors Influencing Cells in the Blood

Stage of Disease. There has, been general agreement that, circulating cancer cells are more likely to be found as the disease becomes more advanced (Engell, 1955; Fisher and Thurnbull, 1955; Roberts et al., 1958; Engell, 1959; Long et al., 1960; Pruitt et al., 1962; Sato, 1962; Scheinin and Koivuniemi, 1963). This was true for both peripheral blood specimens and for specimens of local blood draining the tumour in all the types of cancer which have been studies. Investigations in our laboratory, (Potter et al., 1960) on 285 patients showed cancer cells in 9% of the peripheral blood specimens from resectable or early cases and cancer cells in 15% of the blood specimens from non-resectable or advanced cases. The local blood specimens showed a similar trend with circulating cancer cells demonstrable in 30% of the resectable cases and 48% of the non-resectable cases.

Early in the course of studies of cancer cells in the blood, the possibility of screening blood specimens for the early detection of unsuspected cancer was entertained. This idea was quickly dismissed, however, in view of the relatively low cancer cell incidence observed in the peripheral blood of known cancer patients. The possibility of making preoperative diagnosis of moderately advanced cancer of internal organs such as liver, lung, kidney, etc. when a lesion of unknown type exists has not been experimentally studied.

Growth Rate of Primary Tumour. An interesting correlation between the growth rate of melanomas and the detection of cancer cells in the blood was made by Romsdahl et al., 1960). In his study of 42 patients he observed that the detection of tumour cells in the blood corresponded in time with an increased growth rate of the tumour and an increased number of skin metastases. When the size increase in the tumours was 10% or less in one week, 8% of the peripheral blood specimens contained cancer cells. When the size increase in the tumour was 10 to 20% in a week, 25% of the peripheral blood specimens contained tumour cells, and 66% of the blood specimens were positive when there was an increase in the tumour size of more than 20% in one week. The same pattern was seen when comparing the per cent increase in the number of metastases with the finding of cancer cells in the blood.

This observation is of particular interest because it demonstrates the importance of the characteristics of the tumour in the metastatic process. It is true that the characteristics of the host and tumour are inseparable but still Romsdahl's study emphasizes the importance of factors which are related to the release of cells from the primary tumour in contrast to the factors which influence the lodgement and growth of the cells at a distant site in the host.

Characteristics of the Primary Tumour. In addition to the stage of the disease, the histologic grade of the cancer very probably influences the finding of tumour cells in the blood just as the

histologic grade is apparently related to metastasis (Dukes and Bussey, 1958). In 1955, Engell made the first and only study of this correlation. He reported a close parallelism between finding cancer cells in the blood and the histologic grade of carcinoma of the colon and rectum. Cancer cells were detectable in the blood of 35% of the cases with Grade II tumours, 78% of the Grade II tumours and 100% of the Grade IV tumours.

An attempt was made in our laboratory to correlate a variety of characteristics of the primary tumour with the presence of cancer cells in the blood. Seventy-four patients with resectable tumours of the cervix (22), head an neck (19), breast (9), intestine (13), and miscellaneous (13) had their blood examined for tumour cells. The tumours from these patients were examined for differentiation, desmoplasia, lymphocytes, plasma cells, polymorphonuclear leucocytes, eosinophiles, necrosis, nuclear-cytoplasmic ratio, nucleolar-nuclear ratio and mitosis. Each of these parameters was divided into a roughly quantitative category of "high", "much", "increased", etc..., or "low", "little", "decreased", etc.... A comparison was then made between patients with an increased amount and those with a decreased amount of each parameter as to whether or not tumour cells were found in their blood.

The patients with a tumour classified as poorly differentiated had a 10% higher incidence of cancer cells in the blood than did the patients with well-differentiated tumours. The patients with little fibrous tissue in their tumours had a 6% higher incidence of cancer cells in their blood. The presence of many lymphocytes was associated with an 8% higher incidence of tumour cells in the blood while the presence of many polymorphonuclear leucocytes was associated with a 4% higher incidence of tumour cells in the blood. Plasma cells in a high concentration in the tumour seemed to decrease the chance of finding tumour cells in the blood by 14%. On the other hand, the presence of many eosinophils in the tumour was associated with an increase of 22% in the incidence of detectable tumour cells in the blood. The same was true for necrosis where the incidence of tumour cells in the blood was 27% higher in patients whose tumours had necrosis as a prominent feature. The nuclear-cytoplasmic ratio and the nucleolar-nuclear ratio seemed to have little effect. The incidence of tumour cells in the blood was increased by only 3% and 2%, respectively, when these two parameters were higher. Increased mitosis above 8 per 100 cells was associated with an increase of 8% in the incidence of tumour cells in the blood.

Thus, the degree of differentiation, the number of eosinophils and necrosis seemed to be the most significant factors influencing the presence of cancer cells in the blood. If one equates necrosis and lack of differentiation with rapid growth, this would be further evidence in support of ROMSDAHL's observations that the more rapidly proliferating tumours produce more metastasis and have a higher incidence of circulating cancer cells.

Cell Type and Organ of Origin. The data from studies of cancer cells in the blood has also been analyzed in terms of the significance of cell type and organ of origin. In general, cancer cells are most often seen in the blood of patients with sarcoma. Circulating malignant cells are seen less often in patients with adenocarcinoma and least often in patients with squamous cell carcinomas (SALGADO et al., 1959; POTTER et al., 1960; PRUITT et al., 1962). This observation is in accord with the clinically observed metastatic potential of these tumours.

When analyzed in terms of the organ of origin certain organs such as breast seem to be frequently associated with cancer cells in the blood-stream while in other studies, gastrointestinal tract malignancies seem to be less often associated with cancer cells in the blood (SALGADO et al., 1959; POTTER et al., 1960; PRUITT et al., 1962).

Collection Site. Studies in which both peripheral blood and blood from veins draining the tumour were examined showed that the likelihood of finding cancer cells was greater in the local blood than in the peripheral blood (SANBDERG and MOORE, 1957; REISS, 1959; SALGADO et al., 1959; POTTER et al., 1960; NIGOGOSYAN and McDONALD, 1961; PRUITT et al., 1962; SATO, 1962; SCHEININ and KOIVUNIEMI, 1963). In addition, the number of cancer cells recovered was greater in local blood specimens (MALMGREN and POTTER, 1959; PRUITT et al., 1962). This decrease in cancer cells detectable in a given volume of blood might very well be explained by the "dilution" that occurs after the blood leaves the tumour. However, the lodgement of cancer cells in various tissues may also account for this decrease, and how much of this decrease may be due to cell loss by filtration as the blood passes through the lungs, liver or other organs before becoming available to the peripheral circulation is not certain. It would be interesting to know what the filtration efficiency of different organs is, but under the circumstances which exist in the human cancer patient, too few cells pass through the circulation at any one time to permit sampling the arterial and venous side of an organ to acquire this information.

Manipulation. ROBERTS et al. (1958) and LONG et al. (1960) have emphasized the importance of manipulation in the dissemination of cancer and have stressed the importance of this hazard to the patient when various diagnostic and therapeutic procedures are being conducted. They have described finding a shower of prostatic cancer cells in the inferior vena cava of 4 of 11 patients at the time of rectal massage of a prostatic carcinoma (JONASSON et al., 1961). They have also found cancer cells in the blood of 5 patients with endometrial cancer during curettage while the blood specimens from 3 patients with benign lesions and 2 with squamous cell carcinoma of the cervix were negative (ROBERTS et al., 1960). In addition, cancer cells were recovered from the inferior vena cava of 9 out of 25 patients during transurethral resection for bladder or prostatic cancer (ROBERTS et al., 1962).

ENGELL (1955) on the other hand, was unable to demonstrate any relationship between cancer cells in the blood and manipulation, and the results in our laboratory tend to support his observation. WEST (1964) while investigating patterns of tumour cell embolization, studied nearly 10,000 ml of blood taken from patients at various times during a 24-hour period and during various phases of surgery. He found that the number of cancer cells detectable was very small and that they were mainly present in the early morning (8:30 a.m.) specimen. That this happens to coincide with the time during which surgical procedure and manipulation frequently occur is worth noting. In addition, a breakdown of the time of surgery into 5 phases revealed that a slightly higher percentage of the blood specimens was positive during the induction of the anesthesia phase than during the period when manipulation of the tumour occurred.

It is unfortunate that the effect of manipulation on cancer cell dissemination has not been settled by these studies because the avoidance of manipulation, if manipulation does produce an increased number of circulating cancer cells, is one positive action the clinician can take in the treatment of malignancy. On the other hand, if manipulation does not increase tumour cell embolization, its avoidance should not be urged lest the clinician also avoid the degree of examination and surgery consistent with the best possible treatment.

Viability of Circulating Cancer Cells. One of the factors associated with metastasis which several investigators have thought to be significant is the degree of viability of the released cells. To study this point MOORE et al. (1959) attempted to grow cancer cells isolated from blood and reported the successful growth of cells in 3 of 64 specimens tested. Six attempts to cultivate cells from the blood in our laboratory were all unsuccessful. This inability to grow the cells in vitro does not definitely indicate that cancer cells in the blood are non-viable, particularly in view of the difficulty of establishing a cell in tissue culture under the best of circumstance, but the ability to grow cancer cells from the blood in tissue culture would have been quite significant.

Single Cells and Cell Clumps. An analysis of the number of single cancer cells and the number of groups of cancer cells observed in the local and peripheral blood of cancer patients was made in our laboratory (MALMGREN and POTTER, 1959). As might be expected, fewer single cancer cells and groups of cancer cells were found in the peripheral blood than in the local blood. An average of 5 single cancer cells and 1.2 groups of cancer cells were seen per positive case of peripheral blood and 7.5 single cancer cells and 4 groups of cancer cells per positive case of local blood. The interesting thing about this is not that the local blood contained more cancer cells than did the peripheral blood, as this would be expected solely on the basis of dilution, but rather that groups of cancer cells were to be seen at all in the peripheral blood. Cells collected from the peripheral vessels must have gone through the vessels of the lungs and the fingers before collection and one is left to ponder why the clumps were not filtered out in this process. Although a number of studies (PRINZMETAL, 1948; ZEIDMAN, 1961; PRESSMAN, 1964) have shown the passage of cancer cells and inert substances of relatively large diameter through organs, it was still surprising to find occasional groups of cells in peripheral blood specimens.

Prognostic Significance. Theoretically, the presence of cancer cells in the blood of a patient suggests that the prognosis for that patient should be worse than for a patient in whose blood no cancer cells can be found. If this supposition were true, examination of the blood would provide a very useful way of separating the good risk from the poor risk patients and treatment could be instituted accordingly. Unfortunately, examination of the blood for cancer cells has not proved to be of value in predicting which patients would develop metastases and which would not (ENGELL, 1955; 1959; CANDAR et al., 1962; DRYE et al., 1962; ROBERTS et al., 1962). The findings in our laboratory corroborate this opinion.

We found that of 74 patients with various types of cancer who were believed to be curable at the time of surgery, 34% developed recurrence of their disease. These patients were followed for 18 to 22 months after treatment. Thirty-two per cent of the patients with cancer cells in the blood developed a recurrence and thirty-six per cent of the patients without cancer cells in their blood developed a recurrence.

Although WATNEY et al. (1961) and ROBERTS et al. (1960) noted a slightly poorer prognosis for patients with cancer cells in their blood the difference was not highly significant. Clearly then, the care of cancer patients should not be influenced by the blood findings.

The lack of correlation between cancer cells in the blood and the development of metastasis points up the fact that many of the cancer cells which gain access to the blood stream must perish. This conclusion then emphasizes the importance of the factors which influence cell lodgement and growth in contrast to the importance of the factors which permit the cells to enter the bloodstream in the first place.

Summary

Intensive studies of the vascular dissemination of cancer have been carried out during the past decade and the following conclusions seem to be indicated. Cancer cells are demonstrable in the blood of cancer patients and this has been the case more often with rapidly growing, far advanced tumours than with early, slow growing cancer lesions.

No correlation has been clearly demonstrated between the presence of cancer cells in the blood and the subsequent development of metastasis, suggesting that factors other than cancer cell entry into the vascular system are essential in the formation of metastasis.

Discussion

Questions put to R. A. Malmgren

H. Sato: Is there any correlation between the number of cancer cells appearing in the circulating blood and the prognosis?

R. A. Malmgren: Analysis of our data has failed to reveal any correlation between the number of cancer cells found in the blood of cancer patients and the prognosis.

R. E. Madden: I would like to say that I agree with Dr. Malmgren's conclusion as to the lack of prognostic significance in the finding of circulating tumour cells. When reports on circulating tumour cells first appeared, considerable prognostic importance was attached to them, and this was a matter of great concern to us, in particular, as surgeons. It was felt that operation caused showers of tumour cells and perhaps aggravated the patient's condition. This is possible. However, the significance of circulating tumour cells in blood samples taken at random times is very difficult to assess statistically. Animal experiments have shown that the half-life of these cells varies from a few minutes to a few hours. The occurrence of a positive blood sample — that is to say, one in which tumour cells are cytologically demonstrated — would have to be almost fortuitous.

R. A. Malmgren: Dr. Madden is theoretically correct. One would not expect to find cancer cells in the blood of a cancer patient except occasionally and in "showers". The studies of West *et al.* (1964) bear out this idea to a certain extent.

However, these studies do indicate a tendency for tumour cells to appear in the blood-stream more often in the morning than at other times of the day.

D. Schwartz: Judging from the results reported by Dr. Malmgren and from the literature to which he has referred, it would seem, first, that there is probably no relationship between the presence of circulating cancer cells and the prognosis, and, secondly, that there is, by contrast, a perfectly admissible relationship between the presence of circulating cancer cells and the degree of "extension" of the cancer.

Do not these two findings contradict each other to some extent?

R. A. Malmgren: The inconsistency which Mr. Schwartz has pointed out is due to the fact that different groups of patients were used for the data on the relationship of cancer cells in the blood and prognosis. The studies concerned with a correlation between cancer cells in the blood and the stage of the disease included all cancer patients — those with very early cancer, as well as those with far advanced, inoperable disease. On the other hand, when evaluating the prognostic significance of finding cancer cells in the blood, only patients with cancer which was considered operable at the time the blood study was made, were included, since the prognosis for the cases with far advanced, inoperable cancer was already known.

S. Wood: Concerning the biological half-life of blood-borne embolic cancer cells, may I summarize briefly the recent and unpublished studies my colleagues and I have carried out with the ascitic V 2 carcinoma of the rabbit? We have employed a *bioassay* to determine the presence of cancer cells in cardiac blood serially after the intravenous inoculation of a standard dose of cells (approx. 10^8). Tumour cells are quite infrequently present during the initial 30 minutes. By the third hour, as many as 80% of the animals have circulating cancer cells. Then carcinoma cells vanish, but reappear after 1 day and may be found in almost all instances until the animal dies (after 30—33 days) from pulmonary metastases.

Our interpretation of these data is that the original tumour cells are briefly arrested by adhesion within the pulmonary blood vessels [cf. Ann. N.Y. Acad. Sci. **63**, 938 (1956); Aust. J. exp. Biol. med. Sci. **37**, 489—498 (1959) and Canad. Cancer Conf. **4**, 167—223 (1961)], then appear in the blood, and perish after 3 to 4 hours. Subsequently, cells reappear owing to a continuous repopulation of the blood from the growing metastatic foci [cf. Canad. Cancer Conf. **4**, 167—223 (1961) and Bull. Swiss Acad. Med. Sci. **20**, 92—121 (1964)].

B. Halpern: Is the low degree of invasiveness of tumours containing plasma cells in some way related to the well-known immunological properties of this type of cells?

R. A. Malmgren: Although I do not know why tumours with many plasma cells should be associated with a decreased incidence of tumour cells in the blood

stream, it is tempting for those of us who are interested in immunology and cancer to postulate that a plasma-cell-mediated immunological response is involved.

B. Halpern: What is the significance of the malignant cells found circulating in normal subjects?

R. A. Malmgren: I do not know the significance of the rare finding of "cancer-like cells" in the blood of a normal patient. I am personally aware of only three such cases out of about 350 normal patients who were examined by several different investigators. One of these patients returned to the hospital about 5 months later with a clinically evident squamous-cell carcinoma. The other two patients are still alive and well to the best of my knowledge. It is of course not possible to say whether they actually had clinically unrecognized cancer which they were able to control by their own defence mechanism or whether the cytological examination produced false positive results.

References

ASHWORTH, T. R., A case of cancer in which cells similar to those in the tumors were seen in the blood after death. *Med. J. Aust.* **14**, 146 (1869).

CANDAR, Z., RITCHIE, A. C., HOPKIRK, J. F., and LONG, R. C., The prognostic value of circulating tumor cells in patients with breast cancer. *Surg. Gynec. Obstet.* **115**, 291—294 (1962).

DRYE, J. C., RUMAGE, W. T., and ANDERSON, D., Prognostic import of circulating cancer cells after curative surgery. *Ann. Surg.* **155**, 733—739 (1962).

DUKES, C. E., and BUSSEY, H. J. R., The spread of rectal cancer and its effect on prognosis. *Brit. J. Cancer* **12**, 309 (1958).

ENGELL, H. C., Cancer cells in the circulating blood. *Acta chir. scand., Suppl.* 201 (1955).

— Cancer cells in the blood. *Ann. Surg.* **149**, 457—461 (1959).

ERIKSSON, O., Method for cytological detection of cancer cells in blood. *Cancer (Philad.)* **15**, 171—175 (1962).

FAWCETT, D. W., and VALLE, B. L., Studies on the separation of cell types in serosanguinous fluids, blood, and vaginal fluids by flotation on bovine plasma albumin. *J. Lab. clin. Med.* **39**, 354—364 (1952).

FISHER, E. R., and TURNBULL jr., R. B., The cytologic demonstration and significance of tumor cells in the mesenteric venous blood in patients with colorectal carcinoma. *Surg. Gynec. Obstet.* **100**, 102—108 (1955).

FOSS, O. P., MESSELT, O. T., and EFSKIND, L., Isolation of cancer cells from blood and thoracic duct lymph by filtration. *Surgery* **53**, 241—246 (1963).

JONASSON, O., LONG, L., ROBERTS, S., McGREW, E., and McDONALD, J., Cancer cells in the circulating blood during operative management of genitourinary tumors. *J. Urol. (Baltimore)* **85**, 1 (1961).

KUPER, S. W. A., BIGNALI, J. R., and LUCKCOCK, E. D., A quantitative method for studying tumor cells in blood. *Lancet* **1961 I**, 852—853.

LONG, L., JONASSON, O., ROBERTS, S., McGRATH, R., McGREW, E., and COLE, W., Cancer cells in blood. *Arch. Surg.* **80**, 910—920 (1960).

— ROBERTS, S., McGRATH, R., and McGREW, E., Simplified technique for separation of cancer cells from blood. *J. Amer. med. Ass.* **170**, 1785—1788 (1959).

MALMGREN, R. A., and POTTER, J. F., Cancer cells in the circulating blood. *Sth med. J. (Bgham, Ala.)* **52**, 1359—1362 (1959).

— PRUITT, J. C., DEL VECCHIO, P. R., and POTTER, J. F., A method for the cytologic detection of tumor cells in whole blood. *J. nat. Cancer Inst.* **20**, 1203—1213 (1958).

MOORE, G., MOUNT, D. T., and WENDT, A., The growth of human tumor cells in tissue culture. *Surg. Forum* **9**, 572 (1959).

NEDELKOFF, B., CHRISTOPHERSON, W. M., and HARTER, J. S., A method for demonstrating malignant cells in the blood. *Acta cytol. (Philad.)* **5**, 203—205 (1961).

NIGOGOSYAN, G., and McDONALD, J. R., Occurrence and significance of tumor cells in the blood. *Harper Hosp. Bull.* **19**, 11—18 (1961).

PIMENTA DE MELLO, R., The detection of cancer cells in peripheral blood by means of a flurochrome-ultraviolet microscopic method. *Hospital (Rio de J.)* **57**, 119—124 (1960).

POOL, E. H., and DUNLAP, G. R., Cancer cells in the blood stream. *Amer. J. Cancer* **21**, 99 (1934).

POTTER, J. F., LONGENBAUGH, G., CHU, E., DILLON, J., ROMSDAHL, M., and MALMGREN, R. A., The relationship of tumor type and resertability to the incidence of cancer cells in blood. *Surg. Gynec. Obstet.* **110**, 734—738 (1960).

PRESSMAN, J. J., BURTZ, M. V., and SHAFER, L., Further observations related to direct communication between lymph nodes and veins. *Surg. Gynec. Obstet.* **119**, 984—990 (1964).

PRINZMETAL, M., ORNITZ jr., E. M., SIMKIN, B., and BERGMAN, H. C., Arteriovenous anastomosis in liver, spleen and lung. *Amer. J. Physiol.* **152**, 48 (1948).

PRUITT, J. C., HILBERG, A. W., MOREHEAD, R. P., and MENGOLI, H. F., Quantitative study of malignant cells in local and peripheral circulating blood. *Surg. Synec. Obstet.* **114**, 179—188 (1962).

REISS, R., Demonstration of carcinoma cells in the blood stream. *J. Mt Sinai Hosp.* **26**, 171—176 (1959).

ROBERTS, S., JONASSON, O., LONG, L., McGREW, E. A., McGRATH, R., and COLE, W. H., Relationship of cancer cells in the circulating blood to operation. *Cancer (Philad.)* **15**, 231—239 (1962).

— LONG, L., JONASSON, O., McGRATH, R., McGREW, E., and COLE, W. H., The isolation of cancer cells from the blood stream during uterine curettage. *Surg. Gynec. Obstet.* **111**, 3—11 (1960).

— WATNE, A., McGRATH, R., McGREW, E., and COLE, W. H., Technique and results of isolation of cancer cells from the circulating blood. *Arch. Surg.* **76**, 334—346 (1958).

ROMSDAHL, M. M., POTTER, J. F., MALMGREN, R. A., CHU, E. W., BRINDLEY, C. O., and SMITH, R. R., A clinical study of circulating tumor cells in malignant melanoma. *Surg. Gynec. Obstet.* **111**, 675—681 (1960).

SALGADO, I., HOPKIRK, J. F., LONG, R. C., RITCHIE, A. C., RITCHIE, S., and WEBSTER, D. R., Tumor cells in the blood. *Canad. med. Asso. J.* **81**, 619—622 (1959).

SANDBERG, A. A., and MOORE, G. E., Examination of blood for tumor cells. *J. nat. Cancer Inst.* **19**, 1—11 (1957).

SATO, H., Cancer cells in the circulating blood. *Bull. Wld Hlth Org.* **26**, 675—681 (1962).

SCHEININ, T. M., and KOIVUNIEMI, A. P., Factors influencing the occurrence of circulating malignant cells in lung cancer. *Cancer (Philad.)* **16**, 639—645 (1963).

SEAL, S. H., Silicone flotation: A simple quantitative method for the isolation of free-floating cancer cells from the blood. *Cancer (Philad.)* **12**, 590—595 (1959).

— A sieve for the isolation of cancer cells and other large cells from the blood. *Cancer (Philad.)* **17**, 637—642 (1964).

SPRIGGS, A. I., and ALEXANDER, R. F., An albumin gradient method for separating the different white cells of blood, applied to the concentration of circulating tumor cells. *Nature (Lond.)* **188**, 863—864 (1960).

STEIN, A. A., HARDING, R., and MAURO, J., A simple method for identification of circulating cancer cells. *Acta cytol. (Philad.)* **6**, 273—277 (1962).

WATNE, A. L., SANDBERG, A. A., and MOORE, G. E., The prognostic value of tumor cells in the blood. *Arch. Surg.* **83**, 190—195 (1961).

WEST, J. T., HIRME, R., and KINDURYS, A., A one step filtration technique for recovery of tumor cells from blood. *Amer. J. clin. Path.* **41**, 27—32 (1964).
— MALMGREN, R. A., and CHU, E. W., An unsuccessful attempt to demonstrate diurnal patterns of tumor cell embolization. *Surg. Synec. Obstet.* **119**, 83—91 (1964).
ZEIDMAN, J., The fate of circulating tumor cells in passage of cells through capillaries. *Cancer Res.* **21**, 38—39 (1961).

Immunological Tolerance and Host-Tumour Relationship

Michael Feldman and David Nachtigal

Section of Cell Biology, Weizmann Institute of Science, Rehovoth, Israel

One of the unique properties of mouse sarcomas induced by polycyclic hydrocarbons is that they are non-metastatic. This is particularly manifested in tumour grafts. Syngeneic transplants of chemically induced tumours grow only at the site of transplantation. The non-manifestation of detectable metastases elsewhere in the organism could have been attributed to the early death of the animals caused by rapid growth of the primary implant, before metastases could develop. Our finding, however, that the removal of primary implants of benzpyrene-induced sarcomas permits survival of the host, and nevertheless there is no development of metastases, excludes this interpretation. The very fact that such mouse sarcomas are non-metastatic has limited the experimental approach to the problem of tumour invasion. Yet it appears that this negative characteristic may suggest some new approaches to the problem, through analysis of the factors which may determine the metastasibility of tumour cells. One such approach would be to test whether non metastasizing tumours possess any specific property which may be causally related to their non-metastasizibility. A phenomenon firmly established in recent years, namely, that sarcomas induced by polycyclic hydrocarbons such as methylcholanthrene or benzpyrene possess specific tumour antigens, must be considered here. The question is whether the antigenicity of the sarcoma cells may determine host tumour interactions, of which the probability of metastases may be an important parameter. Evidently, any attempt to study possible correlations between tumour antigenicity and invasion should be based on the antigenic properties of the tumour cells.

Following reports of Folley (1953), Prehn (1957) provided unequivocal evidence that tumours produced in mice by methylcholanthrene possess specific antigens. Tumour antigenicity was demonstrated by the isograft reaction; isogenic animals grafted with the test tumours produced an immune response which was manifested by the rejection of second grafts of the same tumours. Further studies in our and other laboratories have shown that sarcomas produced by other polycyclic hydrocarbons, e.g., benzpyrene, also contain tumour-specific antigens (Prehn, 1960; Old, 1962; Feldman, 1963; Globerson, 1964). Analysis of the antigenic pattern of such tumours showed that each of the sarcomas produced by the same carcinogen, in animals of the same genetic constitution (same strain), had a different tumour antigen (Prehn, 1957; Globerson, 1964). None, or very little, cross reactivity could be found between tumours produced by the same carcinogen in different animals of the same strain. We were, in fact, able to demonstrate different antigenic properties in the tumours produced in a single animal by the same carcinogen (GLOBERSON, 1964). When immunogenic effects in syngeneic recipients were tested, no cross reactivity could be detected in pairs of tumours produced in individual mice by two simultaneous injections of benzpyrene into two subcutaneous sites of the organism (GLOBERSON, 1964).

when grafted onto radiation chimeras (Tables I, II from FELDMAN, 1959, 1962). It appears that lymph node metastases of mouse sarcomas are more susceptible to the immunological reactivity of the recipient than is the original implant. Thus, sarcoma C 10 (Table I), originally produced in C3H mice by benzpyrene, formed metastases when grafted onto syngeneic chimeric hosts, i.e. X-irradiated C3H animals which were repopulated

Table I. *Tumour metastasis produced in radiation chimeras by sarcmoas C10 and MC1M*

Expt. group no.	Tumour	Host	Growth of primary graft	Growth of metastasis
1	C10	Foetal C3H→C3H	+	+
2	C10	Spleen C3H→C3H	+	+
3	C10	Foetal C57BL→C57BL	+	−
4	C10	Spleen C57BL→C57BL	−	−
5	C10 from expt. 2	Normal C3H	+	−
6	C10 metastasis from expt. 2	Normal C3H	+	−
7	MC1M	Foetal C57BL→C57BL	+	+
8	MC1M	Spleen C57BL→C57BL	−	−
9	MC1M from expt. 7	Normal C3H	+	−
10	MC1M metastasis from expt. 7	Normal C3H	+	−

In regard to the question whether the antigenicity of mice sarcomas be causally related to the lack of metastasizing properties of such tumours, experiments were carried out in our laboratory in which four different "non-metastatic" tumours were tested for their growth properties in immunologically deficient recipients, i.e., in radiation chimeras of various degrees of immunological reactivity (FELDMAN, 1959, 1962). Tumours which did not form progressive metastases when grafted either subcutaneously or intramuscularly in normal, non-irradiated mice, produced metastases in the lymph nodes (inguinal, brachial or axillary),

after exposure with either spleen or foetal liver cells of C3H origin. However, when grafted onto allogeneic hosts, i.e. irradiated C57BL animals repopulated following exposure with C57BL foetal liver cells, the original implant grew progressively, but no metastases appeared. Similar results were obtained with a tumour of C57BL origin, sarcoma SBL1. Here, metastases were formed not only in syngeneic chimeric hosts but also in one allogeneic combination, i.e. in irradiated C3H mice protected by C3H foetal liver cells. However, when grafted onto a slightly different, immunologically more reactive, allogeneic combination, i.e., irradiated C3H animals protected with C3H spleen cells, the original implant grew, but without the appearance of metastases (Table II).

The formation of metastases in X-irradiated isologous systems could be attributed to either of the following processes: (1) the destruction of the lym-

at various time intervals following grafting, and nodal cell suspensions from individual hosts were injected intramuscularly into other isologous normal animals. It was found that re-inoculation of lymph node cell suspensions from each of the primary hosts 25 days following subcutaneous transplantation of SBL1 resulted in tumour growths in all sec-

Table II. *Tumour metastasis produced in radiation chimeras by sarcoma SBL 1 and mammary adenocarcinoma S 2*

Expt. group no.	Tumour	Host	Growth of primary graft	Growth of metastasis
1	SBL1	Foetal C3H→F1(C3H×C57BL)	+	+
2	SBL1	Foetal C57BL→F1(C3H×C57BL)	+	+
3	SBL1	Foetal C57BL→C3H	+	+
4	SBL1	Foetal C3H→C3H	+	+
5	SBL1	Spleen C3H→C3H	+	−
6	SBL1 from expt. 4	Normal C57BL	+	−
7	SBL1 from expt. 4	Normal C3H	+	−
8	SBL1 metastasis from expt. 4	Normal C57BL	+	−
9	SBL1 metastasis from expt. 4	Normal C3H	+	−
10	S2	Foetal C3H→C3H	+	+
11	S2	Spleen C3H→C3H	+	+
12	S2 from expt. 10	Normal Swiss	+	−

phatic tissue by X-irradiation furnishes favourable physiological conditions for tumour cell migration, which is restricted in animals with normal lymphatic tissue; or (2) that cell migration from the original implant, via the lymphatics, does take place in normal animals, but that the progressive growth of the tumour cells is suppressed within the normal lymph nodes; X-irradiation reduces the inhibition exerted by the organized lymph nodes. To test which of these two possibilities is operative, tumours were grafted subcutaneously into isologous C57BL animals, the lymph nodes were extirpated

ondary hosts (Feldman, 1959, 1962). Hence, metastatic migration takes place even in non-irradiated normal animals, but within the organized normal lymph nodes the progressive growth of such tumour emboli is suppressed. This suppressive effect is abolished by X-irradiation.

The formation of metastases in radiation chimeras was also noted by Barnes et al. (Barnes, 1957). In non-irradiated animals, cortisone was found to activate the formation of metastases in otherwise non-metastatic tumours (Agosin, 1952; Baserga, 1954). Furthermore, Baserga

(1954) has shown that cortisone, like X-irradiation, has elicited the progressive growth of pre-existing metastatic emboli. In view of the similarity between the effects of cortisone and X-rays on the lymphatic system and the immune mechanism, one is tempted to speculate further on the possible role of resistance to metastasis in controlling metastatic development.

While there is no direct indication that an immunological mechanism participates in controlling the formation of metastasis of the primary tumour, or of the isologous tumour graft, the above experiments do suggest that, at least for the types of tumours studied, host resistance, probably of an immunological nature, determines the probability of production of tumour metastases. If this is so, the question arises whether one can increase the host immune reactivity towards the tumour cells, and thereby aim at controlling growth and metastasis formation.

The question is particularly crucial as regards autochthonous tumours, i.e. for animals in which the tumours have originated. It is common that such animals do not acquire a detectable level of immunity following the growth of their tumours; only following a complicated schedule of immunization could KLEIN et al. (KLEIN, 1960) demonstrate some immunizing effect of autochthonous tumour cells in the carrier mice. More recently, experiments carried out on rats (P. ALEXANDER, personal communication), seem to indicate that rats can acquire an immune response towards their original tumours. It appears, however, that in general the reactivity of autochthonous animals towards their tumours is considerably less than the reactivity of syngeneic mice to isografts of the same tumours. It seems possible that such animals may have acquired a partial

immunological tolerance towards the specific antigens of their tumours. The acquisition of specific immunological tolerance towards their tumour antigens is comprehensible in view of a) the suppressing effect of carcinogenic polycyclic hydrocarbons on the immunological reactivity of the organism, which may make the animal susceptible to the tolerogenic effects of the tumour antigens and b) the accumulation of a massive dose of tumour-specific antigens in the growing sarcomas, which may be instrumental in inducing and maintaining immunological tolerance.

In order to approach the question whether immunological tolerance towards tumour antigens could be experimentally broken down, a system of tolerance towards a defined protein antigen, induced in X-irradiated adult animals has been developed and analysed. The induction of tolerance breakdown by immunizing the tolerant animal with a hapten conjugate of the tolerogenic protein was studied (NACHTIGAL, 1963, 1964), using as a model system adult rabbits, exposed to 550 r total body irradiation. The animals were injected after irradiation with human serum albumin (HSA) at dose levels which were immunogenic in normal non-irradiated rabbits, and challenged repeatedly with the same antigen at two-weekly intervals. After recovery from the general effect of irradiation, the rabbits were found to be completely unresponsive to further injections of HSA, although they did respond immunologically to non-related antigens, i.e. human γ-globulin (HGG) (NACHTIGAL, 1963). Thus, the injection of a protein antigen to adult rabbits exposed to total body X-irradiation at sublethal doses conferred specific immunological tolerance. Whether the specificity of immunological recognition of such experimentally tolerant animals is identical with that of animals naturally tolerant towards their own serum proteins was examined by comparing the types of antibodies produced in rabbits made tolerant to HSA and immunized with sulphanil HSA, with those produced in normal rabbits immunized with sulphanil rabbit serum albumin (RSA). The pattern of antibodies obtained in these two systems was found to be completely identical, strongly suggesting that natural and induced tolerance are based on the same mechanism (14). Two types of antibodies were produced by each of the two sulphanil-proteins. One showed complete identity when reacting with the two conjugates, and therefore seemed to be directed to the haptenic component; the other was specific to the homologous conjugate, and seemed to be directed towards an antigenic determinant comprising the hapten and part of the protein carrier. However, upon further immunization of HSA-tolerant animals with sulphanil HSA, antibodies reacting with HSA were produced. Thus, immunization of HSA-tolerant rabbits with sulphanil-HSA appeared to have terminated the tolerant state towards HSA. Further analysis has indicated that the anti-HSA antibodies in HSA-tolerant animals which appear following immunization with the azo-conjugates are not identical with the antibodies to HSA produced in normal rabbits immunized with native HSA. The formation of anti-HSA in these experiments reflects only the immunogenic effect of the conjugated molecule; one cannot infer that the tolerant animal has regained its original capacity to recognize the native HSA immunogenic determinants reactive in non-tolerant animals. Only such a recognition would represent a real restoration of immunological reactivity. To test whether such a restoration does, in fact, take place, the animals which had produced anti-HSA antibodies following immunization with sulphanil-HSA, were untreated for 75 days and then immunized with native HSA. Under these conditions, antibodies of a high titer were produced, showing a complete identity with anti-HSA formed in normal animals (NACHTIGAL, 1965). This indicates that animals which have acquired specific immunological tolerance towards protein antigens, can regain their original capacity to respond to the native tolerogen if properly immunized with hapten protein conjugates. It should be noted here, in relation to the further implications of these findings as regards aspects of host-tumour relationships, that the breakdown of tolerance was achieved only when the sulphanil-HSA conjugate was injected in the absence of native HSA. The immunization of tolerant animals with the hapten conjugate admixed with native HSA failed to break tolerance to HSA (NACHTIGAL, 1965).

Further studies have indicated that polypeptidyl HSA can also terminate tolerance to HSA (SCHECHTER, 1964). We have demonstrated that the chemical nature of the hapten determines whether the conjugate will or will not terminate tolerance to the carrier protein. Polytyrosyl-HSA did, whereas poly-alanyl-HSA did not break tolerance to HSA. This is of particular interest with regard to the capacity of polytyrosin to confer antigenicity on otherwise non-antigenic or weakly antigenic protein molecules (SELA, 1960).

What then are the implications of this model system of tolerance breakdown as regards the host-tumour relationship? We have previously indicated that immune responses may partially control the formation of metastases. Metastasis appears to be more susceptible to the immunological reactivity of the host than is the original tumour mass. We have further suggested that the deficient immune reactivity of an animal towards its own tumours may reflect a state of partial yet specific immunological tolerance towards the tumour antigens. We have demonstrated that actively acquired tolerance can be experimentally terminated by immunizing the tolerant animals with the proper hapten conjugates of the tolerogenic protein. This leads to the suggestion that an induced alteration in host-tumour relationship should be attempted by immunizing tumour-bearing animals with hapten conjugates of tumour antigens or cell components containing the tumour antigens (cell membranes).

Such immunization might perhaps terminate the state of partial immunological tolerance which the animal seems to have acquired towards its autochthonous tumours. The immune response towards tumour antigens evoked by such conjugates may elicit resistance of the animal to the autochthonous tumour cells; such expected resistance might be particularly effective towards lymph-node metastases. In view of the results of our studies on tolerance breakdown to HSA, where the native antigen was found to obviate the effect of the antigen conjugate, any attempt at immunization with hapten conjugates of tumour components should be carried out only in animals from which the tumour mass has been removed. An excess of the native tolerogen may inhibit the capacity of conjugates to terminate tolerance. The fact that spontaneous tumours may have weak antigens or be non-antigenic when tested by presently available methods, does not invalidate the suggested approach, since attachment of polytyrosin to weakly antigenic molecules was shown to have increased the antigenicity of the carrier protein (i.e. gelatin) (SELA, 1960).

Conclusions

Tumour metastases in mice were discussed in relation to the antigenic properties of sarcoma cells. It was suggested that the lack of metastases in mouse sarcomas, particularly those induced by polycyclic hydrocarbons, may be a function of their immunogenic properties among other factors. Some non-metastasizing tumours, when tested in radiation chimeras of various combinations, formed metastases in the recipients' lymph nodes. The distribution of metastases in the various groups of chimeric hosts showed an inverse relationship to the expected immunological reactivity of the chimera towards the tested tumour. Since mice show a deficient reactivity towards their autochthonous tumours, it was argued that this may be attributed to a state of partial tolerance towards the tumour antigens. Experiments carried out on the experimental induction of tolerance breakdown to protein antigens by hapten conjugates of the tolerogens suggest an approach to an experimental alteration of host reactivity towards tumour cells, which may be particularly active towards cells of tumour metastases.

Discussion

Questions put to M. FELDMAN

J. Harel: You have demonstrated that two tumours induced from identical cells by the same carcinogenic agent in the same animal are immunologically different. Is this difference temporary, or does it persist after a certain number of serial passages in isologous animals?

M. Feldman: We found with our benzpyrene-induced tumours that the immunogenicity, i.e. the capacity to elicit an immune response, decreases as a function of successive transplantations, but the antigens are not completely lost from the tumour cells (A. Globerson and M. Feldman, 1964). Thus, following 7 transplant generations, tumours may no longer be capable of evoking a detectable immune reaction, yet they are susceptible to such a reaction produced by grafts of earlier transplant generations of the same tumour.

C. Southam: I was impressed by Dr. Feldman's demonstration of a breaking down of immunological tolerance by administration of an altered but cross-reacting antigen, and his suggestion that this observation might have a therapeutic application to cancer if it be assumed that the cancer patient is immunologically tolerant to his cancer antigen and if most of the tumour mass could be eliminated.

Dr. Arthur Levin and I are at present carrying out a clinical experiment which may represent a crude clinical parallel to Dr. Feldman's beautiful experiments in rabbits.

We have taken leukaemic cells from untreated patients with acute leukaemia, prepared saline extracts from these cells, irradiated them with ultra-violet light and stored them at $-70°$ C until the patient is in hematological remission. I postulate that the UV treatment may slightly alter antigenic structure and hence perhaps be comparable to Dr. Feldman's chemical treatment. The patient who is in complete hematological remission has had his tumour mass reduced to an undetectable minimum.

We then administer the autogenous, irradiated, leukaemia-cell extract to the patient. To date, we have treated only 6 patients, and want only to report that all 6 have developed positive, immediate-type skin tests. (Skin tests were negative before treatment.) One of our patients

had an episode of anaphylactic shock following the fourth weekly intravenous injection — a particularly convincing demonstration of immunological reaction to the autogenous extract.

An obviously pertinent question is whether this reaction is directed only against the irradiated extract, or also against the unirradiated leukaemic extract, or even against normal leucocyte auto-antigens. The extract contains no antibiotics or any other additives. We did not have the foresight to keep unirradiated extract at first so as yet we have only one study with unirradiated extract. In that patient there is a positive skin reaction to both irradiated and unirradiated extracts, but a significantly greater reaction to the former. We have not yet had an opportunity to use normal autologous leukocyte extracts, nor have we as yet carried out serological studies.

S. Wood: Dr. Feldman, in the animal in which you have induced tumours with carcinogenic hydrocarbons, did you identify a tumour-specific antigen and antibody and did you find that the latter acts to inhibit metastasis?

If this finding has general validity, why in man does metastasis occur in the case of lung cancer associated with chromate exposure or cigarette smoking, bladder tumour in aniline dye workers, and other carcinogen-associated neoplasms? If you cannot generalize, what are the fundamental differences that exist between metastasis formation from induced, transplanted, or spontaneous neoplasms in animals or man?

M. Feldman: Tumours produced in mice by polycyclic hydrocarbons (in our experiments by 3—4-benzpyrene), possess tumour-specific antigens. The immunogenic properties of these antigens are manifested not by circulating antibodies, but by the isograft reaction, i.e. by the rejection of secondary grafts folowing the immunizing effect of primary grafts. Such tumours in mice, i.e. sarcomas produced by polycyclic hydrocarbons, do not produce metastasis. Dr. YAFFE and I have found that some non-metastatic tumours did, however, produce lymph-node metastasis in radiation chimeras of low immunological reactivity. I have made no attempt to make any generalizations regarding possible correlations between the immunological response of the host and arrest of metastasis. Furthermore, I do not maintain that even in mice tumour antigenicity is the sole or main factor which determines the probability of metastasis. Yet, I do not know of any evidence that in man lung cancer associated with chromate exposure or cigarette smoking, or bladder tumours possess tumour-specific antigens that elicit a host response.

G. A. Voisin: There were several points in Dr. FELDMAN's presentation with which I am in full agreement, but his views on the possible relationships between tumour invasion and immunological reactivity differ in some respects from my own.

The points on which I agree with him include in particular the following:

I am convinced that lymph-nodes and immunological reactions play an active part in the fate of metastases, which are much less numerous than embolisms of living cancer cells.

One may even go further and say that early immunological reactions probably help to determine the fate and even the clinical manifestation of the primary tumour.

Moreover, I was much impressed by Dr. FELDMANS' experiments on immunological tolerance to purified proteins. Of particular interest here was the fact that this tolerance was interrupted by means of a method identical to that employed by WEIGLE, and that interruption of the tolerant state by the antigen associated with sulphonyl was prevented by the addition of a tolerogenic antigen; this is an experimental finding of considerable theoretical importance.

The points on which my views do not coincide with those of Dr. FELDMAN concern the immunological mechanisms which may play a part in the presence or absence of metastases with various tumours in relation to their particular antigenic capacity.

Dr. FELDMAN believes that the anti-tumour immunological reaction would tend to inhibit the formation of metastases, whereas the establishment of a state of immunological tolerance towards the tumour antigens could permit these metastases to develop. Dr. FELDMAN puts forward the hypothesis that such a state of tolerance would be easy to obtain in respect of *autochthonous tumours* owing to the massive accumulation of antigens in the growing tumour. We do not believe that this is the case because if these autochthonous tumours contained such an abundance of antigens as would confer a state of immunological tolerance on the animal, they should have immunized the animal at an earlier stage, when they were still small and releasing a smaller quantity of antigens; logically, this immunization would inevitably have led to the rejection of the tumour. Furthermore, small quantities of metastasizing autochthonous tumours (of the order of the quantities employed for transplants) should have a very marked immunizing capacity following transplantation into isogenic hosts. In actual fact, the very opposite is observed: it is precisely the non-metastasizing tumours (i.e. those which, according to Dr. FELDMAN's hypothesis, are relatively less tolerogenic) which have the greater immunizing capacity and, apparently, are richer in antigens.

Moreover, the idea that every active immunological reaction must be directed against the growth of metastases (or even against the growth of the tumour itself) fails to take account of the existence of the paradoxical facilitating phenomenon of active immunization, or "enhancing phenomenon", which has the effect of facilitating the growth of the tumour and sometimes of the metastases, and thus opposes the immunological reaction of rejection. The part played by this reaction is of fundamental importance as regards the fate of homo-transplanted tumours which invariably provoke an immunological reaction on the part of the host. The fact that induced indigenous tumours often possess their own antigenic properties which can be demonstated today, and the possibility that spontaneous tumours may also possess such properties, suggests that these tumours might be subject to immunological reactions no different from those with which we are already familiar in the case of homo-transplanted tumours. Immunological reactions of the immunotoxic (cytotoxic) type and of the facilitating (enhancing) type have in fact both been demonstrated by GORAN MOLLER in cases of methylcholanthrene-induced tumours. Finally, the fact, stressed by Dr. FELDMAN, that metastases appear to be more susceptible than the primary tumour to the immunological reaction of the host puts one very much in mind of the experiments described by NATHAN KALISS, in which a first homo-transplant took in an animal treated in such a way as to ensure passive immunological enhancement; this first transplant, however, immunized the recipient so that a second homo-transplantation from the same tumour, performed 1—2 weeks later, was rapidly rejected, while the first continued to proliferate and finally killed the allogenic host. Thus, KALISS's first and second transplant behaved, respectively, like Dr. FELDMAN's primary tumour and metastasis.

In conclusion, I should like to draw attention to the risk of attempting to immunize human cancer patients with the aim of combating the development of the tumours and their metastases immunologically. If these attempts are carried out blindly (and it is difficult to control them properly), they may in fact be not only useless but even harmful, for they may induce an enhancing immunization which will facilitate the development of the tumour and its metastases.

M. Feldman: I very much appreciate your comments, Dr. VOISIN. I would not, however, predict that primary antigenic tumours should have been rejected by the host immune response, instead of inducing immunological tolerance. Rejection of an antigenic cell population will take place only if a certain ratio of antibody to antigen is achieved. At levels of excess of antigenic cells, rejection will not take place, since the tumour will resist the immune response. In the early stages of tumour growth the immunological competence of the animal may have been reduced owing to the treatment with the carcinogenic hydrocarbons (R. PREHN: J. Nat. Can. Inst. **31**, 791—805, 1963). The reduction in the immunological reactivity of the host, coinciding with the increase in antigen mass, can then result in tolerance, with or without a prior temporary state of immunity.

I agree with Dr. VOISIN that one can conceive of an immune reaction towards autochthonous tumours which may result in tumour growth, i.e. in "immunological enhancement". I share Dr. VOISIN's view that in any attempt at immunizing patients against their own tumours, one should consider the possibility of inducing enhancing antibodies, rather than tumour rejection. However, a distinction should be made between tumour growth which involves no immune response or which involves immunological tolerance, and tumour growth due to enhancing antibodies. The latter, i.e. enhancement, involves the production of antibodies and should be *transplantable* by antiserum. To my knowledge it has not so far been demonstrated that the host produces antibodies during the "normal" growth of the primary tumours, nor that serum from animals with primary tumours has an enhancing effect.

F. Lacour: Does Dr. FELDMAN have any idea of the number of tumour cells in the lymph nodes which he removed from tumour-bearing mice on the 25th day of development and which, when retransplanted into a normal, irradiated host, gave rise to a tumour?

Apart from lymph nodes, did Dr. FELDMAN remove from the tumour-bearing mice any other tissue — e.g. pulmonary tissue — and transplant it into other hosts?

Dr. FELDMAN has postulated the existence of a certain state of tolerance in the animal towards its own tumour, and he believes it desirable to attempt to interrupt this tolerance. On the basis of the results obtained by Dr. FELDMAN in another model — tolerance induced in the rabbit towards a protein and interruption of this tolerance by injection of a protein combined with sulphonyl — interruption of the animal's tolerance towards the tumour would call for the injection of an antigen-protein combination or the like in the absence of autochthonous tumour cells.

Hence, it would perhaps be necessary to know how many tumour cells may remain in the organism even after removal of the tumour.

M. Feldman: Your question, Mrs. LACOUR, regarding the number of tu-mour cells arrested within the lymph nodes, is a very important one. It is, as you have pointed out, particularly pertinent with regard to the suggested approach of tolerance breakdown, which is inhibited by an excess of the native antigen. Unfortunately, we do not at present have an answer to this question.

R. A. Malmgren: The experiment performed by Dr. FELDMAN in which he produced two tumours in the same animal with a chemical carcinogen and found them to be immunologically distinct was also undertaken by Dr. DONALD MORTON and myself with the same results.

An attempt to evaluate the effect of immunization with methylcholanthrene tumours upon the ability to produce metastasis with the same tumour has been carried out in our laboratory. Our methods have been somewhat different from those described by Dr. FELDMAN. In particular, we were testing pulmonary metastasis following intravenous injection of the tumour rather than lymph node metastasis. To date, we have not been able to detect a significant difference in the number of metastatic nodules in the lungs of the immune and control animals.

G. Barski: In your paper you suggest that there is a relationship between the antigenicity of tumours and their incapacity to produce metastases, which is the case in tumours produced by synthetic carcinogens.

It seems doubtful, however, whether this generalization is true of human cancer or of experimental cancer.

We should like to refer, by way of example, to pulmonary cells of C57BL mice which have become malignant *in vitro*. These cells produce sarcomas which grow very rapidly and prove fatal, but which never metastasize. In recent experiments we have succeeded in proving that these tumours are only very slightly antigenic, if at all.

M. Feldman: I would like to re-emphasize, with regard to the interesting observation of Dr. Barski, that I have made no claim that the antigenicity of tumours is the only factor which determines the probability of metastasis formation. Dr. Yaffe and I have found that for mouse tumours that we tested, the host's immune reactivity seemed to be associated with the inhibition of lymph node metastasis. Although in Dr. Barski's cases some other factors may have determined the lack of metastasis, I would hesitate to draw final conclusions regarding the non-antigenicity of his tumours from the experimental methods available so far for testing tumour antigenicity.

C. Southam: The phenomenon of enhancement is of great fundamental interest and cannot be ignored when considering possible methods of immunological treatment of cancer, as we have just been reminded by Dr. Voisin. There are several reasons, however, for doubting its practical importance at the clinical level.

1. The few examples of immunological enhancement of autochthonous cancer are not particularly impressive and are counterbalanced by the numerous examples of immunological resistance to autochthonous cancer.

2. What little evidence we have of host resistance in clinical cancer points to cellular rather than humoral mechanisms.

3. In addition to the studies of leukocyte effects on human cancer autotransplants, we have studied mixtures of autogenous serum and cancer cells. Inhibition by serum was infrequent, and enhancement was never observed.

Finally, in most clinical situations in which the use of experimental immunological treatment of cancer would be considered, the disease is predictably progressive and the theoretical possibility of therapeutic effects is of greater importance than the theoretical possibility of tumour enhancement.

D. B. Amos: As we have shown in our experiments in patients with cancer (Amos, Hattler, and Shingleton, 1965) and in animals treated with methylcholanthrene (Amos and Tsuhi, unpublished), there is a very marked increase in the transplantability of skin taken from a tumourous donor. An abstract of the animal experiments will appear in the text, but it is essential to realize that we have not yet shown that the increased transplantability is the result of an antigenic *loss*. Studies carried out in collaboration with Dr. Peacocke suggest that patients with leukaemia have relatively normal amounts of iso-antigen on their white cells. Studies in a few patients with cancer also suggest a normal antigenicity of the leukocytes. We do not yet know about skin, but there does not appear to be any complete loss of antigen. An alternative explanation, of course, would be enhancement.

P. Grabar: May I emphasize that when an immunserum is used in experiments of this kind, the type of antibody involved must be clearly stated, for we know very well now that there are several families of heterogeneous immunoglobulins possessing different properties (complement-fixing or non-complement-fixing, provoking histamine release, etc.). Moreover, the quantities of antibody used must also be indicated. It has been known for a very long time that opposite effects may be observed with different amounts of immunos rum.

References

AGOSIN, M., CHRISTEN, R., BADINEZ, O., GASIC, G., NEGHME, A., PIZARRO, O., and JARPA, A., Cortisone-induced metastases of adenocarcinoma in mice. *Proc. Soc. exp. Biol. (N.Y.)* **80**, 128—131 (1952).

BARNES, D. W. H., FORD, C. E., ILBERY, P. L. T., KOLLER, P. C., and LOUTIT, J. F., *J. cell. comp. Physiol.* **50**, Suppl. 123 (1957).

BASERGA, R., and SHUBIC, P., The action of cortisone on transplanted and induced tumors in mice. *Cancer Res.* **14**, 12—16 (1954).

FELDMAN, M., GLOBERSON, A., and YAFFE, D., Immunological properties of chemically induced sarcomas. *Acta Un. int. Cancr.* **19**, 65—72 (1963).

—, and YAFFE, D., Immunogenetic studies on X-irradiated mice treated with hematopoietic cells and grafted with tumor tissues. *J. nat. Cancer Inst.* **23**, 109—132 (1959).

— — Immunogenetics of tumours grown in radiation chimeras. *In: Ciba Foundation Symposium on Transplantation*, p. 163—184.

FOLEY, E. J., Antigenic properties of methylcholantrene-induced tumors in mice of the strain of origin. *Cancer Res.* **13**, 835—837 (1953).

GLOBERSON, A., and FELDMAN, M., Antigenic specificity of benzo (a) pyrene induced sarcomas. *J. nat. Cancer Inst.* **32**, 1229—1243 (1964).

KLEIN, G., SJOGREN, H. O., KLEIN, E., and HELLSTROM, K. E., Demonstration of resistance against methylcholanthrene induced sarcomas in the primary autochthonous host. *Cancer Res.* **20**, 1561—1572 (1960).

NACHTIGAL, D., and FELDMAN, M., Immunological unresponsiveness to protein antigens in rabbits exposed to X-irradiation or 6-mercaptopurine treatment. *Immunology* **7**, 616—625 (1964).

— — The immune response to azoprotein conjugates in rabbits unresponsive to the protein carriers. *Immunology* **7**, 616—625 (1964).

NACHTIGAL, D., ESHEL-ZUSSMAN, R., and FELDMAN, M., Restoration of the specific immunological reactivity of tolerant rabbits by conjugated antigens. *Immunology* **9**, 543—551 (1965).

OLD, L. J., BOYSE, E. A., CLARKE, D. A., and CARSWELL, E. A., Antigenic properties of chemically induced tumors. *Ann. N.Y. Acad. Sci.* **101**, 80—106 (1962).

PREHN, R. T., Tumor specific immunity to transplanted dibenz (A.H.) anthracene-induced sarcomas. *Cancer Res.* **20**, 1614—1617 (1960).

—, and MAIN, J. M., Immunity to methylcholanthrene induced sarcomas. *J. nat. Cancer Inst.* **18**, 769—778 (1957).

SCHECHTER, I., BAUMINGER, S., SELA, M., NACHTIGAL, D., and FELDMAN, M., *Immunochemistry* **1**, 249 (1964).

SELA, M., and ARNON, R., Studies on the chemical basis of the antigenicity of proteins. I. Antigenecity of polypeptidyl gelatins. *Biochem. J.* **75**, 91—102 (1960).

The Role of the Cell Surface in Tumour Invasion

E. J. Ambrose

Chester Beatty Research Institute, Institute of Cancer Research, Royal Cancer Hospital, London, S.W. 3, Great Britain

Introduction

The pioneering work of Coman (1944) provided evidence for some decrease in the adhesiveness of cells during carcinogenesis. Using micromanipulation, Coman was able to show that cells in carcinoma tissue required less force to pull them apart than those in normal epithelium. More recent studies in this field have made use of tissue culture (Abercrombie and Heaysman, 1953; and Abercrombie and Ambrose, 1958). The movements of migrating fibroblasts in culture are regulated by contact with neighbouring cells. This contact inhibition, as it has been called by Abercrombie, is lost in anaplastic sarcoma cells. The cells move freely over each other and their direction of migration is not controlled by cell contacts. Time lapse filming with the interference microscope has shown that this change in social behaviour is determined largely by alterations in the properties of the cell membrane in regions of contact. When the membranes of normal fibroblasts come into contact a stable adhesion between the membranes is formed in this region. These stable adhesions are not formed between the membranes of anaplastic sarcoma cells. Later studies have shown that this loss of contact inhibition can be observed in a number of instances where strictly comparable normal and homologous tumour cells have been compared under similar conditions. This loss of adhesiveness of the tumour cell membrane must clearly be related to a change in the structure of the cell surface. Such changes have been investigated by a number of physical, biochemical and immunological methods. The purpose of the present paper is to define as far as possible the properties of the cell surface in precise terms and to consider the extent to which these properties play a role in the invasiveness of tumours.

The Movements of Isolated Tissue Cells

When an isolated fibroblast in tissue culture is examined by time lapse filming using the interference microscope, it can be seen that the cell membranes are in constant activity. Wave-like movements occur particularly at the leading edge of an advancing pseudopodium. These ruffles arise on the leading edge and travel backwards towards the cell nucleus. Measurements with the interference microscope indicate that the waves may reach a considerable height; up to 5μ in some cases, i.e., several times the thickness of the cell in this region. These movements have also been studied using a surface contact microscope. In this microscope light is totally internally reflected within a 60° glass prism. When viewed from above through the microscope objective no light penetrates and a dark field is seen. If a cell is making contact with the glass the critical angle is not reached in this region and this part of the cell is illuminated, as in a dark field system. Using this technique it is possible to show that the ruffled movements of the cell membrane are taking place over the whole area of the cell where it is in contact with the glass. This gives rise to intermittent contact with the glass, so that the cell moves forward by these peristaltic waves, arising at the membrane surface. The movement is rather like that of an earthworm, except that a single cell is involved instead of the coordinated movements of groups of muscle cells. This type of movement differs from that occurring in the large Amoeba, Amoeba proteus. In this organism the cytoplasm flows forwards continuously down the centre of the cell. The membrane appears to expand on the leading edge as the cytoplasm flows forward into the expanding pseudopodium. No such general flow of cytoplasm occurs in mammalian tissue cells. If anything, there is a predominant movement of cytoplasm backwards from the leading edge of the cell towards the nucleus. Some work has also been done on the possible motive force responsible for these ruffled movements of the tumour cell membrane (AMBROSE and GOLDACRE, 1964). Indirect evidence has been obtained which suggests that membrane potentials generated by ionic pumps may produce electroosmosis and give rise to flow of cytoplasm near the membrane surface. But it is hardly appropriate to go into the details of this hypothesis in this article. What is of importance from the point of view of tumour invasion is that when tumour cells in culture are examined under similar conditions, it becomes apparent that the basic mechanism of locomotion is similar to that of the normal cells. Undulations of the membrane are taking place continuously both on the leading edge of the cell and over the whole area in contact with the glass. The behaviour depends to some extent on the type of tumour. With more differentiated tumours, a limited number of fan-like pseudopodia occur and the movements of the membranes are to some extent coordinated. In anaplastic tumours the cells assume a more rounded form: there are many fine microvillae and membrane movements occur largely at random.

From the considerable amount of evidence obtained both *in vitro* and *in vivo* it now seems reasonable to suggest that tumour invasiveness takes place because the membranes are generating these peristaltic waves. The tumour cells migrate through the tissues by active locomotion, due to intermittent contact between their membranes and those of other cells, connective tissue fibres, etc. in basically the same way as they move on a glass surface.

Cell Contacts

If this view of tumour invasion is correct, then the problem is not to explain why tumour cells invade, but to explain why normal tissue cells do not invade. Normal connective tissue and epithelial cells generally form stable adhesions between their membranes on contact in culture. These adhesions can only be broken after considerable tension has been generated in the region of contact. When these adhesions form, the ruffling activity of the membrane ceases. In other words, normal cell movements are controlled by contact inhibition which operates partly by the formation of intercellular adhesions so that the cells are immobilised, and partly by the switching off of the locomotory mechanism in the region of contact. The normal tissue cells of the body are immobilised in an organised manner partly by intercellular contacts, whereas the tumour cells are able to break away from this contact and migrate actively due to the active movement of their membranes.

Chemical Constitution of the Tumour Cell Surface

A decrease in the mutual adhesiveness of the tumour cell membranes implies a change in their chemical constitution. Various approaches have therefore been made to an analysis of the surface material, particularly with the help of cell electrophoresis.

In this technique the cells are suspended in a suitable medium and their velocity in an electric field of known strength is determined. This technique makes possible a wide range of investigations similar in type to those which have been used so successfully in the study of protein structure using the method of TISELIUS. With cell suspensions the mobility depends on the density of electric charge carried by the cell surface, i.e. the charge per unit area; it is almost independent of the cell size. When this technique was first applied to a study of solid tumours using controls of normal tissues from which the tumour was derived, it became apparent that the net negative surface charge was higher on the tumour than the normal cell. This was the case when a stilboestral-induced kidney tumour of cortical origin was compared with normal cortical kidney cells and when hepatoma cells were compared with normal liver cells. Since that time a number of other systems have been examined in which the same condition exists. With the principal type of transformation produced by polyoma virus in culture, a similar increase in mobility can be observed when the sarcoma cells are compared with the normal fibroblasts (FORRESTER, STOKER and AMBROSE, 1964).

RUHENSTROTH and FUHRMANN (1961) have obtained similar results in both granulocytic and myeloid leukemia. In granulocytic leukemia the normal granulocytes are replaced by cells of higher mobility, while in lymphatic leukemia the normal lymphocytes are replaced by cells of higher mobility. It has not proved possible to carry out this comparison with all types of tumours because in many cases the actual normal cells from which the tumour cells originate are not available or cannot be isolated in quantity. But so far, the evidence for a general increase in the net surface charge during carcinogenesis is good. In some cases it has been possible to compare a series of sublines of a tumour which shows, in biological terms, a progressive increase in capacity to form ascites tumours and to produce infiltrating metastases (PURDOM, AMBROSE and KLEIN, 1958). In general it is found that ascites tumours, which are extremely non-adhesive and will invade the organs adjoining the peritoneum at any early stage of growth, have the highest known charge for cells derived from solid tissues.

The chemical constitution of the material responsible for this surface change has also been investigated by cell electrophoresis. Experiments with model suspensions of purified phospholipids have made it possible to determine the pH mobility curves and ion adsorption of these substances. By these methods the presence of exposed phospholipids on the surface of the cell can be recognised. In addition, it is possible to treat the cell surface directly with enzymes without destroying the intact membrane. For example, in the case of human erythrocytes, 90% of the surface charge per unit area can be removed by treatment with neurominidase. This observation indicates that most of the surface charge on this cell is due to the carboxyl groups of sialic acid. Phospholipids have a considerable affinity for calcium ions, while the human erythrocyte has no appreciable affinity for these ions. It is therefore possible to distinguish between sialic acid and phospholipid on the cell surface by alternative treatment with neurominidase and with calcium ions. Using this method on various types of tumour cells it can be shown that, in some cases, e.g. EL 4 leukemia, the charge is almost entirely due to sialic acid, whereas in other cases, e.g. Ehrlich carcinoma cells, exposed phosphate groups of phospholipid are also present.

It is clearly important to know which type of material changes most characteristically during the malignant transformation. Information on this point has been obtained by studying the transformation of C^{13} hamster fibroblasts with polyoma virus. The cells are cloned from a single cell and the mobility measured when the cultures have been grown to produce a sufficient number of cells for measurement. The transformed cells, when a stable culture had been obtained, showed an increase in mobility in comparison with the normal cells and also a much larger standard deviation (FORRESTER, AMBROSE and MACPHERSON, 1962). Treatment of the two cell types with calcium reduced the mobility but a difference between the normal and tumour cells could still be observed. But when the two cell types were treated with neurominidase the mean values and standard deviations for the two cell types became identical. This observation strongly suggested that the sialic acid component of the tumour cell surface played a major role in bringing about alterations of cell surface charge. A detailed analysis of this material has therefore been carried out. The material was removed from the surface of the ascites tumour cells by tryptic digestion, in such

a way that the membrane was not disrupted, according to staining tests with Lissamine green. The material so isolated proved to be a sialo mucopeptide, containing sialic acid as a terminal group and one other sugar, N-acetyl glactosamine (LANGLEY and AMBROSE, 1964). There are indications that the sugar portion may be linked to the peptide by glutamic acid. The peptide itself has an amino acid composition rather similar to collagen, with much proline, glycine and alanine and very few large side chains; such an amino acid composition will be favourable to the formation of an *extended* polypeptide chain rather than a coiled α chain and will lie satisfactorily on the outer surface of the cell membrane. It would be of interest to know whether the increased amount of sialo mucopeptide on the tumour cell surface is due to the formation of a new substance, or simply to an increased proportion of a material already present on the normal cell surface. In the hope of finding a specific change in the structure of tumour cells, a detailed sugar and amino acid sequence determination, both on normal and tumour cell surfaces, is clearly desirable.

Recent studies of viral carcinogenesis have revealed the presence of new antigens in the transformed cells. These appear to be surface antigens according to serological methods used for their detection. It is therefore distinctly possible that the sialo-mucopeptides, or other mucopeptides closely related to them, form part of the new tumour antigens. But it would be unwise to assume that the entire alteration in the tumour cell surface occurs in the sialomucopeptides. For example, a change in the quantity or structure of the surface mucoproteins and proteins might make new lipid sites available on the cell surface without any change in the composition of the phospholipids. But the work of Rapport on cytolipin H and the Japanese work on maligno-lipin have shown that quantitative changes in the lipid phase of the tumour cells do take place. AMBROSE, EASTY, CORMACK and DUDGEON (1960, 1962) studied the effect of a wheat germ lipase preparation and showed that it acted selectively in inhibiting the growth of tumour cultures *in vitro*. By the use of fluorescent labels attached to the enzyme it was possible to show that this material adsorbed on the cell membrane. EASTY, and AMBROSE (1961) found evidence for some slight selectivity against tumour cultures, using RUSSEL's viper venom, which contains phospholipases. Recently, BRAGANZA and AMBROSE (1965) have obtained a striking selectivity against ascites tumour cells, using a nontoxic fraction isolated from Cobra venom. This fraction is more than 100 times less toxic for whole animals than crude venom, but shows a strikingly selective cytic action on YOSHIDA sarcoma cells, being effective at a $30 \times$ times lower concentration than any normal cells so far tested, including erythrocytes, bone marrow, lymphocytes and gastric mucosa.

Adhesive Forces between Cells

So far we have been thinking almost entirely in terms of the negative charges on the cell surface and their relationship to the repulsive forces between cell surfaces. But whether adhesions occur between cells depends on the attractive forces and the extent to which these are able to overcome the repulsive forces. Alterations in the cell surface during the malignant change can involve changes in the repulsive forces, in the attractive forces, or in both. What has become fairly clear from present work is that the cell surface is a mozaic. In some types of tumour a change has occurred in some regions of the cell membrane, while others retain their normal adhesive properties. There is evidence for this from electron microscopic studies of cell contacts. It may not always be possible to detect these minor changes by cell electrophoresis, which gives an average value for the surface properties. In one type of transformation, the type II transformation produced by polyoma virus, it is not possible to detect a change in electrical mobility. But this type of transformation is not particularly stable and, after a few cell generations, reverts to a type I transformation. From observations in tissue culture it looks as though the initial contacts between cells are over small areas, due to the development of microvillae, which presumably contain areas of adhesive material at their tips. A complete understanding of the behaviour of cells on contact must clearly involve an understanding of the nature of the attractive forces. It has become fairly clear that the adhesive material contains protein. The standard procedure for separation of cells for tissue culture, either from tissues or from monolayers, involves the use of weak trypsin. In embryos, calcium ions play a major role. Addition of EDTA, which removes calcium by chelation, causes disaggregation of the embryos. On replacing in calcium containing medium, the cells reaggregate and can pass through a number of stages of development. But in adult tissues the need for proteolytic enzymes to separate cells is much more marked (EASTY and MUTOLO, 1960). So it looks as though an increased secretion of protein takes place between the membranes in adult tissues. Some studies by DUMONDE and FORRESTER (1967) and by SHEPLEY and AMBROSE (1967) have shown an interesting difference between sensitised and non-sensitised macrophages, which may have some bearing on this problem. When placed in the presence of the antigen these cells stick together, but time-lapse filming shows that the membranes are still extremely active and the cells are moving continuously, although certain regions of the membranes are firmly adhering together, i.e., the presence of the antigen in the medium enables the cells to adhere firmly together, although there is no toxic action of the antigen. This adhesion prevents migration of the cells, but in the presence of trypsin the rate of migration increases once more. In the presence of neuraminidase the rate of migration is reduced. These results suggest that sensitised macrophages carry an antibody-like protein on their surface. This protein is digested by trypsin so that the adhesiveness in the presence of antigen is reduced. But neurominidase removes sialic acid from the cell surface, so reducing the repulsive forces due to negative charge and the adhesiveness is increased once more. But clearly, much more detailed biological and biochemical analysis of the cell surface will be required before a complete picture of the nature of the adhesive material on the cell surface is obtained. This material probably provides the key to our understanding of the true nature of the tumour cell surface which leads to its invasive properties.

The Interactions between Cells and Stroma

Much emphasis has been placed in this account on the nature of the cell surface and on the interactions between cells. But another factor must be taken into account when we consider the nature of the invasive process in tumours. The cells will be coming into contact with non cellular surfaces such as fibrous structures formed by collagen and elastin, basement membranes etc.

Some recent studies of the movement of normal and tumour cells on such surfaces may throw some light on this problem (AMBROSE and ELLISON, in course of publication). We have studied the behaviour of BHK 21 fibroblasts of the cells after transformation with polyoma virus on various surfaces. We have used glass surfaces of various texture, i.e. (1a) smooth glass, (2a) fine sintered glass and (3a) coarse sintered glass. Also (1b) smooth cellulose acetate (made by casting Millipore material from solution in ethyl acetate), (2b) fine Millipore (0.2μ porosity), (3b) medium grade Millipore (0.6μ porosity) and (4b) coarse Millipore (0.8μ porosity).

The interesting point here is that the tumour cells are able to spread and migrate on all these surfaces irrespective of their texture. The BHK 21 cells which do not form tumours, show a very different behaviour depending on the surface texture. On smoothe glass they also spread and produce a monolayer when confluent. But on fine sintered glass (2a) or fine Millipore (2b) the cells coalesce into colonies. They finish up as dense aggregates separated by large spaces on the Millipore surface. There may be 1,000,000 cells in an aggregate. On surfaces (3a), (3b) and (4b) the untransformed cells are able to attach to the surface and on (3a) and (4b) they once more produce monolayers as on smooth glass or cellulose acetate.

These experiments show that the transformed cells shows a more generalised adhesion to surfaces of varying texture than do the untransformed cells. We have been able to demonstrate that this difference is due to the more frequent and irregular appearance of undulating membranes over the tumour cell surface, so that the cell is able to acquire purchase on almost any surface.

So we can see that the changes in the physical and chemical properties of the malignant cell surface may go a long way towards explaining the ability of these cells to disseminate into normal tissues. Not only have they lost or partially lost the specific interactions between neighbouring cells which enable them to show contact inhibition but they have acquired a more versatile surface which may enable them to spread along channels provided by connective tissue fibres etc. by contact guidance as first demonstrated by PAUL WEISS. Such a behaviour is in line with the known behaviour of tumours. Cases where the cells spread in a diffuse form throughout the normal tissues are not so common as those in which a mass of tumour cells migrates along some region of apparent weakness within the normal tissue structure.

Acknowledgement

I wish to thank Sir ALEXANDER HADDOW. F.R.S. for his interest in this work and to acknowledge the great help received from my colleagues Dr. J. A. FORRESTER, Dr. N. K. LANGLEY, Miss K. SHEPLEY and Miss M. ELLISon. This work has been supported by grants to the Chester Beatty Research Institute (Institute of Cancer Research: Royal Cancer Hospital) from the Medical Research Council, the British Empire Cancer Campaign for Research and by the Public Health Service Research Grant No, CA-03188-10 from the National Cancer Institute, U.S. Public Health Service.

Discussion

Questions put to E. J. AMBROSE

E. J. Ambrose: As a cell biologist, I have faith in the idea that a change in the properties of the cell is the primary cause of cancer. This is the reason why a colloquium of this kind is so valuable for those who are endeavouring to explain the nature of cancer in terms of the atoms and molecules of the cell, because it clarifies the biological properties we are trying to understand. Much is now known from molecular biology about the storage of information by RNA and DNA and their relation to genetic properties. So far as cancer is concerned, there is now a considerable measure of agreement that changes in the cell surface are to some extent involved in the invasive process, in interactions leading to the control of growth and morphogenesis, and finally in immunological reactions. If we can express these changes in precise physico-chemical and immunological terms, we may come a great deal closer to finding an interpretation for the associated molecular changes within the cells.

K. E. Hellström: You mentioned that there was sometimes no overall increase of the cell surface charge during the early stages of malignant transformation following polyoma infection of normal cells. You suggested that the surface charge of such cells was changed only in certain spots. Do you have any experimental evidence showing that this is so, or do you know of any method by which it is possible to demonstrate a change of surface charge within a small part of the cell membrane?

E. J. Ambrose: Studies of cell contacts seen in the light microscope and in the electron microscope provide experimental evidence in favour of the view that local changes in the cell surface are involved in the early stages of carcinogenesis. Small areas of the cell membranes remain in stable contact, but where they do attach, the contacts look like normal cell contacts and may in some cases form desmosomes. Cell electrophoreses gives a measure of the average change in density on the cell surface. Dr. FORRESTER, Dr. DUMONDE, and I have studied the effect of adding heterologous antiserum to cells. γ-globulin is then absorbed on the surface. The pH mobility curve obtained is similar to that of γ-globulin, and not to that obtained with cell surfaces. By the use of an antiserum, specific to an altered local region of the tumour cell surface, it should therefore be possible to detect local changes by a combination of immunological methods and cell electrophoresis.

M. Feldman: Dr. AMBROSE, you have demonstrated interesting differences in the mobility of different cell types in an electric field. In order to get an indication of the relevance of such *in vitro* differences to *in vivo* phenomena, it would be of interest to test *in vitro* embryonic cells which are known to manifest *in vivo* differences in rate of migration within the developing embryo. Thus, cells originating in the neural crest migrate over long distances in the organism and reassociate later in various areas to form the sympathetic ganglia, part of the adrenals, etc. Will such cells, when tested *in vitro,* show a higher mobility in an electric fields, as compared with other embryonic cells which *in vivo* do not show such a high rate of motility?

My second question is related to the effect of antigen on the aggregation of sensitized cells which you have demonstrated. Were the "sensitized" cells macrophages, or were they lymphocytes?

E. J. Ambrose: I agree with Dr. FELDMAN that an electrophoretic analysis of migrating embryonic cells is most desirable. Technically, this is very difficult in view of the small numbers of cells available. With present techniques we need at least 100,000 cells to make measurements. But I am sure that it will be possible to do these experiments eventually.

The sensitized cells which I demonstrated in the film were macrophages

obtained from guinea-pigs showing delayed hypersensitivity and were prepared by Dr. DUMONDE.

P. Sträuli: If you investigate the electrophoretic behaviour of cells of solid tumours — e.g. hamster kidney tumours — how do you prepare the necessary single cell suspensions?

E. J. Ambrose: For the preparation of cells from solid tissues, low concentrations of chelating agents in calcium-free, TYRODE's solution has been used. In some cases, the animals have been perfused with this medium. We have always treated the normal tissues and the tumour tissues with the same medium and used similar degrees of mechanical agitation. For separating tissue cultures from glass, we have used the low concentration of trypsin that is employed in standard tissue culture procedures. Experiments with cells which grow naturally in suspension, using the concentration of trypsin, have shown that there is no effect on cellular mobility.

R. E. Madden: On of your text you refer to the removal of sialic acid from the cell surface, stating that this may reduce negative-charge repulsive forces and increase adhesiveness. GASIC and GASIC (1962) have furnished evidence that treatment of intravenously injected cells, as well as of the animal itself, with neuraminidase lessened the incidence of lung metastases. These authors felt that this was due to loss of stickiness between cell and endothelium.

E. J. Ambrose: Treatment of macrophages with neuraminidase decreases their rate of migration and appears to increase *intercellular* adhesiveness. But in the formation of metastases the initial process involves the adhesion of cells to a surface which in this case may be coated with mucoid material. The mucoid substances on the cell surface may assist the first stage by increasing adhesion. We need to distinguish in this field between adhesions to glass or other solid substrate and the more specific stable intercellular contacts. This was first pointed out by COMAN. The two types of adhesion do not necessarily change in the same sense. In some cases they may be inversely related. In fact, FORRESTER and DUMONDE have shown that treatment with neuraminidase reduces the adhesiveness of tumour cells to glass although it increases the *intercellular* adhesiveness which arrests migration.

D. F. H. Wallach: In connection with Dr. MADDEN's comments, I should like to point out that the relation of electrophoretic mobility to sialic acid is not a simple one. Thus, in Ehrlich ascites carcinoma there is a rather constant diminution in the amount of sialic acid owing to its removal by sialidase. By contrast, the removal of similar amounts of sialic acid from MCIMs sarcoma produces no change in electrophoretic mobility. In $MCIM_{AA}$ *ascites* sarcoma, the removal of a small proportion of sialic acid reduces electrophoretic mobility to a striking extent, but the further action of sialidase causes no further electrokinetic change. We have discussed some

of the possible mechanisms involved in a previous paper [Biochim. Biophys. Acta *83*, 303 (1964)].

E. J. Ambrose: Electrophoretic measurements at 0.14 M ionic strenght only detect the surface of the cell to a depth of 10Å, i.e. that region of the cell which makes contact with the exterior and probably plays the main part in intercellular contacts. But other sialic acid groups are present which are below this level and are masked in cell electrophoresis.

Z. Brada: From the point of tumour cell behaviour, what significance do you attach to the differences between Type I and Type II fibroblast transformation by polyoma virus?

E. J. Ambrose: I think that the cell surface charges in the Type II transformation may be more local than they are in the Type I, and are therefore not detected in the average mobility measured by cell electrophoresis. It might therefore be expected that the Type II cells would be less invasive, but without a quantitative measure of early invasiveness (not metastasis) *in vivo* it is not possible to test this hypothesis.

References

ABERCOMBIE, M., and AMBROSE, E. J., Interference microscope studies of cell contacts in tissue culture. *Exp. Cell Res.* **15**, 332 (1958).

—, and HEAYSMAN, J. E. M., Social behaviour of cells in tissue culture. I. Speed of movement of chick heart fibroblasts in relation to their mutual contacts. *Exp. Cell Res.* **5**, 111 (1953).

AMBROSE, E. J., DUDGEON, J. A., EASTY, D. M., and EASTY, G. C., The inhibition of tumour growth by enzymes in tissue culture. *Exp. Cell Res.* **24**, 220—227 (1961).

—, and SOLDACRE, R. J., *Int. Biophysics Meeting Abstract.* Paris 1964.

BRAGANCA, B. M., BADRINATH, P. G., and AMBROSE, E. J., A highly selective carcinalytic agent isolated from cobra venom. *Nature (Lond.)* **207**, 534—535 (1965).

COMAN, D. R., Decreased mutual adhesiveness, a property of cells from squamous cell carcinomas. *Cancer Res.* **4**, 625—629 (1944).

CORMACK, D., EASTY, G. C., and AMBROSE, E. J., Interaction of enzymes with normal an tumour cells. *Nature (Lond.)* **190**, 1207—1208 (1961).

CURTIS, A. S. G., Cell contacts; some physical considerations. *Amer. Naturalish* **94**, 37 (1960).

EASTY, DOROTHY M., and AMBROSE, E. J., *Brit. Empire Cancer Compaign Rep.* p. 58 (1961).

FORRESTER, J. A., Microelectrophoresis of normal and polyoma virus transformed hamster kidney fibroblasts. In: *Cell electrophoresis* (ed. E. J. Ambrose), p. 115. Churchill, 1965.

Forrester, J. A., and Ambrose, E. J., In Preparation 1967.

— —, and Macpherson, J. A., Electrophoretic investigations of a clone of hamster fibroblasts and polyomatransformedcells from the same population. *Nature (Lond.)* **196**, 1068—1070 (1962).

—, —, and Stoker, M. G. P., Microelectrophoresis of normal and transformed clones of hamster kidney fibroblasts. *Nature (Lond.)* **201**, 945—946 (1964).

—, Dumonde, D. C., and Ambrose, E. J. The effects of antibodies on cells. II. Changes in the electrophoretic mobility of ascites tumour cells treated with antibodies and complement. *Immunology* **8**, 37—48 (1965).

Langley, N. K., and Ambrose, E. J., Isolation of a mucopeptide from the surface of Ehrlich ascites tumour cells. *Nature (Lond.)* **204**, 53—54 (1964).

Purdom, L., Klein, S., and Ambrose, E. J., A correlation between electrical surface charge and some biological characteristics during the step-wise progression of a mouse carcinoma. *Nature (Lond.)* **181**, 1586—1587 (1958).

Rueff, F., Fuhrmann, G. S., and Ruhenstroth-Bauer, G., Cell electrophoresis in clinical diagnosis. Electrophoretic studies of blood, lymph node and tumour cells of recently obtained specimens. *Münch. med. Wschr.* **105**, 1242—1250 (1963).

Ruhenstroth-Bauer, G., Haemocytopherograms of man. In: *Cell electrophoresis* (ed. E. J. Ambrose), p. 67. Churchill 1965.

Ruhenstroth, G., Straub, E., Sachtleben, P., and Fuhrmann, G. F., Die elektrophoretische Beweglichkeit von Blutzellen beim Gesunden und bei Kranken. *Münch. med. Wschr.* **103**, 794—797 (1961).

Shepley, K., and Ambrose, E. J., In Preparation (1967).

— —, and Kirby, K., Alterations of hamster cells by nucleic acid *in vitro*. *Nature (Lond.)* **208**, 1072—1074 (1965).

Steinberg, M. S., On the chemical bonds between animal cells. A mechanism for type-specific association. *Amer. Naturalist* **92**, 65 (1958).

Tyler, A., An auto-antibody concept of cell structure growth and differentiation. *Growth* (6th Symp. Suppl.) **10**, 7—19 (1947).

Ward, P., and Ambrose, E. J. (in course of publication).

Weiss, P., The problem of specificity in growth and development. *Yale J. Biol. Med.* **19** 235—278 (1947).

Wheatley, D. N., Ambrose, E. J., and Easty, G. C., Infiltration of intraabdominal organs by ascites tumours. *Nature (Lond.)* **199**, 188—189 (1963).

Yamada, T. (in course of publication).

An in vitro Model of the Mechanism of Invasion

M. Abercrombie

University College London

This paper is intended to direct attention to a tissue culture model of malignant invasion, or at least of malignant infiltration, which is one aspect of invasion. The ability of malignant cells to infiltrate persistently into the adjacent normal tissues is rightly regarded as a character that is as near diagnostic of malignancy as any. It is distinctive because normal cells (other than leucocytes), even when in a state of proliferation, rarely show anything like the same ability to infiltrate amongst their normal neighbours. Correspondingly, in the tissue culture model, cancer cells are shown to infiltrate a population of normal cells, in circumstances where normal cells will not.

The model, as it concerns the behaviour of normal cells, is as follows. Two primary explants of fibroblast-producing tissue are placed close together, but not touching, in a drop of liquid medium on a plane surface. Cells emigrate from the explants, by individual locomotion on the substrate, to form a spreading halo around each explant. In the gap between the explants the two radiating populations meet in head-on collision. When this happens, the locomotion of the cells is here sharply checked. The populations do not proceed with their migration in such a way as to produce a mutual infiltration (Abercrombie and Heaysman, 1954).

When however certain malignant and normal cells are confronted in the same way, by placing near together a fragment of a sarcoma and a fragment of fibroblast-producing tissue, the outcome is different. When the collission occurs, a sharp check to locomotion is not observed. The two populations proceed, and there is mutual infiltration (Abercrombie, Heaysman and Karthauser, 1957).

An analysis of the change in locomotory behaviour that follows the collision between the two normal populations has been made in terms of contact inhibition of movement (Abercrombie and Heaysman, 1954; Abercrombie and Ambrose, 1958). When a fibroblast collides with another during its movement on a plane surface, it usually ceases to move in a direction that would carry it over the surface of the other cell. A cell thus inhibited is not prevented from deflecting its movement in a new direction, provided this is free of cells; and a certain proportion of collisions escape the inhibition altogether. The term contact inhibition was used because the inhibitory effect is only observed when visible contact has been made between the cells. Because fibroblasts in culture form a meshwork (though a dynamic one) by mutual adhesion, no individual fibroblast can move far relative to its neighbours without undergoing contact inhibition. Between the two explants no cell can escape, and all are reduced to small-scale oscillations. The sarcoma cells that have been tested in the model system are defective in their contact inhibition by normal fibroblasts (and vice versa); in other words there is a much reduced, but not necessarily zero, probability that collision will result in inhibition.

We have then a certain parallelism between the infiltrative behaviour in general of normal malignant cells within the organism, and the behaviour of those normal and malignant cells that have been tested in the model system *in vitro*. An analysis of behaviour in the model system is to some extent available, in terms of contact inhibition; and if the model is a good one, the same analysis should be applicable to the behaviour *in vivo*. There is incidentally an additional parallelism, which encourages one to examine the model seriously. Leucocytes, in general terms, can invade normal tissues; certain leucocytes also fail to show contact inhibition by certain normal fibroblasts in the model system (OLD-field, 1963).

In assessing the value of the model there are many points that can be raised about the comparability of the *in vivo* and *in vitro* situations. The crucial assessment, however, seems to be to put the parallelism on a quantitative basis. Not all tumours are equally invasive; the impression is that there is every degree of invasiveness, as there is any other property of tumours. Nor is any one kind of tumour equally invasive of all kinds of normal tissue. On the other hand contact inhibition as assessed in culture also varies quantitatively, according to the cell types concerned, in the frequency with which it is the outcome of a collision. Insofar as the model is useful, there should be, for both tu-

mour and normal cells, a correlation between the degree of contact inhibition by a given population of cells *in vitro* and the degree of invasion into a population of the same cells *in vivo*. The quantitation of what we want to measure on either side of this correlation is difficult, and has not yet been achieved; but it should not be impossible.

I should like, however, to add a note of caution, in view of some recent discussions of the relation of contact inhibition to malignancy. Much of the recent important work on virus-transformed cells, insofar as it has dealt with contact inhibition of movement rather than of mitosis, is probably not concerned with the parallelism I have described. The degree of contact inhibition of malignant cells by other cells of the same kind is not relevant to an assessment of the value of the model, or rather is not yet known to be relevant. The intensity of this contact inhibition may turn out to be of interest in reflecting changes in the cell surface which themselves affect infiltration into normal tissues, as well as other properties of malignant cells (ABER-CROMBIE and AMBROSE, 1962). But at present there are no grounds for expecting a close correlation between contact inhibition by homologous and by heterologous cells. Equally, ability to grow as a tumour when transplanted does not yet rank as an adequate test of invasiveness. Because the contact inhibition of malignant cells has recently been discusses from so many points of view, it has seemed worthwhile to restate the case for the restricted model originally proposed.

Discussion

Questions put to M. Abercrombie

J. Leighton: Would you, please, answer two questions:

1. Do you suppose that one mechanism of invasion may be the transport by normal fibroblasts of cancer cells "stuck" to the surface of normal cells?

2. Would you please distinguish between two cells that are "stuck" and two that are "contact-inhibited"?

M. Abercrombie: 1. It had never occurred to me that this might be a mechanism of invasion. It cannot be excluded.

2. In contact inhibition the two cells involved seem to stick together, so I do not think one can make the distinction.

M. Stoker: Could Prof. Abercrombie comment on the possible relationship between contact inhibition and cell division? I ask this because of the very dramatic development of contact inhibition in virus-transformed cells which have ceased to divide and have developed into giant cells, either spontaneously or as a result of irradiation.

M. Abercrombie: The relationship has exercised us for a long time, because of the association in malignant cell populations of a deficiency in contact inhibition with increased mitosis. It is conceivable that both are affected by the same surface change. Cells actually in mitosis have deficient contact inhibition. It is evident, however, that mitotic rates in a population of normal cells can increase without appreciably diminishing contact inhibition, though I have argued that there is an associated change in the "mobilization" of the locomotor machinery of the cells.

E. J. Ambrose: In considering the effect of cell contacts on mitosis, we may have to take note of two types of contact, those between tumour cells and those between tumour and normal cells. It is unfortunate that Dr. Vasiliev was not here to present his paper. As you have read in the manuscript, a limited number of tumour cell to tumour cell contacts seems to favour an increased growth rate. This may depend on the maintenance of a microclimate favourable to growth in the neighbourhood of the cells, this climate being maintained by cellular reaction. On the other hand, the work of Prof. Stoker indicates that in his system, contact of transformed cells with a layer of untransformed cells leads to a decreased mitotic rate.

P. Vigier: As Prof. Abercrombie has so rightly said, it is extremely important to distinguish between homologous and heterologous contact inhibition. In collaboration with Mrs. Golde, we have studied this problem in embryonic chicken cells transformed by several known Rous viruses. In the case of the high-titre Bryan strain of virus [RSV (RAV)], the transformed cells display a clear-cut homologous contact inhibition. On the other hand, they show little inhibition in respect of non-transformed embryonic fibroblasts, inasmuch as isolated zones of Rous cells may develop on a confluent layer of fibroblasts; in this latter case, however, the transformed cells usually remain grouped together. By contrast, cells transformed by virus isolated from transformed cells of the XC rat strain (Svoboda) generally disperse round the central zones they form. They are therefore more mobile and, apparently, still less inhibited by normal cells than those transformed by RSV (RAV). The behaviour of cells transformed by Schmidt-Rappin virus is midway between that of the other two types of cells.

To sum up, cells transformed by Rous virus may display both a clear-cut homologous inhibition and a reduced heterologous inhibition (in respect of normal cells). The degree of heterologous inhibition may vary according to the transforming virus used.

M. Abercrombie: I find these results of very great interest. They underline the difficulty of assigning a single overall value to the diminished contact inhibition of tumour cells.

G. Barski: The great merit of Prof. ABERCROMBIE's film is that it draws attention to the fundamental difference in the dynamic behaviour of cells, depending on whether they are normal or malignant.

The original concept that contact inhibition exists between normal cells but not in malignant cells should, however, be viewed in the light of other observations and considerations.

Prof. ABERCROMBIE bases his ideas chiefly on observations of normal fibroblasts confronted with mouse sarcoma cells. The behaviour of other types of normal and malignant cells towards each other should also be taken into account. In our experiments, malignant cells had difficulty in passing through the endothelium, and this example proves that the results of the interaction between normal and cancer cells are by no means uniform.

I should like to add that a study of the nature and degree of mobility of cells in relation to their invasive capacity might be most informative. We believe that this mobility is increased in malignant cells, and we are trying to measure this increase in the case of both "free" cells and cells in contact with others.

J. Harel: I should like to make a very provocative comment. If loss or absence of contact inhibition is to be regarded as the essential feature of a malignant cell, the feature which determines its invasive capacity, is not the lymphocyte the model of a malignant cell? The excellent presentations we saw here, and other documents such as Dr. ALICE MOORE's recent film, show not only that there is little, if any, contact inhibition between lymphocytes and other cells — whether normal or malignant — but also that lymphocytes are capable of invading other cells, even of penetrating into their nucleus and re-emerging without any great damage being caused to either. I therefore wonder whether, in our studies of this phenomenon, it would not be preferable to compare the properties of tumour cells with those of immunologically competent cells, such as the lymphocytes, rather than with the properties of normal cells having the same origin as the malignant ones.

M. Abercrombie: In our tissue culture system, lymphocytes, and also granulocytes and macrophages, show a highly deficient contact inhibition by normal fibroblasts. A study of their surfaces might well give important information about the nature of malignant invasiveness.

P. Vigier: At this point in the discussion it may be useful to relate the problem of contact inhibition and, in particular, growth arrest following the collision of cells to the model of the replicon proposed by JACOB. It is, in fact, probable that the division of animal cells, like that of bacterial cells, is controlled by a system of genes, which is repressed when the cells do not divide. It is thus conceivable that contact between inhibited cells activates the repressive system and that this activation does not occur when the inhibition is reduced of suppressed, as in the case of contact between cancer cells and normal cells.

The activation of the repressive system might be due either to blockage of certain specific sites on the cell membrane at the moment of contact, or to the passage of a chemical messenger from one cell to the other after contact. In this connection, Mrs. HAREL has recently obtained particularly interesting results.

References

ABERCROMBIE, M., and AMBROSE, E. J., Interference microscope studies of cell contacts in tissue culture. *Exp. Cell Res.* **15**, 332—345 (1958).

— — The surface properties of cancer cells: A review. *Cancer Res.* **22**, 525—548 (1962).

—, and HEAYSMAN, J. E. M., Social behaviour of cells in tissue culture. II. Monolayering of fibroblasts. *Exp. Cell Res.* **6**, 293—306 (1954).

ABERCROMBIE, M., AMBROSE, E. J., and KARTHAUSER, H. M., Social behaviour of cells in tissue culture. III. Mutual influence of sarcoma cells and fibroblasts. *Exp. Cell Res.* **13**, 276—291 (1957).

OLDFIELD, F. E., Orientation behavior of chick leucocytes in tissue culture and their interactions with fibroblasts. *Exp. Cell Res.* **30**, 125—138 (1963).

Fluorescent Antibodies to Methylcholanthrene Sarcomas

L. A. Zilber, O. M. Lejneva and E. S. Ievleva

Department of Immunology and Oncology of Gamaleya Institute, Moskow, U. S. S. R.

Specific humoral antibodies have been regularly detected in mice leukemias (Slettenmark, 1962; Wahren, 1963; Boyse, 1962; Old, 1963; Klein, 1966), but attempts to find similar antibodies in other neoplastic diseases gave negative results (Old, 1962). Only in some experiments with tumours induced by carcinogenic substances were antibodies revealed (Bubenic, 1962).

In our experiments we tried to reveal humoral antibodies to mouse syngeneic sarcomas, induced by methylcholanthrene (MC) technique of fluorescent antibodies.

C57BL/10Sn and CC57W inbred strains were used. These strains were maintained by strict brother × sister mating in our laboratory. According to Egorov's date (Egorov, 1966), with skin transplants homozygosity of the strain C57BL/10Sn is not lower than 99.8 per cent. The experiments proving the homozygosity of the strain CC57W are still in progress: 120 skin transplants for 120—180 days were observed. No transplants were rejected during this period of time.

The following tumours have been examined: MC-6 C57BL/10Sn and MC-8 CC57W — polymorphous cell sarcomas induced by MC. We used the 32nd and 28th generations of these tumours. The first of these lost the strain specificity from generation 34 and began to grow in I R-line.

Two-month-old mice were immunized with syngeneic tumours. The tumours were cut with scissors into very small fragments and treated with X-rays (15,000 r). Seven to nine inoculations of irradiated suspension were given subcutaneously and bilaterally at intervals of 3 to weeks. Each dose was 0.1—0.2 ml. 13 and 35 days after the last inoculation blood was collected from the retro-orbital sinus from 2 to 6 mice. The pooled sera were stored at −30° C.

Rabbit anti-mouse serum was obtained by immunisation of the rabbits with mouse γ-globulin, extracted from serum of mice which were inoculated with plasmacytoma X 5563 12—14 days before bleeding. γ-globulin fraction of rabbit sera was conjugated with fluorescein according to Riggs (1958). A free dye was removed by filtration through sephadex g-25 M. One ml of the conjugated serum is usually absorbed by once for an hour at room temperature with 40 mg of acetone powder of mouse liver prepared according to Coons (1958).

Cell suspensions were obtained by trypsinisation of solid sarcomas. For staining the cells we used 3 variants of the indirect technique:

1. Möller's method: Möller (1961) developed for the demonstration of mouse isoantigens in suspension of living cells. Our process of staining living cells was the same as that of Möller. Smears were then prepared from the cell

suspension and included in 50% glycerol solution.

2. The staining of tissue sections which were washed in abundant Ringer's solution just after thawing.

surface, 2. A fluorescence of single dots, 3. A fluorescence of vacuoles due to pinocytosis of fluorescent dye.

Living cells pretreated with mouse antiserum and subsequently exposed to

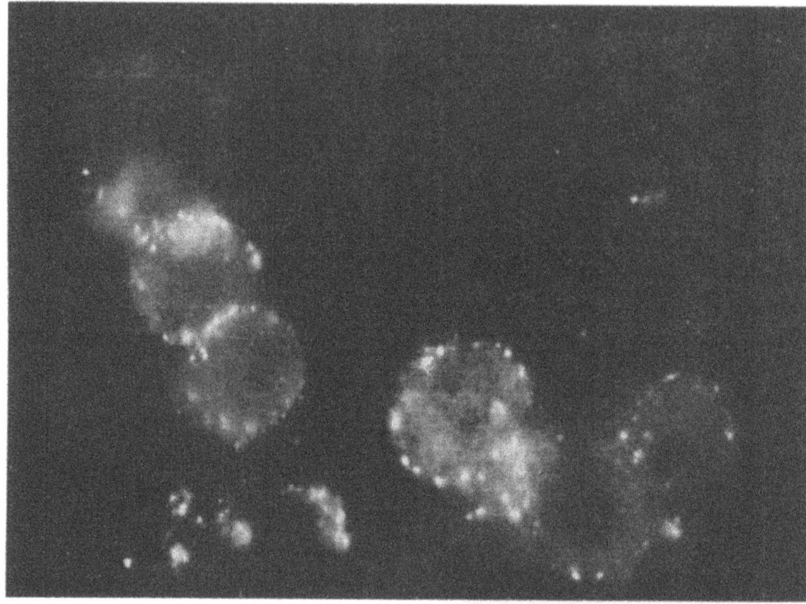

Fig. 1

3. The staining of dead cells in smears. Both tissue sections and smears were subsequently treated with 0.25 ml of test serum and 0.25 ml fluorescein-conjugated rabbit antimouse serum for 15 minutes and washed three times in Ringer's solution. The follwing controls were used: 1. The mouse antiserum was replaced by normal mouse serum. 2. The cells of tumour DBA C57BL/10Sn induced by dibenzanthracene were treated with the serum against MC-induced tumours.

The best results were acheived in experiments with living cells. 1. In all experiments a green-yellow fluorescence of three types were observed: 1. A fluorescence of many dots on the whole cell the fluorescent rabbit anti-mouse serum demonstrated, as a rule, the fluorescence of the first type which was considered as

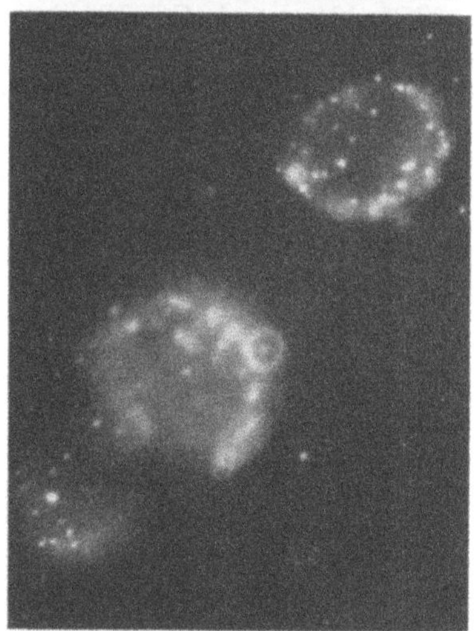

Fig. 2

Figs. 1 and 2. Cells of MC-8CC57W treated with mouse antiserum. Dotted fluorescence along the periphery of cells

specific (Figs. 1 and 2). The proportion of fluorescent cells in some experiments

Table I. *Fluorescent staining of target cells by rabbit anti-mouse globulin after exposure with mouse antisera*

Designation	Immunization with syngeneic tumour	Number of inoculation	Mice bled at	Targets cells	Index
275 * undiluted	MC-6 C57 BL/10 Sn ♂	7	13 days	MC6 C57 BL/10 Sn	0.30
288 * undiluted	MC6 C57 BL/10 Sn ♂	8	35 days	MC6 C57 BL/10 Sn	0.21
311 ** undiluted	MC-6 C57 BL/10 Sn ♂	9	35 days	MC6 C57 BL/10 Sn	0.64
311 ** undiluted	MC-6 C57 BL/10 Sn ♂	9	35 days	MC6 C57 BL/10 Sn	0.58
311 ** undiluted	MC-6 C57 BL/10 Sn ♂	9	35 days	MC6 C57 BL/10 Sn	0.27
311 ** undiluted	MC-6 C57 BL/10 Sn ♂	9	35 days	MC6 C57 BL/10 Sn	0.47
311 ** undiluted	MC-6 C57 BL/10 Sn ♂	9	35 days	DBAC57 BL/10 Sn	0.02
311 ** 1:2	MC-6 C57 BL/10 Sn ♂	9	35 days	MC6 C57 BL/10 Sn	0.40
311 ** 1:4	MC-6 C57 BL/10 Sn ♂	9	35 days	MC6 C57 BL/10 Sn	0.37
310 ** undiluted	MC-8 CC57 W ♂	9	35 days	MC8 CC57 W	0.42
310 ** undiluted	MC-8 CC57 W ♂	9	35 days	MC8 CC57 W	0,38
310 ** undiluted	MC-8 CC57 W ♂	9	35 days	MC8 CC57 W	0.78
310 ** undiluted	MC-8 CC57 W ♂	9	35 days	DBAC57/BL 10 Sn	0.08
310 ** 1:2	MC-8 CC57 W ♂	9	35 days	MC8 CC57 W	0.52
310 ** 1:4	MC-8 CC57 W ♂	9	35 days	MC8 CC57 W	0.29

* Sera from 2 ♂♂.
** Sera from 6 ♂♂ and ♀♀.

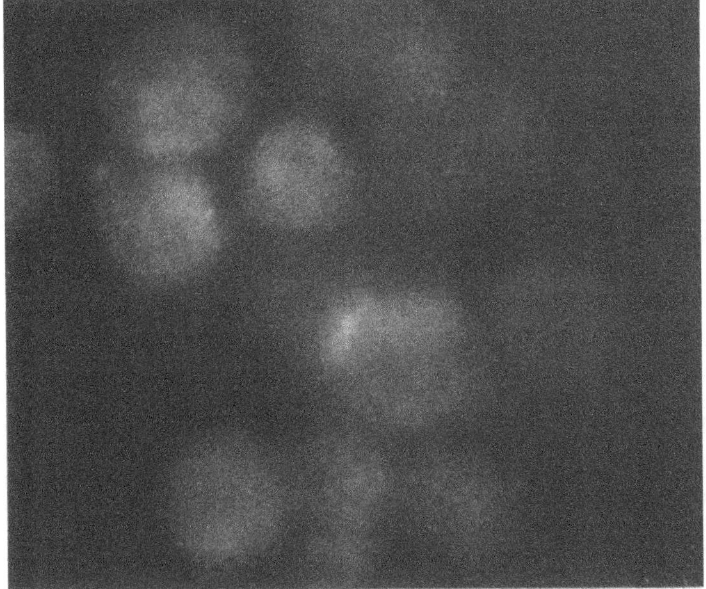

Fig. 3. Control. Cells of MC-8 CC57 W treated with normal mouse serum. No fluorescence

was about 85 per cent. To estimate the results of the experiments a fluorescence index (fi) was calculated. For this 200 to 300 cells, except those showing a diffuse fluorescence, were counted. Fluorescence of the first and third types were taken to the positive group, since sometimes it was difficult to distinguish the fluorescence of cells due to pinocytosis from the specific one.

We did not observe cross-reactions with DBA C57BL/10Sn sarcoma induced by dibenzanthracene (fi = 0.08). It should be noted that in all examined tumours some cells had a tendency to be stained after exposure with normal mouse serum, the amount of stained cells was about 1.7—18 per cent. Data of experiments are summarized in Table I.

Activity of sera produced both in males and in females was identical. The antisera tested did not react with isologous erythrocytes and those of A strain of mice in Gorer's hemagglutination test (1954). They were not cytotoxic to normal lymphocytes of A strain (Gorer, 1956). However these data do not exclude the difference in "weak" histocompatibility antigens.

We are at present carrying out analogous experiments with primarily MC-induced sarcoma.

Since preparing of this manuscript we have received *Nature* with the paper by G. Möller (IIa) who obtained similar results in experiments with methylcholanthrene-induced mouse sarcomas.

References

Boyse, E. A., Old, L. J., and Stockert, E., Some further data on cytotoxic isoantibodies in the mouse. *Ann. N.Y. Acad. Sci.* **99**, 574—587 (1962).

Coons, A. H., *General Cytochemical methods*, p. 399. New York: Academic Press 1958.

Egorov, J. K., and Medvedev, N. N., Homosygosity of C57BL/10ScSn, C57L/S, CC57BR and CC57W mouse strains as studied by the skin transplantation method. *Genetika* (USSR) **2**, 130—136 (1966).

Gorer, P. A., and Mikulska, Z. B., The antibody response to tumour inoculation improved methods of antibody detection. *Cancer Res.* **14**, 651—655 (1954).

—, and O'Gorman, P., The cytotoxic activity of isoantibodies in mice. *Transplant. Bull.* **3**, 142—143 (1956).

Klein, E., and Klein, G., Antigenic properties of lymphomas induced by the moloney agent. *J. nat. Cancer Inst.* **32**, 547—568 (1964).

Möller, G., Demonstration of mouse isoantigens at the cellular level by the fluorescent antibody technique. *J. exp. Med.* **114**, 415—434 (1961).

Möller, G., Effect on tumour growth in syngeneic recipients of antibodies against tumour-specific antigens in methylcholanthrene induced mouse sarcomas. *Nature (Lond.)* **205**, 846—847 (1964).

Old, L. J., Boyse, E. A., Clarke, D. A., and Carswell, E. A., Antigenic properties of chemically induced tumors. *Ann. N.Y. Acad. Sci.* **101**, 80—106 (1962).

— —, and Lilly, F., Formation of cytotoxic antibody against leukemias induced by Friend virus. *Cancer Res.* **23**, 1063—1068 (1963).

Riggs, I. L., Seiwald, R. I., Burckhalter, I. H., Kowns, C. M., and Metcalt, T. G., Isothiocyanate compounds; fluorescent labelling agents for immune serum. *Amer. J. Path.* **34**, 1081—1098 (1958).

Slettenmark, B., and Klein, E., Cytotoxic and neutralization tests with serum and lymph node cells of isologous mice with induced resistance against Gross lymphomas. *Cancer Res.* **22**, 947—954 (1962).

Wahren, B. J., Cytotoxic assays and other immunologic studies of leukemias induced by Friend virus. *J. nat. Cancer Inst.* **31**, 411—423 (1963).

Le système reticulo-endothélial et l'invasion tumorale

B. N. Halpern, G. Biozzi et C. Stiffel

Collége de France, Institut d'Immunobiologie, Paris, France

Une tentative en vue de déterminer le rôle du système réticulo-endothélial (S.R.E.) dans la défense tumorale se heurte à plusieurs obstacles. Le premier résulte de la difficulté de la définition même du S.R.E. et de l'identification des cellules qui y sont intégrées. A cet égard s'offre le choix entre une définition restrictive et une définition élargie. L'interprétation restrictive inclut, dans le S.R.E., les cellules littorales des sinusoïdes sanguins et lymphatiques. Ces cellules se trouvent au contact direct avec les humeurs circulantes et jouent, de ce fait, un rôle primordial dans les phénomènes d'épuration. C'est, en somme, la définition proposée par Aschoff (1924). Considéré dans le sens le plus large, le S.R.E. englobera toutes les cellules mésenchymateuses primitives qui forment la communauté réticuloconjonctivo-histiocytaire.

La seconde difficulté provient du polymorphisme des cellules réticulo-histiocytaires. Ces cellules revêtent les formes les plus variées selon leur situation anatomique, leur degré de différenciation, leur activité fonctionnelle. Leur origine même et leurs relations de filiation avec les autres cellules du mésenchyme deviennent incertaines, depuis que Howard (in press) a montré que les lymphocytes du canal thoracique sont susceptibles de se transformer en cellules de Küpffer.

Aucune définition morphologique, anatomique, ni même cytogénétique n'étant possible, il paraît prudent d'adopter, à titre provisoire, une définition purement *fonctionelle*. Selon cette dernière, on englobe, dans le S.R.E., toutes les cellules qui sont impliquées dans la prise et l'incorporation intracellulaire des matériaux macromoléculaires, des particules organisées ou inertes par un mécanisme similaire à la phagocytose. Il est toutefois évident que, si on limitait à la phagocytose l'activité essentielle des cellules R. E., on les amputerait de toute une série d'autres fonctions qui sont probablement aussi importantes, pour ne pas dire plus importantes: captation de l'antigène, élaboration de l'information, synthèse des protéines, synthèse d'enzymes puissantes et variées impliquées dans la bactério- et la cytolyse, etc. Mais, à l'heure actuelle, l'activité phagocytaire est la seule qui soit susceptible d'être explorée sur une base quantitative (Biozzi, 1953; Halpern, 1954; Benacerraf, 1957).

Réaction histiocytaire au cours de l'invasion tumorale

C'est à la lisière où la cellule cancéreuse affronte le tissu normal qu'il convient de rechercher un des mécanismes de la résistance de l'hôte à l'invasion tumorale.

Les études concernant l'intervention du S.R.E. dans ce processus ont abouti à des résultats encore indécis. Nous nous efforcerons, dans les lignes qui suivront, de faire une synthèse critique de cet important problème.

S.R.E. et propension à la tumorigénèse

En l'absence de données cliniques on est réduit à l'analyse des résultats expérimentaux. Existe-t-il une relation entre le potentiel d'activité du S.R.E. et l'incidence des tumeurs spontanées?

Dans une longue série de recherches qui s'étendent sur plus de dix ans, Kurt Stern (1960) a étudié l'activité du S.R.E. chez des lignées de souris à faible et à forte incidence de tumeurs mammaires et de leucémies. Les résultats indiquent un potentiel d'activité du S.R.E. plus élevé chez les premières que chez les secondes. Bien plus, à l'intérieur de la même lignée où l'incidence des affections malignes est liée au sexe, cette même différence a été notée.

Davidsohn et Stern (1949) ont, en outre, montré que la réponse immune à l'injection d'un antigène hétérologue est sensiblement parallèle à celle de la granulopexie réticulo-endothéliale.

Ces résultats méritent d'être pris en considération. L'introduction récente de méthodes plus quantitatives a montré que, si les écarts dans l'activité de base du S.R.E. chez différentes lignées génétiques de souris sont faibles, la capacité de réagir à une invasion microbienne ou tumorale connaît, par contre, des différences considérables (Halpern, 1964a; Biozzi, 1964; Old, 1961). Il convient également de mentionner les différences observées, à cet égard, en fonction des hormones génitales (Halpern, 1960).

S.R.E. au cours de la tumorigénèse

Il faut distinguer, à cet égard, les réactions locales et les réactions à distance.

Beshford (1908), Murphy (1961) ont consacré à la réaction cellulaire locale des études qui sont demeurées classiques. Lorsqu'on examine la chronologie de ces événements au niveau du greffon tumoral, on retrouve, à quelques variantes près, les mêmes modifications cytologiques dans le tissu environnant. Après la vague éphémère des polynucléaires, on note un afflux de lymphocytes qui s'installent en grand nombre autour du greffon. Mais l'élément dominant devient rapidement les histiocytes qui se différencient et se multiplient pour former une couronne péritumorale, à mailles plus ou moins serrées. Cependant, outre que cette réaction cellulaire n'a rien de spécifique, elle ne constitue qu'un des éléments de l'environnement péritumoral qui est, en quelque sorte, la vague de front qui précède l'implantation et l'invasion tissulaire de la tumeur maligne. Car d'autres modifications de nature biochimique se produisent au voisinage immédiat de la cellule tumorale: modifications vasculaires, libération d'enzymes protéolytiques, accumulation de métabolites en excès, altération de la substance fondamentlae, etc.

Pour notre part, nous nous sommes efforcés, depuis plusieurs années, de scruter les répercussions à distance de l'invasion tumorale sur le S.R.E.

L'étude des modifications du S.R.E. dans les néoplasies humaines reste encore à faire. La méthode est maintenant à la portée de chacun. Le problème comporte, certes, des embûches car une foule de facteurs, agissant d'une manière non spécifique, sont susceptibles d'interférer: état physiologique du sujet, nature de la tumeur et son évolutivité, importance des métastases, etc.

La situation est moins complexe au niveau expérimental, et les renseignements recueillis dans ce domaine sont d'un intérêt certain, bien que leur signification ne soit pas encore claire.

Nous avons étudié (Biozzi, 1958, 1959) les modifications de l'activité du

S.R.E. dans toute une série d'affections malignes spontanées ou induites.

Dans la leucémie AKR, transmise en série isologue, qui aboutit régulièrement à la mort de l'animal receveur, la fonction phagocytaire est peu modifiée au début et nettement déprimée au moment où la leucémie s'établit. La greffe de cellules leucémiques à des lignées de souris naturellement résistantes s'accompagne, par contre, d'une stimulation intense de cette fonction. A cet égard, il est intéressant de rapporter ici le travail récent de KAMPFSCHMIDT et ses collaborateurs (1961). Utilisant notre méthode de mesure de l'activité du S.R.E., ces auteurs en ont étudié les modifications au cours de l'hépatocarcinose expérimentale, provoquée chez le rat soit par l'administration perorale de certains colorants azoïques, soit par celle de la DL-ethionine. Les résultats peuvent se résumer ainsi:

Chez les animaux recevant le 3′ Me-DAB on observe, dès la 2° semaine, une augmentation importante de l'activité phagocytaire du S.R.E., qui se maintient jusque vers la 7° semaine et décroît ensuite. Chez les animaux recevant l'homologue peu cancérigène, le 4′ Me-DAB, à la même dose, les modifications observées sont insignifiantes. La stimulation provoquée par le 3′ Me-DAB correspond à la période prénéoplasique, car les premiers nodules tumoraux n'apparaissent que vers la 8° semaine, c'est à dire au moment où les indices commencent à fléchir.

Dans le groupe des animaux recevant l'ethionine les modifications observées sont très similaires. L'addition de methionine à l'alimentation supprime, à la fois, le pouvoir hépatocarcinogène de l'ethionine et la stimulation du S.R.E.

On sait que l'hypophysectomie supprime la formation des tumeurs par le 3′ Me-DAB. Or, chez les animaux hypophysectomisés, l'administration du co-lorant azoïque ne détermine aucune modification des indices phagocytaires. Mais lorsqu'on administre aux animaux hypophysectomisés de l'ACTH, on voit s'établir la stimulation du S.R.E. chez les animaux recevant le 3′ Me-DAB.

Ces résultats sont intéressants à plusieurs égards: Il s'agit d'une tumeur pratiquement autologue, c'est à dire dépourvue de propriétés antigéniques à l'égard de l'hôte; la stimulation du S.R.E. est surtout marquée au cours de la période prénéoplasique, ce qui permet d'écarter l'action possible des protéines de résorption; la dépendance hormonale de cette tumeur permet d'établir, au gré de l'expérimentateur, une relation certaine entre le développement de la tumeur et la stimulation du S.R.E.

D'autres résultats obtenus avec des tumeurs greffées abondent dans le même sens, bien que des différences considérables s'observent selon la nature de la tumeur. Ainsi, nous avons observé une stimulation vigoureuse du S.R.E. après une greffe de l'épithéliome atypique de Guérin chez le rat (BIOZZI, 1958). Cette activation du S.R.E. est précoce et atteint souvent la valeur maximale dans les jours qui suivent l'implantation. Elle n'est pas sensiblement accrue au cours de l'évolution ultérieure, malgré le développement souvent considérable de la masse tumorale et l'envahissement métastatique généralisé. Ainsi, comme dans le carcinome d'origine chimique, la mise sous tension du S.R.E. est maximale au moment de l'implantation de la tumeur, c'est à dire à la phase préinvasive. On ne peut se défendre contre le sentiment que cette phase est probablement cruciale pour le sort de la tumeur.

La tumeur T_8 est une tumeur, dont l'évolution maintenant stéréotypée est pratiquement invariable. Elle détermine la mort de l'animal dans 100 p 100 des cas. Il était intéressant d'étudier, à cet égard, une tumeur dont le degré de malignité, autrement dit la résistance de l'hôte, dépend des caractères génétiques de celui-ci. La tumeur J de Betz (1959) se prête à une telle étude car ce sarcome manifeste un degré de malignité inégale, selon la lignée génétique de l'hôte. Isolée

l'hôte à l'invasion tumorale, est reflétée par la réponse du S.R.E.

Les résultats sont résumés dans la figure 1.

Une stimulation vigoureuse et quasiment parallèle à la croissance de la tumeur s'observe chez la souris C₅₇Bl. Or,

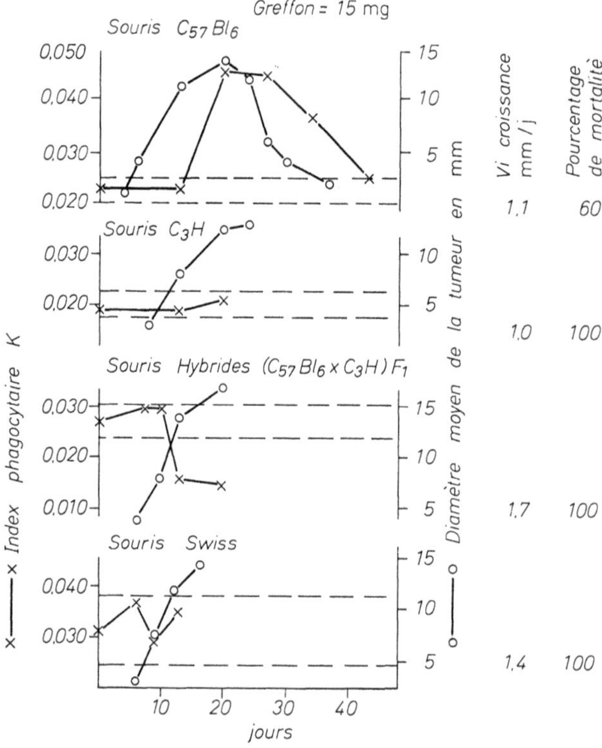

Fig. 1. Modifications de la fonction phagocytaire du S.R.E. (index phagocytaire K) au cours du développement du sarcome J chez des souris de lignées différentes

par Betz d'une souris C₅₇Bl, cette tumeur est transmissible par greffe sous-cutanée en lignée isogénique, chez les hybrides F₁ issus de cette lignée, mais aussi chez d'autres lignées d'histocompatibilité éloignée. Cependant, la vitesse de croissance de la tumeur transplantée et sa virulence varient chez ces différentes lignées d'animaux. Il nous a paru légitime d'étudier dans quelle mesure la différence dans la croissance tumorale, qui exprime en fait le degré de résistance de

cette lignée de souris, qui est isogénique de la tumeur, est relativement résistante à la tumeur puisqu'on observe 40 p 100 de régressions spontanées.

Chez la souris C₃H, la vitesse de croissance du sarcome J est très similaire à celle de la lignée précédente mais, chez elle, la mortalité est de 100 p 100. Or, la stimulation du S.R.E., chez cette lignée, est à peu près nulle. La souris Swiss présente un comportement très similaire.

Il est intéressant de relever les faits observés chez l'hybride $F_1(C_{57}Bl—C_3H)$. Cette lignée oppose la résistance la plus faible à l'invasion tumorale, à en juger par la vitesse de croissance du greffon. Or, chez elle, le développement de la tumeur non seulement ne détermine aucun effet stimulant mais, bien au contraire, une dépression du S.R.E. (HALPERN, 1966a)).

Les relations entre la réaction du S.R.E. et la résistance de l'individu à l'invasion tumorale nous paraissent suggestives, bien que le mécanisme fondamental de ce phénomène biologique et sa signification nous échappent. S'agit-il d'une réaction du type homogreffe? Cette hypothèse doit être envisagée du fait que, dans la plupart des affections malignes spontanées, ou transmissibles rigoureusement en série isologue, l'activation du S.R.E. est, le plus souvent, minime ou nulle. Il faudrait admettre que nous avons affaire ici à une réaction du type «greffon contre hôte» qui, seule, détermine une stimulation du S.R.E. (HOWARD, 1964), ce qui n'est pas démontré.

Dans l'état actuel des recherches l'activation du S.R.E., en réponse à l'invasion tumorale, mais qui est observée également dans toute une série d'agressions infectieuses ou immunologiques, est un phénomène biologique positif, dont la portée demande encore à être précisée.

Stimulation du S.R.E. et invasion tumorale

Si la stimulation spontanée du S.R.E. reflète de quelque manière une mobilisation des éléments de défense, dont s'ensuit une résistance accrue de l'organisme à l'invasion tumorale, on devrait logiquement pouvoir amplifier cet effet en agissant expérimentalement sur ce système cellulaire.

Ce fut l'objectif d'une longue série de recherches, entreprises par nous depuis près de 10 ans (HALPERN, 1964a, 1959; BIOZZI, 1959; OLD, 1960) et encore poursuivies à l'heure actuelle. Elles nous ont permis d'accumuler de multiples observations sur l'implication du S.R.E. dans la résistance naturelle de l'individu contre l'invasion tumorale, dont nous ne rapporterons ici que quelques exemples.

Les substances qui stimulent le S.R.E.

Les méthodes quantitatives de mesure de l'activité du S.R.E. que nous avons proposées (BIOZZI, 1953; HALPERN, 1954; BENACERRAF, 1957) ont permis de constater qu'une stimulation du S.R.E. s'observe régulièrement au cours de diverses infections: infections à germes Gram négatif, BCG, infections virales, etc. Parmi les bactéries étudiées les *Mycobactéries* et les *Corynebactéries anaérobies* se sont montrées, à cet égard, particulièrement actives (BIOZZI, 1957, 1960; HALPERN, 1964b). Mais on connaît des substances non bactériennes douées de propriétés de stimuler le S.R.E.: triglycérides (STUART, 1960), zymosan (BENACERRAF, 1959), hormones sexuelles (BIOZZI, 1957).

Dans la bactérie le pouvoir stimulant revient à certains constituants dont la nature exacte n'est pas encore connue. Entre nos mains, un extrait isolé de *Mycob. phlei,* germe non pathogène, s'est montré plus actif que la bactérie entière (HALPERN, 1964a).

Effet de la stimulation du S.R.E. sur le développement de quelques tumeurs expérimentales

Il ressort de toute une série de données, obtenues dans notre laboratoire et confirmées depuis par d'autres (OLD, 1961; BIOZZI, 1959; OLD, 1964), que l'administration de certains substrats microbiens, dont l'effet se traduit par une stimulation de diverses fonctions biologiques des cellules R.E., a pour résultat une augmentation de la résistance de l'hôte à l'invasion tumorale.

1. La figure 2 montre l'effet de l'extrait mycobacterien Wxb 3148 sur le sarcome 180 chez la souris Swiss.

Cette tumeur transplantée détermine régulièrement, chez certaines lignées de

L'extrait, administré à la dose de 400 µg 8 jours auparavant, exerce un effet inhibiteur sur la croissance tumorale et détermine, chez 40 p 100 des animaux, une régression totale de la tumeur avec survie définitive des animaux. Une seule injection suffit pour obtenir un tel résultat. Pour que le traitement soit efficace il faut que l'extrait bactérien soit administré avant ou simultanément avec la trans-

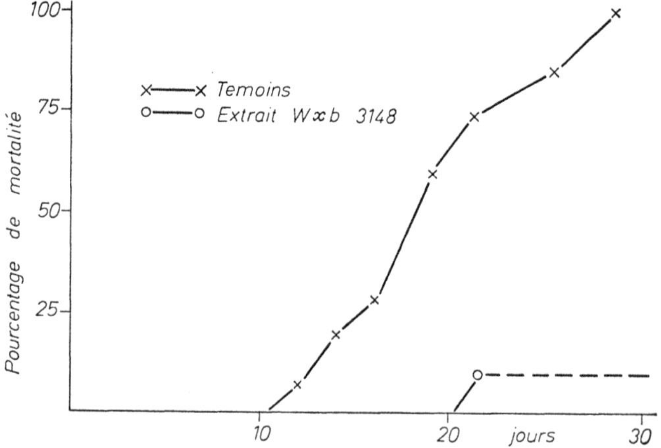

Fig. 2. Evolution de la mortalité chez deux groupes de souris de la même lignée après transplantation du sarcome 180. Groupe témoin: 100 p 100 de mortalité; groupe traité avec l'extrait Wxb 3148: 10 p 100 de mortalité

souris, une mortalité voisine de 100 p 100, en 3 à 4 semaines. Lorsque la tumeur a été greffée chez des animaux ayant reçu, plusieurs jours auparavant, soit du BCG, soit un extrait obtenu de *Mycob. phlei,* désigné ici sous le nom Wxb 3148, les animaux rejettent la tumeur et survivent dans une proportion de 90 p 100.

2. Le sarcome J de Betz est particulièrement virulent chez la souris Swiss. L'inoculation sous-cutanée d'un greffon de 30 mg produit une mortalité de 100 p 100, s'échelonnant entre 16 et 30 jours après la greffe. La figure 3 montre l'effet de l'injection de l'extrait de *Mycob. phlei* sur la croissance du greffon tumoral et la mortalité.

plantation de la tumeur. Ceci pourrait s'expliquer par la nécessité de faire coïncider l'activation du S.R.E. avec le moment où le greffon s'implante dans les tissus.

3. Des résultats similaires ont été observés avec le *Corynebacterium anaérobie.* Cette bactérie, isolée par M. Prevot chez l'homme (Halpern, 1964a), est doué d'un pouvoir stimulant sur le S.R.E. qui est plus intense que celui exercé par les Mycobactéries (Halpern, 1964b). La bactérie est injectée par voie veineuse, à la dose moyenne de 250 µg/20 g, sous forme d'un vaccin tué par la chaleur et formolé.

Les résultats concernant l'effet de la Corynebactérie sur la croissance du sar-

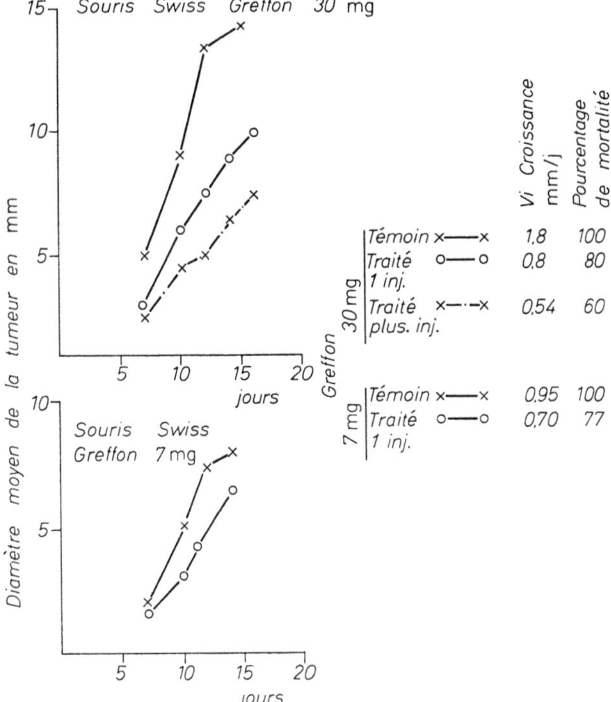

Fig. 3. Action de l'extrait microbien Wxb 3148 sur la vitesse de la croissance du sarcome J et sur la mortalité provoquée par cette tumeur chez la souris » Swiss«

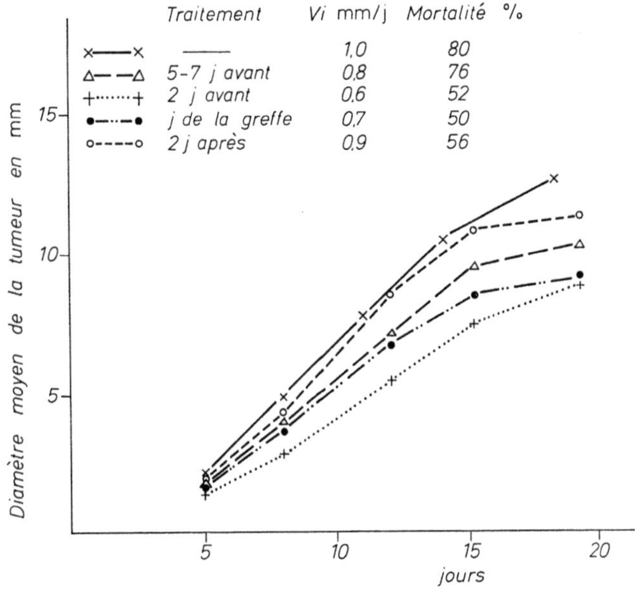

Fig. 4. Influence du traitement avec *Corynebacterium parvum*, administré à des périodes différentes par rapport au moment de la greffe, sur la croissance de la tumeur et sur la mortalité

come J et sur le taux de mortalité sont consignés dans la figure 4.

Il en résulte que la vitesse de la croissance de la tumeur se trouve diminuée chez les animaux traités et que, chez 50 p 100 des animaux, la tumeur régresse définitivement. Ces résultats toutefois ne peuvent être obtenus que si la bactérie est administrée 2 à 4 jours avant ou après la greffe. Comme dans le cas des Mycobactéries, l'augmentation des doses ou la

d'Ehrlich protège efficacement les animaux contre cette tumeur. L'ascite ne se développe pas et les cellules tumorales transplantées disparaissent. La mortalité, qui est de 100 p 100 chez les témoins, est réduite pratiquement à zéro.

Cette action remarquable des Corynebactéries ne s'obtient que lorsqu'elles sont introduites dans la cavité péritonéale, c'est à dire dans le lieu même où s'implante la tumeur ascitique. D'autre part,

Tableau I. *Action protectrice des Corynebactéries contre la tumeur ascitique d'Ehrlich.*
(Les Corynebactéries ont été administrées par voie péritonéale)

Dose de cellules néoplasiques	Dose de Coryneb. μg/20 g	Modalité du traitement	% de mortalité	Temps moyen de survie en jours
	néant	—	100	24
	250	2 jours avant	80	25
	250	le jour même	30	—
	250	1ère le jour même, puis 2 par semaine pendant 3 semaines	10	—
$5 \cdot 10^5$	1000	2 jours avant	60	43
	1000	le jour même	20	—
	1000	1ère le jour même, puis 2 par semaine pendant 3 semaines	10	—

répétition des injections n'apportent pas d'amélioration sensible des résultats.

4. La tumeur ascitique d'Ehrlich ne s'accompagne pas d'une stimulation significative du S.R.E. D'autre part, l'administration du BCG, par voie veineuse, n'affecte que peu l'évolution de cette tumeur épithéliale (Biozzi, 1959). Les résultats ne sont guère meilleurs avec la Corynebactérie administrée par voie veineuse.

Par contre, la Corynebactérie exerce des effets protecteurs tout à fait remarquables lorsqu'elle est administrée par voie péritonéale, dans certaines conditions expérimentales (Halpern, 1966). Les résultats de ces expériences sont résumés dans le tableau I.

Ainsi l'administration de Corynebactéries à des animaux auxquels on vient d'implanter une tumeur ascitique

contrairement à ce qu'on observe dans les autres exemples où le traitement n'est efficace que s'il précède de plusieurs jours la greffe néoplasique, ici l'action est maximale lorsque la bactérie est administrée simultanément ou quelques jours après la greffe.

La Corynebactérie étant dépourvue de toute action propre sur les cellules néoplasiques, il faut admettre qu'elle agit par un mécanisme général.

Mécanismes impliqués

L'introduction de la méthode de mesure quantitative de l'activité phagocytaire du S.R.E. a rendu possible une étude des corrélations entre le potentiel d'activité de cette population cellulaire et le degré de résistance opposé par l'organisme à l'invasion tumorale.

Les avis sont unanimes pour reconnaître que l'implantation de certaines tumeurs cancéreuses s'accompagne rapidement d'une activation du S.R.E. Cette modification biologique a été observée avec divers sarcomes, après inoculation du virus de la leucémie de Friend, après administration de substances cancérigènes *per os*. Cependant, ce phénomène fait défaut dans la plupart des cancers spontanés : leucémie AKR, tumeurs mammaires, etc.

Si l'on considère maintenant l'action de divers agents qui stimulent le S.R.E. sur les divers types de tumeurs, on constate que ceux-ci sont doués de propriétés inhibitrices plus ou moins puissantes à l'égard de toutes les tumeurs dont le développement détermine précisément une activation du S.R.E. Il semble y avoir une relation assez constante entre ces deux phénomènes. Ainsi, les Mycobactéries et les Corynebactéries n'affectent que peu les tumeurs spontanées ou celles qui sont transmissibles spécifiquement en série isogénique. Cette constatation est à l'origine de plusieurs hypothèses quant au mode d'action de ces substances. Une des hypothèses est que les substances activatrices du S.R.E. agiraient par leurs propriétés adjuvantes, en exaltant une réponse immunologique à l'égard des antigènes présents dans le greffon tumoral. Cette thèse n'explique pas tous les faits expérimentaux. En effet, l'extrait de *Mycob. phlei,* Wxb 3148, qui s'est montré aussi efficace dans les diverses tumeurs, est dépourvu de toute propriété adjuvante. Il serait également difficile d'expliquer, sur cette base, l'action sur les tumeurs induites par ingestion de substances cancérigènes, ou encore l'effet remarquable des Corynebactéries dans les tumeurs ascitiques, qui est plus intense lorsque le vaccin est administré après l'inoculation de la tumeur qu'avant.

Les résultats que nous avons rapportés par ailleurs (HALPERN, 1964a) indiquent que, chez les animaux préimmunisés avec la tumeur, l'administration des substrats actifs ne renforce pas l'effet de la préimmunisation. Il est donc malaisé de rattacher ces effets à une action dite adjuvante, autrement dit à la majoration de la réponse immunologique humorale ou tout au moins à elle seule.

Le rôle des anticorps humoraux dans l'immunité antitumorale paraît négligeable. MITCHISON (1955) à montré qu'il est impossible de conférer passivement l'immunité antitumorale à l'aide du sérum. Par contre, les cellules ganglionnaires régionales, prélevées chez un animal guéri, protègent le receveur contre la prise d'une tumeur du même type. L'interprétation qui nous paraît la plus plausible est que les agents qui activent le S.R.E. renforcent les facteurs de défense cellulaires. L'attaque cellulaire contre l'intrus est plus intense. Ceci se traduit non seulement par la multiplication des cellules réticulo-histiocytaires, mais aussi par l'exaltation de leur pouvoir phagocytaire et cytolytique. Nos recherches ont montré, en effet, que la stimulation du S.R.E. se traduit par l'augmentation parallèle de l'activité phagocytaire et de l'activité enzymatique de ces cellules (BIOZZI, 1959).

Cette augmentation de la résistance n'est pas spécifiquement dirigée contre les tumeurs. Les animaux ainsi traités manifestent simultanément un accroissement de leur résistance à l'égard d'autres agressions : infections bactériennes et virales, choc traumatique. Les deux ordres de phénomènes coïncident dans leur chronologie et dans leur développement. L'illustration la plus remarquable de cet état de choses est la récente constatation (BIOZZI, 1965) concernant la réaction greffon contre hôte chez les hybrides F_1. On sait que les hybrides F_1

sont incapables de rejeter la greffe de cellules parentales car l'hybride hérite de tous les antigènes d'histocompatibilité des cellules parentales. Si le greffon est constitué de cellules immunologiquement compétentes, celles-ci s'implantent régulièrement chez le receveur. Dans le cas d'une combinaison d'histoincompatibilité «forte», les cellules spléniques réagissent contre les constituants antigéniques hérités de l'autre lignée parentale, ce qui entraine souvent la mort de l'animal, par un syndrôme de «runt disease».

Or, si l'on administre à l'hybride, avant l'implantation des cellules spléniques parentales, une dose adéquate de Corynebactéries, les animaux traités ne manifestent aucun symptôme de «runting» et survivent définitivement. Mettant à profit la présence du marqueur chromosomique T_6 dans les cellules de la souche CBA, Howard (comm. per.) a montré que cette survie des hybrides est due à la destruction par l'hôte des cellules parentales transplantées. Ceci pose un problème immunologique sans précédent puisque, d'après les concepts immunologiques actuels, l'hybride est incapable de réagir contre les cellules parentales en raison de leur identité antigénique. Faut-il admettre qu'il se produit normalement une certaine reconnaissance des cellules parentales par l'hybride, suivie d'une réaction immunologique, trop faible dans les conditions habituelles mais qui devient efficace chez les animaux dont le S.R.E. a été stimulé? C'est l'explication la plus logique des faits.

Si cette interprétation, qui n'est pas conforme aux conceptions immunologiques présentes, s'avère exacte, on pourrait trouver là l'explication du rejet des tumeurs homologues chez les animaux dont le S.R.E. a été stimulé. Pour l'instant, ceci n'est encore qu'une hypothèse.

Pour terminer nous voudrions ajouter que, si les faits sont ce qu'ils sont, leur interprétation demeure encore hypothétique. Ce rapport est une synthèse d'un nombre considérable de recherches personnelles, dans lesquelles nous en avons entrainé d'autres, concernant l'implication du S.R.E. dans la résistance naturelle contre les infections bactériennes et l'invasion tumorale. Hormis quelques exceptions, nous avons observé régulièrement une activation du S.R.E. dans la phase initiale de la plupart des infections bactériennes et dans les néoplasies transmises par greffe. La stimulation du S.R.E. inhibe, d'une manière très importante, la croissance tumorale et en provoque souvent la régression. On ne peut pas ignorer ces faits. Lorsqu'on scrute les processus de l'invasion tumorale, c'est à dire les forces que l'organisme oppose au développement et à l'extension néoplasique, on doit prendre obligatoirement en considération le S.R.E.

Summary

The implication of the reticulo-histiocytic cells system in the antitumoral defence is now well established.

There is a correlation between the propension to cancerigenesis and the activity potential of the R.E.S.

Cancerigenesis whether induced by certain chemical agents or by grafting is accompanied by the activation of the R.E.S. The phenomenon is less evident when the grafted tumour is specifically isologous.

The previous stimulation of R.E.S. by Mycobacteries and their extracts or by heat killed *Corynebacterium parvum* causes a considerable slowing down of the tumour growth and even a rejection of the tumour, followed by definitive recovery.

The fact that the *Corynebacterium parvum* protects the animal against the runt disease induced by graft-versus-host reaction leads to the speculation that the rejection of tumours in animals so treated may be related to a similar mechanism.

Résumé

Le rôle du système réticulo-histiocytaire dans la défense antitumorale a été bien démontré.

Il existe une corrélation entre la propension à la tumorigénèse et le potentiel d'activité du S.R.E.

La cancérigénèse, qu'elle soit liée à l'action de certains agents chimiques ou à la transplantation d'un greffon tumoral, s'accompagne d'une activation du S.R.E. Cette activation est moins importante lorsque la tumeur greffée est spécifiquement isologue.

La stimulation préalable du S.R.E., soit à l'aide de Mycobactéries ou de certains extraits de Mycobactéries, soit à l'aide de Corynébactéries tuées, détermine un ralentissement de la croissance des tumeurs, voire un rejet de la tumeur avec guérison de l'animal.

Le fait que les Corynébactéries protègent l'animal contre la maladie homologue provoquée par la réaction greffon contre hôte permet de spéculer que le rejet des tumeurs isogéniques, sous l'effet de ce traitement, relève du même mécanisme.

Discussion

Questions put to Prof. B. HALPERN

G. Vogt: May I ask Prof. HALPERN if, in his animals, activation of the reticulo-endothelial system produces a morphological effect analogous to that observed in man. What organs were examined? Spleen, regional lymph nodes, or local reticulo-endothelial tissue surrounding the tumour transplants?

S. Wood: Prof. HALPERN, the role of the reticulo-endothelial system in the dissemination of malignant tumours has been discussed in an eloquent and dynamic fashion in your presentation. Its precise role, however, in metastasis formation from blood-borne cancer cells and in the destruction and/or elimination of neoplasic cells from the microvascular system still remains, to me, unclear.

Our laboratory has been interested in the reticulo-endothelial system and in the microvascular system in the rabbit. I would appreciate your comments on the following observations.

1. Ascitic V 2 carcinoma cells were injected intravenously into rabbits that had received a single prior intravenous inoculation (1 or 10 or 18 hours *before* injection of tumour cells) of 10 µg of endotoxin from *E. Coli*. At autopsy 21 days later the frequency of pulmonary metastases was doubled. However, the most prominent increase in the number of metastases was observed in the extrapulmonary organs (EPM), especially the liver, spleen, adrenal, and kidney, the organs most altered by endotoxin (especially the liver) [cf. Bull. Swiss Acad. med. Sci. **20**, 92—121 (1964)].

2. Ten µg of this endotoxin is about one-fifth of the LD_{50} and evokes the characteristic biphasic febrile responses — thrombocytopenia, leucopenia, and marked leucocytic sticking and aggregation with platelet clumping — observed *in vivo* in the rabbit ear chamber. These changes in the microvascular system are precisely those alterations that have previously been associated with an increased frequency and distribution of metastasis formation from blood-borne

cancer cells in the rabbit [cf. Canad. Cancer Conf. **4**, 167—223 (1961)].

3. In addition to the above findings, it may also be noted that the rabbit rendered tolerant by the daily intravenous inoculation of endotoxin for 10—14 days shows a far greater susceptibility to the formation of metastatic carcinoma developing from blood-borne cancer cells.

4. One further point warrants mention. A number of other investigators have suggested that, in addition to the hypofibrinogenia associated with the intravenous inoculation of endotoxin in the rabbit, a significant degree of fibrinolysis may also be induced. Since fibrinolytic enzymes have been shown to reduce the incidence of metastasis formation from blood-borne cancer cells, why does endotoxin not also protect the rabbit, rather than render it more susceptible? It appears that whatever degree of fibrinolysis may occur after endotoxin treatment, it is completely vitiated by the *endothelial stickiness* i) which commences within 15 minutes after endotoxin treatment and continue for at least 18 hours, and ii) which appears from the above studies and references to represent a decisive factor favouring the adhesion, penetration, and growth of blood-borne cancer cells within the microvascular system.

B. Halpern: The endotoxin may act in two ways:

1. We have shown that endotoxins exert a biphasic action on the reticuloendothelial system, starting with a negative phase which lasts 12—24 hours and during which a considerable decrease in RES activity is observed. This negative phase may perhaps facilitate the implantation of neoplasic cells carried by the blood-stream into other organs.

2. The endotoxin helps the cells to stick to the vascular walls. This may be the mechanism by which the endotoxin facilitates the implantation of tumour cells in vascular beds where such implantation would not normally take place.

G. Barski: In a recent study, carried out in collaboration with Dr. Belehradek and Dr. Kawamata, we also concerned ourselves with the effect of RES stimulation on malignant growth. We used an ascites tumour and RES stimulation was effected by means of intraperitoneal injections of glycogen solution. We established that this stimulation exerted only a local effect, that this effect did not depend on the presence of an excessive number of macrophages in the peritoneal cavity, and that the specific immunological reaction was not enhanced in the animals treated with glycogen.

P. Strauli: Following intraperitoneal implantation of the Walker carcinosarcoma 256, we observed the appearance of large "lymphoid" cells in the thoracic duct lymph within the first 24 hours after transplantation. In normal animals, very few of these elements can be seen. Although, this is not an immunological reaction, it must be the expression of a stimulation of the reticulo-endothelial system.

Bibliographie

Aschoff, L., Reticulo-endothelial system. In: *Lectures on pathology.* New York: Hoeber 1924.

Benacerraf, B., Biozzi, G., Halpern, B. N., and Stiffel, C., Physiology of phagocytosis of particles by R.E.S. In: B. N. Halpern (ed.), *Symposium on physiopathology of the R.E.S.*, p. 52. Oxford: Blackwell Sci. Publ. 1957.

Benacerraf, B., Thorbecke, G. J., and Jacoby, D., The effect of zymosan on endotoxin toxicity in mice. *Proc. Soc. exp. Biol. (N.Y.)* **100**, 796—799 (1959).

BESHFORD, E. F., MURRAY, J. A., and HOALAND, M., Resistance and susceptibility to inoculated cancer. III. — Scientific report on the investigations of the Imperial Cancer Research Fund, London 1908, p. 351 and 359.

BETZ, E. H., Immunisation de souris C57Bl par un sarcome spontané provenant d'une souris de même race. In: P. B. MEDAWAR (ed.), *Biological problems of grafting.* Oxford: Blackwell Sci. Publ. 1959.

BIOZZI, G., BENACERRAF, B., and HALPERN, B. N., Quantitative study of granulopectic activity of the reticulo-endothelial system. *Brit. J. exp. Path.* **34**, 441 (1953).

— HALPERN, B. N., BENACERRAF, B., and STIFFEL, C., Phagocytic activity of the reticulo-endothelial system in experimental infections. In: B. N. HALPERN (ed.), *Symposium on physiopathology of the R.E.S.*, p. 204. Oxford: Blackwell Sci. Publ. 1957a.

— — BILBEY, D., STIFFEL, C., BENACERRAF, B., et MOUTON, D., Oestrogènes et fonction phagocytaire du S.R.E. *C.R. Soc. Biol. (Paris)* **151**, 1326—1331 (1957b).

— — et STIFFEL, C., Stimulation du S.R.E. par l'extrait microbien Wxb 3148 et résistance aux infections expérimentales. In: B. N. HALPERN (ed.), *Rôle du S.R.E. dans l'immunité antibactérienne et antitumorale*, p. 205. Paris: C.N.R.S. 1964.

— HOWARD, J. G., MOUTON, D., and STIFFEL, C., Modifications of graft-versus host reaction induced by pretreatment of the host with *M. tuberculosis* and *C. parvum. Transplantation* **3**, 170—177 (1965).

— STIFFEL, C., HALPERN, B. N. et MOUTON, D., Etude de la fonction phagocytaire du S.R.E. au cours du développement de tumeurs malignes expérimentales chez le rat et la souris. *Ann. Inst. Pasteur* **94**, 681—693 (1958).

— — — — Effet de l'inoculation du bacille de Calmette-Guérin sur le développement de la tumeur ascitique d'Ehrlich chez la souris. *C.R. Soc. Biol. (Paris)* **153**, 987—989 (1959a).

— — — — Etude de la fonction métabolique des cellules de Küpffer. *Rev. franç. Étud. clin. biol.* **4**, 427—441 (1959b).

— — — — Recherches sur le mécanisme de l'immunité non spécifique produite par les Mycobactéries. *Rev. franç. Étud. clin. biol.* **5**, 876—890 (1960).

BIOZZI, G., STIFFEL, C., MATHÉ, G., MOUTON, D. et HALPERN, B. N., Activité phagocytaire du S.R.E. chez la souris de lignée pure après greffe de cellules leucémiques isologues ou homologues et au cours du développement de la leucémie spontanée. *Bull. Ass. franç. Cancer* **46**, 781—791 (1959c).

DAVIDSOHN, I., and STERN, K., Natural and immune antibodies in mice of low and high tumor strains. *Cancer Res.* **9**, 426 (1949).

HALPERN, B. N., BENACERRAF, B., BIOZZI, G. et STIFFEL, C., Facteurs régissant la fonction phagocytaire du S.R.E. *Rev. Hémat.* **9**, 621—642 (1954).

— BIOZZI, G. et STIFFEL, C., Action de l'extrait microbien Wxb 3148 sur l'évolution des tumeurs expérimentales. In: B. N. HALPERN (ed.), *Rôle du S.R.E. dans l'immunité antibactérienne et antitumorale*, p. 221. Paris: C.N.R.S. 1964.

— — —, et MOUTON, D., Phagocytic function of the R.E.S. and experimental tumors. In: J. H. HELLER (ed.), *Reticuloendothelial structure and function*, p. 259. New York: Ronald Press Co. 1958.

— — — — Effet de la stimulation du système réticulo-endothélial par l'inoculation du B.C.G. sur le développement de l'épithélioma atypique de Guérin chez le rat. *C.R. Soc. Biol. (Paris)* **153**, 919—923 (1959).

— — — — Inhibition of tumour growth by administration of *Corynebacterium parvum. Nature (London)* **212**, 853—854 (1966).

— PREVOT, A.-R., BIOZZI, G., STIFFEL, C., MOUTON, D., MORARD, J.-C., BOUTHILLIER, Y. et DECREUSEFOND, C., Stimulation de l'activité phagocytaire du système réticulo-endothélial provoquée par *Corynebacterium parvum. J. reticulo-endothelial Soc.* **1**, 77—96 (1964).

— STIFFEL, C., BIOZZI, G. et MOUTON, D., Influence des hormones sexuelles sur la stimulation de la fonction phagocytaire du S.R.E. provoquée par l'inoculation du bacille de Calmette-Guérin (BCG) chez la souris. *C.R. Soc. Biol. (Paris)* **154**, 1994—2001 (1960).

HOWARD, J. G., A study of R.E. function during graft-versus-host reaction in the adult mouse. In: B. N. HALPERN (ed.), *Rôle du S.R.E. dans la défense antibactérienne et anti-tumorale*, p. 369. Paris: C.N.R.S. 1964.

— CHRISTIE, G. H., BOAK, J. L. et EVANS-ANFOM, E., Evidence for the conversion of lymphocytes into liver macrophages during graft-versus-host reaction In: *La greffe des cellules hématopoetiques allogéniques*, p. 95. Paris: C.N.R.S. 1965.

KAMPFSCHMIDT, R. F., CLABAUGH, W. A., and AVIEDONDO, M. I., Phagocytosis of colloidal carbon by the R.E.S. during hepato-carcinogenesis in rats. *Proc. Soc. exp. Biol. (N.Y.)* **108**, 216—219 (1961).

MITCHISON, N. A., Studies on the immuno-logical response to foreign tumor trans-plants in the mouse. I. The role of lymph node cells in conferring immunity by adop-tive transfer. *J. exp. Med.* **102**, 157—177 (1955).

MURPHY, J. B., *The lymphocytes in resistance to tissue grafting, malignant disease and tuberculosis infection*. Monograph of the Rockefeller In-stitute for Medical Research, New York 1961.

OLD, L. J., BENACERRAF, B., CLARKE, D. A., CARSWELL, E. A., and STOCKERT, E., The role of the reticulo-endothelial system in the host reaction to neoplasia. *Cancer Res.* **21**, 1281—1301 (1961).

OLD, L. J., CLARKE, D. A., BENACERRAF, B., and GOLDSMITH, M., The reticulo-endothelial system and the neoplasic process. *Ann. N.Y. Acad. Sci.* **88**, 264—280 (1960).

PREVOT, A.-R., Les corynebactéries anaérobies. *Ergebn. Mikrobiol.* **33**, 1—48 (1960).

STERN, K., The reticulo-endothelial system and neoplasia. In: *Reticulo-endothelial structure and function*, p. 233 (J. H. HELLER ed.). New York: Ronald Press 1960.

STUART, A. E., BIOZZI, G., STIFFEL, C., HAL-PERN, B. N., and MOUTON, D., The stimu-lation and depression of reticulo-endothelial phagocytic function by simple lipids. *Brit. J. exp. Path.* **41**, 599—604 (1960).

WEISS, D. W., BOUHARG, R. S., and DEOME, K. B., Protective activity of fractions of tubercle bacilli against isologous tumours in mice. *Nature (Lond.)* **190**, 889—891 (1961).

Rôle de la Facilitation Immunologique dans le Développement des Tumeurs Cancéreuses

Guy André Voisin

Centre d'Immuno-Pathologie de l'Association Claude-Bernard (Directeur: Professeur R. Kourilsky), Hôpital Saint-Antoine, Paris 12éme, France

Il a été démontré depuis longtemps (Bride, 1907), surtout par Casey (1932—34) et par Kaliss (1951—55) qu'une injection de tissus tumoraux lyophilisés, loin souvent d'entraîner une immunisation du receveur, peut augmenter sa susceptibilité à l'injection de cellules vivantes de la même tumeur. Cette augmentation de susceptibilité, due au phénomène de Facilitation Immunologique (Enhancement Phenomenon) se traduit par une augmentation du pourcentage de prise des tumeurs et du volume des tumeurs qui prennent; par une augmentation du nombre et du volume des métastases, apparemment sans modification de leur répartition relative; enfin par une augmentation de mortalité chez les animaux homogreffés traités.

Ces faits suffisent à montrer qu'une étude du mécanisme de l'invasion dans le cancer ne peut ignorer le phénomène de Facilitation Immunologique.

Notre dessein est:

1. de rappeler l'essentiel des faits concernant l'action de la facilitation dans les tumeurs homotransplantées. Notre travail personnel dans ce domaine est encore préliminaire.

2. De montrer que ce phénomène déborde largement le cadre des tumeurs homogreffées: c'est à ce problème que nous avons consacré plusieurs travaux expérimentaux.

3. D'envisager enfin certains des problèmes soulevés par l'existence de ce phénomène ainsi que son rôle éventuel dans le développement et l'invasion des tumeurs autologues.

I. La Facilitation Immunologique dans les Tumeurs Homotransplantées

L'essentiel de ce que l'on en connaît aujourd'hui provient des travaux de plusieurs chercheurs: Casey d'abord qui a appliqué au phénomène la qualificatif de enhancement puis l'a dénommé phénomène XYZ, ce qui mettait l'accent sur son caractère, déroutant (Casey, 1932—59). Kaliss ensuite, au cours d'importants travaux portant avant tout sur le Sarcome I des souris de lignée Ajax a précisé la nature immunologique spécifique du phénomène et plusieurs de ses éléments essentiels Kaliss, 1951—62. Enfin il faut retenir les travaux de Snell. 1948—52, ceux de Gorer, 1955—59; Kandutsch, 1962; de Mitchison, 1955a et b; et, plus récemment, ceux de Möller.

De ces travaux, il ressort essentiellement que: 1. Lorsque l'on injecte à une souris future receveuse des cellules vivantes (tumorales ou normales) provenant d'une souris de lignée allogénique future donneuse, cette souris réagira à une greffe tumorale de même origine par une réaction de rejet accéléré de 2ème set (Fig. 1 et 2). Par contre, si l'on prépare

11*

la souris receveuse par des extraits, des broyats ou des lyophilisats d'origine allogénique, souvent la greffe tumorale de

dans notre laboratoire (Kinsky et Voisin, données non publiées) que des souris $B_{10}D_2$, porteuses de Sa I facilités, pré-

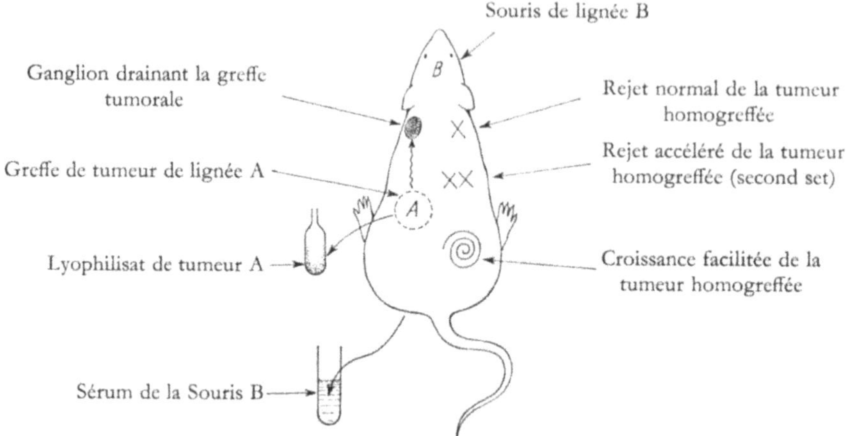

Fig. 1. Légendes des figures 2 à 5

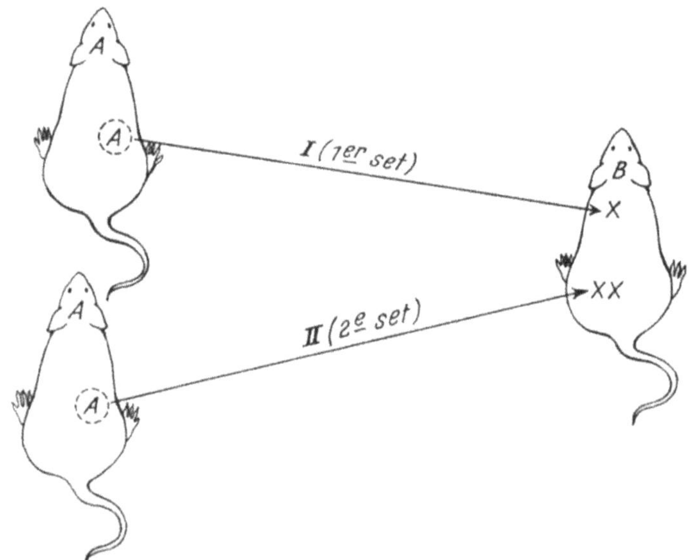

Fig. 2. Représentation schématique de l'immunisation active de rejet: second set

même origine, non seulement ne sera pas rejetée, mais verra sa croissance augmentée (enhanced), sa persistance facilitée, avec métastases plus nombreuses, l'ensemble conduisant souvent à la mort de la souris (Fig. 3). Il a été constaté

sentaient souvent des ascites tumorales. Il faut souligner que, dans des conditions bien particulières de dosage et de temps, chacun des deux traitements précédents peut conduire à des résultats exactement inverses. 2. Il est d'ailleurs possible de dissocier ces deux phénomènes d'immunisation et de facilitation *qui coexistent chez un même animal* ayant teçu une homomunisation, répondant à une 2ème homogreffe tumorale par un rejet accéléré; plusieurs semaines après la 1ère homogreffe,

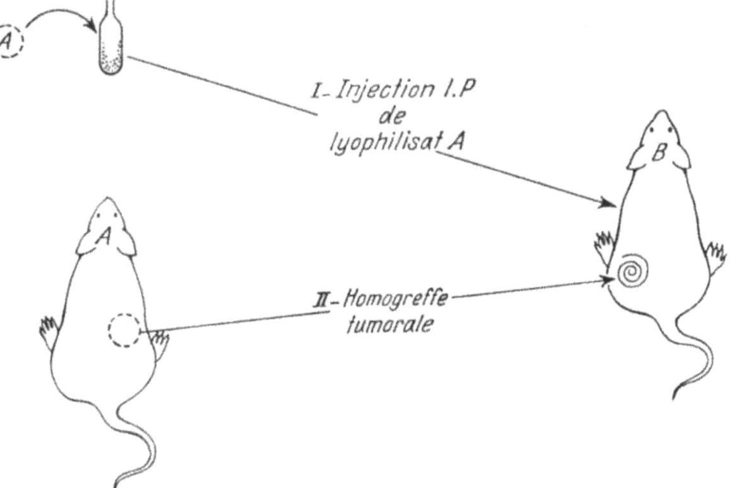

Fig. 3. Représentation schématique de l'immunisation active facilitante ou facilitation active

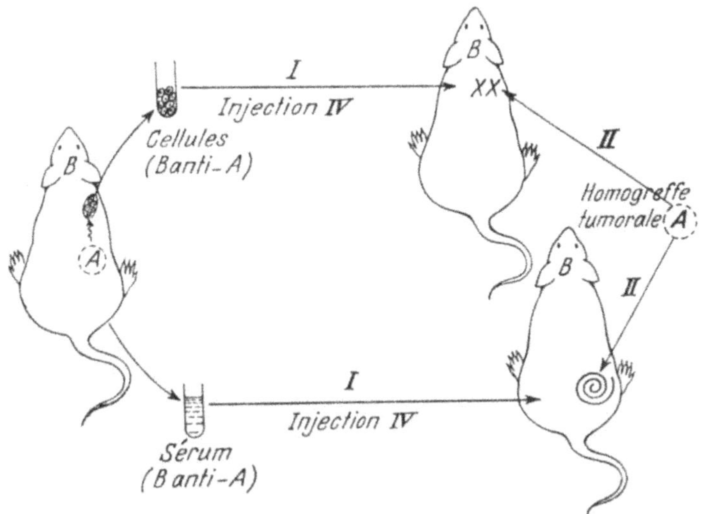

Fig. 4. Dissociation des 2 réactions immunitaires actives de rejet et de facilitation: par transfert cellulaire adoptif (rejet) et transfert sérique passif (facilitation)

greffe de cellules vivantes normales ou tumorales. On peut réaliser cette dissociation au moyen du facteur temps ou du facteur de médiation.

a) *Facteur Temps*, plusieurs jours après la 1ère homogreffe, l'animal est en état d'immunisation, répondant à la 2ème homogreffe tumorale par un rejet accéléré; plusieurs semaines après la 1ère homogreffe, l'animal est, dans certains cas, dans un état de facilitation, répondant à la 2ème homogreffe tumorale pour une acceptation sans rejet, avec prolifération de la tumeur.

b) *Facteur de Médiation* (Fig. 4): les cellules lymphoïdes du ganglion drainant le site de la 1ère homogreffe sont capables de transférer adoptivement à un animal neuf isogénique la capacité de rejeter de façon accélérée une greffe tumorale de même origine (aptitude optimum des cellules vers le 5ème jour); alors que le sérum du même animal peut, à petites doses, transférer passivement à un animal neuf la propriété de ne pas rejeter une

tation aux cellules lymphoïdes et du délai d'immunisation.

4. On sait que les *anticorps* anti antigène H-2 ont une action qui peut être cytotoxique ou facilitante vis-à-vis des cellules tumorales homogreffées. Pendant plusieurs années, on a cru que certaines cellules (leucémiques EL 4 par exemple) étaient susceptibles uniquement à l'ac-

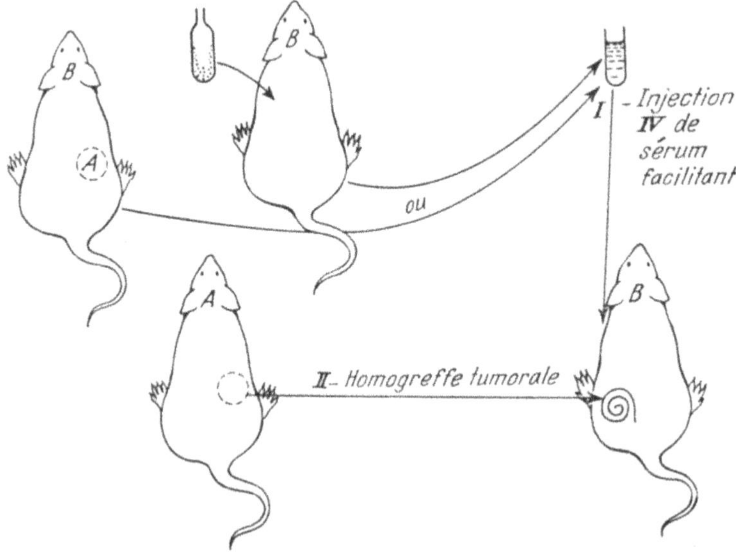

Fig. 5. Représentation schematique de l'immunisation passive facilitante ou facilitation passive

homogreffe tumorale de même origine (aptitude optimum du sérum à partir du 15ème jour) (Mitchison, 1955a et b): des immunoglobulines spécifiques sont responsables de ce phénomène Kaliss, 1956a (Fig. 5).

3. Ces deux phénomènes immunologiquement spécifiques (immunisation et facilitation) sont sous la dépendance d'*antigènes* très proches et vraisemblablement identiques (à détermination génétique H-2 dans le cas des tumeurs de la souris) (Snell, 1957; Gorer, 1961). Le type de réaction (immunisation ou facilitation) est sans doute sous la dépendance de la dose d'antigène administrée, de la voie d'introduction, du mode de présen-

tion cytotoxique des anticorps H-2 alors que d'autres cellules (telles que celles du Sarcome 1 A) n'étaient sensibles qu'à l'action facilitante et que certaines (Sarcome BP 8 par exemple) étaient sensibles aux deux actions (Gorer,1958—61). On sait aujourd'hui que toutes les cellules tumorales étudiées sont, dans certaines conditions, susceptibles aux 2 actions: facilitante aux «doses faibles», cytotoxique aux «doses fortes» d'antisérum. Seule varie la quantité abolue efficace d'anticorps. On sait aussi que plus une cellule tumorale est résistante à l'action cytotoxique «in vitro», plus large sera l'étendue des doses d'antisérum capable d'entraîner la facilitation «in vitro». Ces faits ne précisent pas si le type d'action (cytotoxique ou facilitant) est déterminé par une quantité différente d'un même anticorps ou par deux anticorps différents.

Ce résumé est incomplet; il précise seulement quelques points importants pour la compréhension du phénomène. Plusieurs revues récentes donnent plus de détails sur ces questions: celles de BATCHELOR (1963), de MÖLLER (1963), de

A. Facilitation de Tissus Normaux de Nouveau-Nés. Le premier tissu que nous avons choisi, en raison de ses ressemblances avec le tissu tumoral, est le tissu embryonnaire ou, plutôt, celui du souriceau nouveau-né. On sait que la maladie homologue est une variété particulière de la réaction de transplantation, due au fait que des cellules immunologiquement compétentes, injectées à un hôte allogénique incapable de se défendre

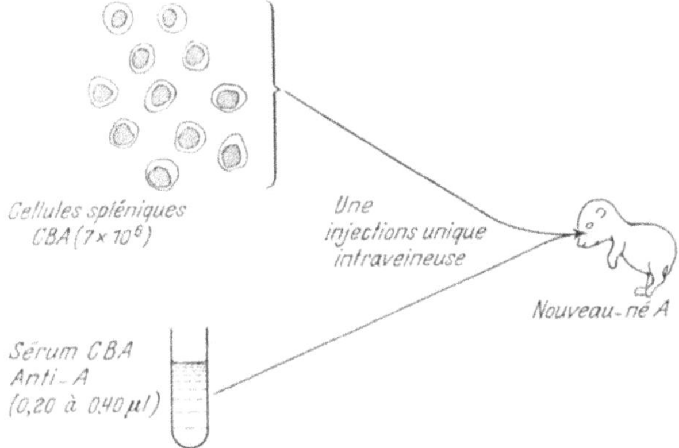

Fig. 6. Schéma des expériences de facilitation passive des souriceaux nouveau-nés contre la maladie homologue

VOISIN (1963); d'autres, moins récentes, demeurent classiques: celles de KALISS (1958), de SNELL (1957) et de GÖRER (1961). Il faut maintenant examiner si un phénomène comparable est retrouvé dans des situations immunologiques autres que celle rencontrée par les homogreffes de tissu tumoral.

II. La Facilitation Immunologique, Expression d'un Mécanisme Général de la Réponse Immunitaire

Lorsque nous avons traduit le mot «enhancement» en français, en 1957, nous avons choisi le terme de «facilitation» immunologique (KALISS, 1958) car des arguments théoriques nous faisaient penser que c'était un phénomène général et nous avons cherché alors à l'appliquer à des tissus non tumoraux.

réagissent immunologiquement contre lui. Nous avons donc essayé de faire bénéficier des animaux nouveau-nés dela réaction de facilitation immunologique pour les protéger contre la maladie homologue des avortons entraînée par l'injection intraveineuse de cellules spléniques allogéniques. Facilitation passive et facilitation active ont été successivement mises en oeuvre.

1. *Expériences de Facilitation Passive* (VOISIN et KINSKY, 1962, Fig. 6). Des souriceaux nouveau-nés Ajax sont divisés en 3 groupes dans chacune de 75 portées: 83 animaux, témoins normaux de portée ne reçoivent rien, 170 animaux témoins reçoivent, dans la veine, 7 millions de cellules spléniques CBA avec, parfois, 0,20 à 0,40 μl de sérum normal CBA (qui ne modifie en rien la réaction:

71% de ces animaux sont morts après 35 jours; 45% seulement, par contre, sont morts parmi les 197 animaux qui ont reçu la même dose des mêmes cellules dose que la dose «facilitante». La quantité d'antisérum injecté semble jouer un rôle.

Ces expériences ont été les premières, en leur temps, à démontrer la possibilité

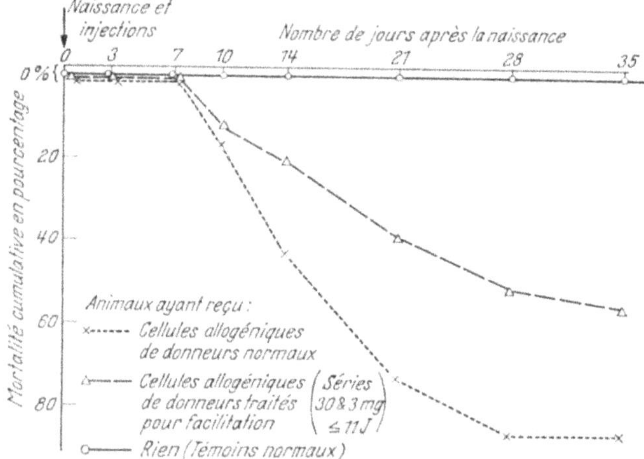

Fig. 7. Facilitation passive des souriceaux nouveau-nés: Courbes de mortalité cumulative. Action d'un sérum très actif. Nombre d'animaux présents le jour 0:18 témoins normaux; 40 animaux protégés; 33 animaux non protégés

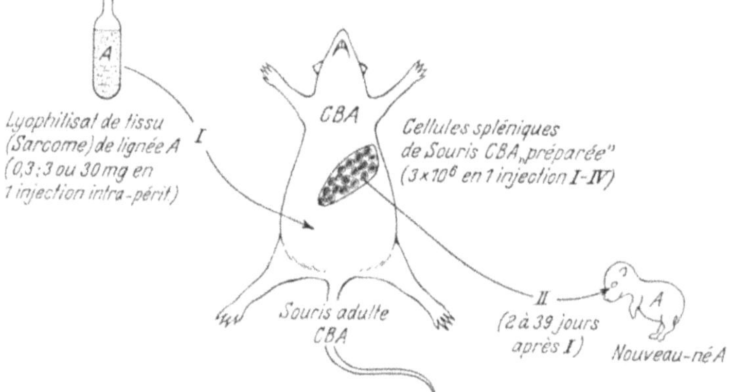

Fig. 8. Schéma des expériences de facilitation active des souriceaux nouveau-nés contre la maladie homologue

CBA additionnées de 0,40 μl (en moyenne) de sérum CBA anti-A. L'activité des divers antisérums est variable (Fig. 7) et fonction de l'immunisation des animaux donneurs, de la présence d'anticorps hémagglutinants et du pouvoir «bréphotoxique» (toxique pour le nouveau-né) de ces sérums employés à plus forte d'appliquer le phénomène de facilitation immunologique à des tissus non tumoraux.

2. *Expériences de Facilitation Active* (Voisin, Kinsky et Maillard, 1964) (Fig. 8). Des souriceaux nouveau-nés A/He sont divisés en 3 groupes dans chacune de 64 portées: 52 animaux,

témoins normaux de portée, ne reçoivent rien; 73 animaux témoins reçoivent, dans la veine, 3 millions de cellules spléniques CBA normales; 136 animaux reçoivent 3 millions de cellules spléniques d'animaux CBA préparés. Cette préparation, faite en vue de facilitation active, consistait à injecter au futur donneur de cellules spléniques

gène): un délai 11 jours se montre actif (Fig. 9) (56% de mortalité au lieu de 87% chez les témoins), un délai 12 jours est inactif et peut-être même immunisant (66% de mortalité contre 57% chez les témoins). Il faut noter qu'il existe une liaison inverse, très significative entre le pouvoir hémagglutinant des sérums CBA anti A et le pouvoir agressif des

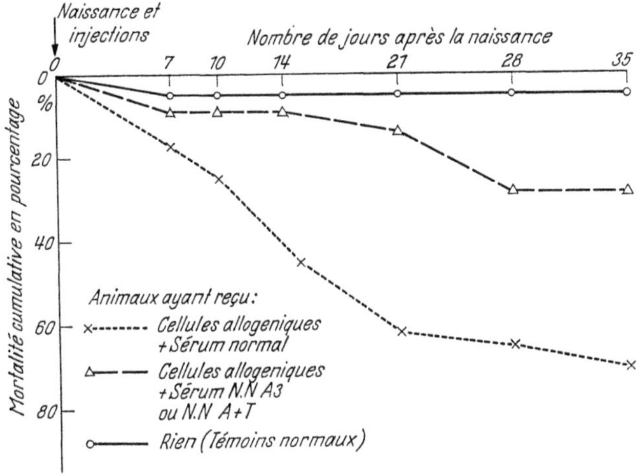

Fig. 9. Facilitation active des nouveau-nés: Courbes de mortalité cumulative. Nombre d'animaux présents le jour 0:21 témoins normaux; 48 souriceaux traités par cellules spléniques provenant de souris CBA préparées depuis moins de 12 jours pour facilitation active envers la lignée A au moyen de 3 ou 30 mg de lyophilisat de Sa 1; 30 souriceaux traités par cellules spléniques CBA normales

des antigènes de lignée A sous forme d'un lyophilisat de tumeur Sa I, procédé connu comme très efficace pour promouvoir une réaction de facilitation envers des tumeurs de lignée A chez des souris allogéniques. Les cellules spléniques CBA provenant de ces animaux ont entraîné chez les nouveau-nés A une mortalité moins importante que celles provenant d'animaux non traités. On a mis en évidence l'importance du rôle de la dose de l'antigène utilisé pour immunisation: 30 mg et 3 mg sont actifs (61% de mortalité au lieu de 71% chez les témoins), 0,3 mg sont inactifs; ainsi que le rôle du délai d'immunisation (après injection de 30 ou 3 mg d'anti-

cellules spléniques provenant des mêmes souris.

B. Facilitation de Tissus Adultes Normaux Transplantés. Puisque des tissus adultes normaux (spléniques par exemple) lyophilisés peuvent induire une réaction de facilitation immunologique, qu'elle est due à des anticorps dirigés contre des antigènes H-2 et que des tissus non tumoraux (souris nouveau-né) peuvent en bénéficier, on doit se demander si des tissus adultes normaux homotransplantés ne peuvent pas en bénéficier également. C'est bien le cas, en particulier pour le tissu ovarien comme le suggéraient fortement les travaux de LINDER (1962) et comme l'a plus récemment démontré Möller (1963.) En ce qui concerne les homogreffes de peau, malgré plusieurs expériences suggestives depuis la description du phénomène de Billingham et Sparrow (1955), la preuve d'une possibilitè de facilitation n'a été apportée de manière démonstrative que récemment par D. S. Nelson (1962) chez le cobaye et par Möller (1963) chez la souris. Nous avons étudié certains aspects du mécanisme de la facilitation des homogreffes de peau chez le lapin Snyder, (1964). Il en sera question plus loin. La question se pose alors de savoir si ce phénomène de facilitation immunologique peut s'appliquer à d'autres situations que celles concernant les réactions de type homotransplantation, c'est-à-dire concerner d'autres antigènes que les antigènes de transplantation. C'est apparemment le cas pour des autoantigènes et d'autres antigènes, en particulier bactériens.

C. Facilitation de Tissus Autoantigéniques. La possibilité en était suggérée par les cas cliniques et expérimentaux d'ophtalmie sympathique où tout semble se passer comme si une réaction d'hypersensibilité de type retardé était liée à la présence de la maladie, les anticorps circulants joueraient un rôle protecteur. Voisin et Toullet (données non publiées) ont essayé sans succès d'empêcher l'apparition d'orchite aspermatogénique auto-immune chez le Cobaye par facilitation passive (injection pendant un mois d'anticorps spécifiques de l'antigène actif). Récemment, par contre Chutna (1964) a pu réaliser une protection impressionnante contre cette affection expérimentale, apparemment par facilitation active. Par ailleurs, Paterson et Harwin (1962) ont pu prévenir l'apparition d'encéphalomyélite expérimentale auto-immune chez le Rat en lui injectant du sérum anti-système nerveux central.

D. Facilitation d'Autres Antigènes. Des bactéries (Salmonella Adelaïde: Möller [1963]), des érythrocytes (Rowley, et Fitch 1964) voire des antigènes protéiques (anatoxines: Uhr et Baumann [1964]) peuvent être l'objet de phénomènes qui sont souvent interprétés comme résultant d'une facilitation immunologique.

Ainsi, il est désormais clair que le phénomène de facilitation immunologique ne s'applique pas seulement aux tissus tumoraux homogreffés et qu'il ne concerne pas que les antigènes de transplantation. Ce fait est capital pour envisager la possibilité du rôle de la facilitation dans le développement de tumeurs autologues. Mais, auparavant, il faut envisager plusieurs problèmes concernant ce phénomène.

III. Problèmes Soulevés

Ces problèmes ne pourrons qu'être évoqués. Les plus importants d'entre eux concernent l'origine des anticorps facilitants, leur nature, la pluralité de la réaction immunitaire aux antigènes, le mécanisme de la facilitation; enfin, l'application possible aux tumeurs autologues.

A. Origine des Anticorps Facilitants. Bien sûr, comme tous les anticorps, les anticorps facilitants doivent être produits par le système lymphoïde. Mais tous les organes lymphoïdes sont-ils particulièrement aptes à les produire ou bien certains seraient-ils plus prédisposés à le faire? Cette deuxième éventualité semble à retenir. Au cours d'expériences concernant la greffe de sarcome DBA_{49} à des souris BALB/c, Prehn (1959) avait constaté que la préimmunisation intraveineuse du receveur avec du sang du donneur à forte dose (0,25 ml) entraînait une augmentation de prise de l'homogreffe tumorale et que la splénectomie faite avant l'immunisation inhibait cette action «facilitante». Nous avons, avec G. SNYDER et R. KINSKY (1964), abordé l'étude de ce problème dans les homogreffes de peau chez le lapin. Nos constatations, très résumées, ont été les suivantes (Fig. 10 et tableau I): chez les témoins normaux, le temps de survie moyen de 58 greffons est de 8,2 jours; la splénectomie faite 5 jours après le sang intraveineux et juste avant la greffe, porte le temps moyen de survie à 13,6 jours donc supérieur à celui observé avec le sang intraveineux seul. Tous ces résultats sont compatibles avec l'hypothèse que le ganglion drainant est le siège principal

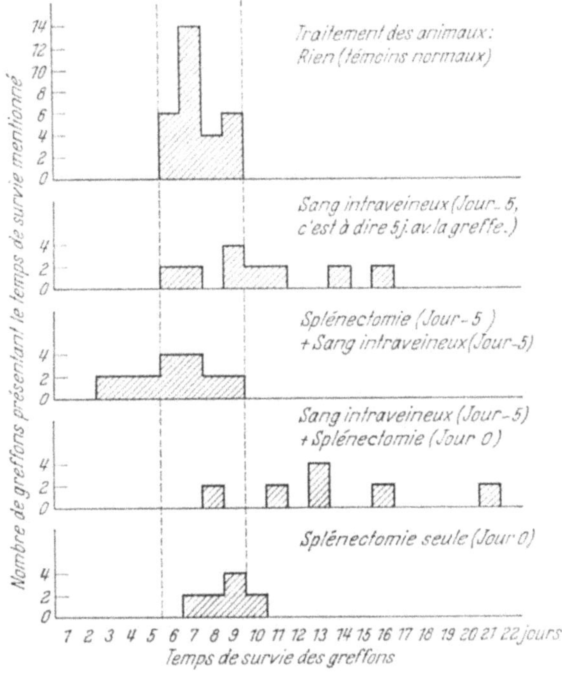

Fig. 10. Facilitation active d'homogreffons cutanés. Origine des anticorps facilitants. Histogrammes de survie des homogreffons pratiqués sur les 2 oreilles de lapins Fauves de Bourgogne à partir des Blancs de Bouscat. Divers traitements des receveurs

chez les animaux prétraités (5 jours avant la greffe) avec le sang du futur donneur, injecté par voie intradermique, on n'observe que des greffes blanches, signe d'extrême immunisation; si l'injection de sang a été faite dans la veine, le greffon survit 11,2 jours en moyenne (3 jours de plus que chez les témoins); la splénectomie faite avant l'injection intraveineuse de sang ramène le temps de survie à 7,8 jours (avec, dans 8/34 cas, un temps de survie inférieur aux temps les plus courts observés chez les 58 greffons témoins); de la réaction de rejet; que la rate est le siège principal de production des anticorps facilitants car, si on l'enlève avant l'injection intraveineuse d'antigène, l'effet facilitant est supprimé; bien plus, dans ce cas, les antigènes injectés, rejoignant parfois les ganglions, ont une action apparemment immunisante; par ailleurs, la splénectomie faite à un moment propice (5 jours après l'injaction de sang intraveineux et le jour des greffes) permet une nouvelle augmentation de survie due sans doute au fait que la rate immunisée n'est pas totalement inactive dans les réactions de rejet (peut-être parce que des anticorps d'un type différent, ou produits à plus forte dose après la pose du greffon agissent en synergie avec les agents de la réaction de rejet d'origine surtout ganglionnaire).

B. Nature des Anticorps Facilitants. Nos connaissances sont encore

traînent des réactions immunitaires diverses de la part du tissu lymphoïde de l'hôte.

D'un point de vue analytique on peut distinguer une réaction cellulaire responsable des phénomènes d'hypersensibilité de type retardé et la formation d'anticorps ou immunoglobulines de types variés (dont trois sont actuelle-

Tableau I. *Facilitation active d'homogreffons cutanés. Origine des anticorps facilitants. Temps de survie moyens des homogreffons pratiqués sur les 2 oreilles de Lapins Fauves de Bourgogne à partir de Blanc de Bouscat et vice-versa. Divers traitements des receveurs*

Traitement des Animaux		Temps moyen de survie des greffons	Nombre de greffons
Jour −5	Jour 0: homogreffe +		
Rien	rien	8,2	2 × 29 *
Splénectomie	rien	8,8	2 × 9
Sang ** S C	rien	8,3	2 × 12
Sang I D	rien	≤ 3 ***	2 × 10
Sang I V	rien	11,2	2 × 21
Sang I V	*splénectomie*	15,1	2 × 11
Splénectomie puis Sang I V	rien	7,8 †	2 × 17

* Chaque animal est porteur de 2 greffons de même origine. Le destin des 2 greffons s'est toujours montré identique.

** Il s'est toujours agi de 1 ml de sang total du futur donneur de peau.

*** Dans tous ces cas, il s'est agi de greffes blanches.

† Un quart des greffons de cette série ont présenté un temps de survie inférieur aux temps les plus courts observés chez les greffons témoins.

plus embryonnaires dans ce domaine. Des suggestions existent que des anticorps incapables de fixer le complément seraient capables de protéger *in vitro* des cellules-cibles contre des anticorps vraisemblablement de même spécificité immunologique mais capables de fixer le complément. Cette manière de voir est suggérée par les expériences de F. Kourilsky (1963) sur l'hémolyse immune et par celles de Chutna (1964), sur la cytotoxicité auto-immune envers des cellules spermatiques.

C. Pluralité de la réponse immunitaire aux antigènes cellulaires. Les antigènes présents dans les cellules en-

ment bien individualisées (Snell, 1960); en particulier certaines immunoglobulines sont capables de fixer les complément, d'autres ne le sont pas.

D'un point de vue pratique, cette réaction a deux conséquences : réaction de rejet des cellules-cibles et réaction de facilitation protégeant ces cellules contre le rejet.

La difficulté surgit lorsqu'il s'agit de rapprocher ces deux points de vue. D'un côté, il est bien établi que l'instrument de facilitation sont des immunoglobulines sériques peut-être d'une certaine catégorie. Par contre l'accord n'est pas fait sur l'instrument du rejet: peut-être cellules sensibilisées, peut-être anticorps cytotoxiques agissant avec l'aide du complément, sans doute les deux agissant synergiquement.

Quoinqu'il en soit, le point le plus important, dans notre opinion, est que ces divers types de réaction coexistent et interagissent et qu'il s'agit d'un phénomène général. Les débats portant sur l'instrument de rejet des cellules-cibles

1. *Inhibition primaire.* La réalité d'un tel mécanisme, quels qu'en soient les rouages (les anticorps facilitants empêchent les antigènes correspondants de se rendre, au moins sous une forme convenable, au niveau des cellules immunologiquement compétentes ou bien les anticorps facilitants empêchent ces cellules de réagir contre les antigènes correspondants) est démontrée par plusieurs expériences: cel-

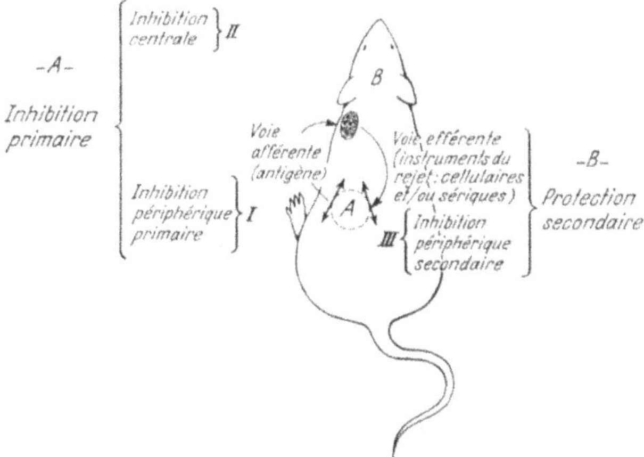

Fig. 11. Représentation schématique des mécanismes possibles d'action de la facilitation immunologique

ne modifient pas sensiblement la position du problème du mécanisme de la facilitation.

D. Mécanisme de la Facilitation Immunologique. Assez complexe, ce problème peut se ramener, sous sa forme la plus simple, à la question suivante: les anticorps facilitants, agents actifs de la facilitation immunologique, agissent-ils par *inhibition primaire,* c'est-à-dire en déprimant d'une manière ou d'une autre la réaction immunitaire aboutissant à l'atteinte des cellules-cibles, ou bien agissent-ils par *protection secondaire,* c'est-à-dire en protégeant d'une manière ou d'une autre les cellules-cibles contre les effets nocifs d'une réaction immunitaire existante? (VOISIN [1965]) (Fig. 11)

les de UHR et BAUMANN (1961) portant sur des antigènes protéiques; celles de NEIDERS et Col. (1962) portant sur des érythrocytes; celles de MÖLLER (1963) portant sur Salmonella Adelaide; celles enfin de SNELL et Col. (1960) portant sur des cellules tumorales.

2. *Protection secondaire:* également démontrée par les expériences de KALISS (1958—62); également par celles de MÖLLER (1963) et de nous-mêmes (VOISIN et KINSKY, données non publiées) montrant que des cellules cancéreuses allogéniques injectées dans le flanc d'une souris sont rejetées alors que des cellules identiques mais préincubées avec du sérum facilitant, injectées en même temps dans l'autre flanc, croissent plus intensément et sont

rejetées plus tard ou pas du tout. La nature de cette protection est sujette à discussion: pour Kaliss, il s'agirait d'une modification «physiologique» de la tumeur (sans modification antigénique); en réalité un tel phénomène ne semble s'observer qu'inconstamment. Pour d'autres, les anticorps formeraient un «écran protecteur» empêchant les agents du rejet immunitaire de parvenir au contact intime des cellules-cibles.

Quelque soit celui des deux mécanismes, inhibition primaire ou protection secondaire, ou encore une action synergique des deux qui soit opérationnel, il faut souligner la spécificité exquise de la facilitation immunologique: pour être totalement efficace, un sérum facilitant doit contenir des anticorps contre tous les antigènes touchés par la réaction de rejet.

E. Application Possible aux Tumeurs Autologues. Il est bien évident que les cancérologistes expérimentaux ne s'intéressent qu'indirectement aux problèmes d'homotransplantation posés par les homogreffes de tumeurs. Il serait souhaitable que la «transplantologie» rendit à la cancérologie les immenses services que cette dernière lui a prêtés. Cette possibilité n'est nullement exclue pour les raisons suivantes: d'abord, nous avons vu que les tissus tumoraux semblent bien les plus aptes à bénéficier efficacement d'une réaction de facilitation immunologique; par ailleurs le phénomène de facilitation peut s'exercer vis-à-vis d'autres antigènes que les antigènes de transplantation; enfin, le nombre s'accroît de tumeurs non transplantées possédant des antigènes particuliers absents des tissus normaux du sujet porteur de la tumeur. Il convient de s'arrêter brièvement sur ces deux derniers points:

1. *Facilitation envers d'autres antigènes que ceux de transplantation.* Une partie de cette présentation a été consacrée à montrer cette possibilité. Plus important ici est le fait que l'on peut induire activement ou passivement une facilitation (aboutissant à une augmentation de prise tumorale) vis-à-vis de tumeurs isotransplantées (et même parfois autotransplantées semble-t-il). Casey (1949—1952) a insisté sur la possibilité d'obtenir de telles facilitations actives sur le carcinome mammaire EO 771 ($C_{57}Bl/6$) et sur la tumeur Z 8352 (C_3H). Plus évocateurs sont les travaux de Möller (1963) montrant que le sérum de souris immunisées avec des sarcomes isologues, induits per méthylcholanthrène, acquérait la propriété de modifier la croissance des mêmes tumeurs chez des hôtes isologues. Cette modification consistait, suivant les tumeurs en une facilitation ou en une inhibition de la croissance tumorale.

2. *Présence d'antigènes particuliers aux tumeurs.* Que de tels antigènes proviennent de mutations cellulaires ou qu'ils soient dus à l'intégration d'ADN viral dans le génome cellulaire, ou à tout autre mécanisme le fait est que leur existence est déjà démontrée dans un certain nombre de cas, mentionnons, pour mémoire: les antigènes (d'origine virale) de certaines leucémies des souris; les antigènes TL (d'origine proprement cellulaire) des leucémies TL; les antigènes (à individualité apparemment spécifique) des sarcomes induits par le méthylcholanthrène; les antigènes des tumeurs induites par les virus du polyome; les antigènes des lymphomes induits par le virus de Gross; les antigènes X de Gorer dont certains relèvent peut-être d'une des catégories précédentes. Beaucoup de ces antigènes (dont certains sont trouvés dans des tumeurs spontanées) sont iso-antigéniques; certains mêmes sont capables d'induire l'apparition d'isoanticorps cytotoxiques.

Dans ces conditions on a le devoir de se demander si ces antigènes propres aux tumeurs ne sont pas capables de jouer chez le sujet porteur d'une tumeur, un rôle analogue à celui que jouerait un antigène d'histocomptaibilité faible. En d'autres termes, ne seraient-il pas capables d'entraîner, chez le sujet hôte, des réactions de nature immunitaire suivant le double type que nous connaissons maintenant: réaction de rejet (immunité cellulaire ou immunoglobulines cytotoxiques ou les deux) et réaction de facilitation (immunoglobulines, peut-être d'un certain type); le destin final de la tumeur dépendant de l'équilibre des deux réactions. Il serait alors logique de supposer que de destin «immunologique» des cellules cancéreuses se jouerait au début, à un moment où la tumeur n'est pas encore cliniquement décelable; mais peut être serait-il encore possible d'influencer le cours de son développement si l'on savait bien manier l'antagonisme entre rejet et facilitation, et les échecs des tentatives d'immunisation ne constituent pas une objection à cette manière de voir, en raison de leur caractère aveugle. Il semble bien, en définitive, qu'il y ait là un domaine intéressant à explorer expérimentalement.

Summary

The present report is divided into three parts:

1. *In the first part,* the essential known facts concerning the *enhancement phenomenon* are briefly summarized . This phenomenon is paradoxical since it leads to *protection* of a homografted tumour by specific antibodies directed *against* the homotransplantation antigens (Figs. 1 to 5).

2. *In the second part,* the phenomenon of immunological enhancement of homografted tumours is broadened to the concept of *immunological facilitation,* meaning that this is a general phenomenon which may concern any kind of antigen and may lead to the protection of target cells which bear the corresponding antigens. Experiments from this laboratory are summarized and relevant experiments from other laboratories are recalled. Experiments from this laboratory were the first to establish unequivocally that immunological facilitation, passively transferred by immune sera, can efficiently counteract immunological rejection directed against normal tissues. Since the runting syndrome (homologous disease induced in newborn mice by allogeneic spleen cells from adults) is triggered by a transplantation rejection reaction and since the enhancement phenomenon is able to counteract such a type of reaction (against tumours), attempts were made to counteract the runting syndrome by considering newborn mice in the same way as tumoural homografts and helping them to "take" by means of immunological enhancement-facilitation, either passive or active. In *passive facilitation-enhancement experiments* (Figs. 6 and 7, reference VOISIN, 1962), newborn mice of A strain received 7×10^6 spleen cells from adult CBA mice plus 0.4 µl of anti-A CBA serum; a striking and highly significant degree of protection was obtained against runting syndrome. Furthermore the "protected" mice were significantly more tolerant toward skin grafts of CBA origin than the were unprotected mice. In *active facilitation-enhancement experiments* (Figs. 8 and 9 and reference VOISIN, 1964), the prospective CBA spleen cell donors were treated by lyophilisates of A origin in order to initiate an active immunological reaction of the enhancing-facilitating type. A significant degree of protection was obtained when the immunizing injection was not older than 11 days. There was a direct relation between the degree of protection and the titer of synergic hemagglutinins in the donors of spleen

cells. The "protected" mice were also found to be more tolerant toward CBA skin grafts. Experiments from this and from other laboratories brought together lead to the concept that immunological facilitation enhancement applies to histocompatibility antigens of tumoural and normal tissues, to autoantigens, to antigens in erythrocytes, in bacteria and, possibly, to soluble protein antigens.

3. *In the third part,* problems raised by this phenomenon are briefly discussed, namely, the origin of facilitating-enhancing antibodies, their nature, the diverse immunological responses to cellular antigens, the mechanism of the facilitation-enhancement phenomenon and, finally, the possible applications to autologous tumours.

Concerning *the origin* of facilitating-enhancing antibodies, experiments from this laboratory performed on skin homografted rabbits previously treated for active enhancement, with or without splenectomy at different intervals of time, suggest that the spleen may play a key role in manufacturing enhancing antibodies (Fig. 10, Table I and reference SNYDER, 1964).

Concerning *the mechanism* of the facilitation-enhancement phenomenon, the two possibilities of primary inhibition and of secondary protection are mentioned (Fig. 11).

Finally, it is emphasized that, since the phenomenon of immunological facilitation-enhancement can concern various antigens, besides the transplantation antigens of homografted tumours, and since tumour-specific antigens are more and more often demonstrated, it is quite feasible that autologous tumours and their metastases are subjected to the antagonistic effects of the two immunological reactions which seem to act in transplantation as well as in auto-immunity, namely the rejection reaction and the facilitation reaction.

Since the submission of this manuscript, we have obtained the following results:

1. Both active and passive facilitation enhancement can be applied to the protection of adult hybrids against homologous disease provoked by parental spleen cells injection (VOISIN, G. A., KINSKY, R., et MAILLARD, J., to be published).

2. We were able to fractionate by curtain electrophoresis the cytotoxic and facilitating-enhancing activities of transplantation immune sera, showing that these two phenomena are under the dependance of different antibodies: cytotoxic antibodies were 75 γ_2, while enhancing-facilitating properties were born by faster migrating Ig (VOISIN, G. A., KINSKY, R., and JANSEN, F., Nature, 1966, **210**, 138).

3. The presence of specific enhancing-facilitating antibodies was demonstrated in the sera of mice tolerant to H_2 antigens by passive transfer (VOISIN, G. A., KINSKY, R., and MAILLARD, J., First International Congress of the Transplantation Society, Paris 1967).

Bibliography

BATCHELOR, J. R., The mechanisms and significance of immunological enhancement. *Guy's Hosp., Rep.* **112**, 345—359 (1963).

BILLINGHAM, R. E., and SPARROW, E. M., The effect of prior intravenous injections of dissociated epidermal cells and blood on the survival of skin homografts in rabbits. *J. Embryol. exp. Morph.* **3**, 265 (1955).

BRIDE, J., Recherches sur le cancer expérimental des souris. *Ann. Inst. Pasteur* **21**, 760 (1907).

CASEY, A. E., A species limitation of an enhancing material derived from a mammalian tumor. *Proc. Soc. exp. Biol. (N.Y.)* **30**, 674 (1933).

CASEY, A. E., Specificity of enhancing materials for mammalian tumors. *Proc. Soc. exp. Biol. (N.Y.)* **31**, 663 (1934a).

— A persistent hypersusceptibility induced in rabbits with an homologus tumor material. *Proc. Soc. exp. Biol. (N.Y.)* **31**, 666 (1934b).

—, and CASEY, J. G., Enhancement tumor transplantability following second transplantation in mouse of original strain. *Cancer Res.* **13**, 737—740 (1953).

— — HATHAWAY, C. O., and DOWLING, E. A., Enhanced tumor homografs following pretreatment of donor mice. *Proc. Soc. exp. Biol. (N.Y.)* **100**, 762—763 (1959).

— DRYSDALE, G. R., SHEAR, H. H., and GUNN, F., Second transplantation of Eo 771 mouse carcinoma and of Brown-Pearce rabbit tumor. *Cancer Res.* **12**, 807—813 (1952).

— MEYERS, L., and DRYSDALE, G. R., Selective blocking of host resistance to malignant neoplasm (Brown-Pearce tumor in New Zealand white rabbits). *Proc. Soc. exp. Biol. (N.Y.)* **69**, 579 (1948).

— ROSS, G. L., and LANGSTON, R. R., Selective XYZ factor in C 57 black mammary carcinoma Eo 771. *Proc. Soc. exp. Biol. (N.Y.)* **72**, 83—89 (1949).

—, and SCOTT, G. M., Experimental enhancement of malignancy in the Brown-Pearce rabbit tumor. *Proc. Soc. exp. Biol. (N.Y.)* **29**, 816—818 (1932).

CHUTNA, J., and RYCHLIKOVA, M., Prevention and suppression of experimental autoimmune aspermatogenesis in adult guineapigs. *Folia biol. (Kraków)* **10**, 177—187 (1964a).

— — A study of the biological effectiveness of antibodies in the development and prevention of experimental auto-immune aspermatogenesis. *Folia biol. (Kraków)*, **10**, 188—197 (1964b).

GORER, P. A., The antibody response to skin homografts in mice. *Ann. N.Y. Acad. Sci.* **59**, 365 (1955).

— Variations dans la réponse aux homogreffes tumorales chez la souris. *In:* C.N.R.S. (ed.), *Coll. Internat. sur la Biologie des Homogreffes*, p. 60, Paris 1958.

— Some reactions of H-2 antibodies *in vitro* and *in vivo*. *Ann. N.Y. Acad. Sci.* **73**, 707—721 (1958).

— Interactions between sessile and humoral antibodies in homograft reactions. *In: Ciba Foundation symposium on Cellular aspects of immunity*, p. 330. London: J. & A. Churchill 1959.

GORER, P. A., The antigenic structure of tumors. *Advanc. Immunol.* **1**, 345—393 (1961).

—, and KALISS, N., The effect of isoantibodies *in vivo* on three different transplantable neoplasms in mice. *Cancer Res.* **19**, 824—830 (1959).

KALISS, N., Regression of survival of tumor homoiografts in mice pretreated with injections of lyophilized tissues. *Cancer Res.* **12**, 379—382 (1952).

— Induced alteration of the normal host graft relationships in homotransplantation of mouse tumors. *Ann. N.Y. Acad. Sci.* **59**, 385—393 (1955).

— Acceptance of tumor homografts by mice injected with antiserum. II-Effect of time of injection. *Proc. Soc. exp. Biol. (N.Y.)* **91**, 118—121 (1956).

— The survival of homografts in mice pretreated with antisera to mouse tissue. *Proc. Soc. exp. Biol. (N.Y.)* **74**, 977 (1957).

— «Facilitation» immunologique d'homogreffes de tumeur chez la souris. Conséquence de l'exposition du greffon à un anti-sérum spécifique. *In:* La biologie des homogreffes, vol. 1, p. 225. Paris: Monograph C.N.R.S. (ed.) 1958a.

— Immunological enhancement of tumor homografts in mice: A review. *Cancer Res.* **18**, 992—1003 (1958b).

— The induction of the homograft reaction in the presence of immunologic enhancement of tumor homografts. *In:* Symposium on *"Mechanisms of immunological tolerance"* p. 413. Prague: Publ. House of the Czechoslovak Academy of Sciences 1962.

—, and BRYANT, B. F., Factors determining homograft destruction and immunological enhancement in mice receiving successive tumor inocula. *J. nat. Cancer Inst.* **20**, 691—704 (1958).

—, and DAY, E. D., Relation between time of conditioning of host and survival of tumor homografts in mice. *Proc. Soc. exp. Biol. (N.Y.)* **86**, 115—117 (1954).

—, and KANDUTSCH, A. A., Acceptance of tumor homografts by mice injected with antiserum. I. — Activity of serum fractions. *Proc. Soc. exp. Biol. (N.Y.)* **91**, 432—437 (1956).

— MOLOMUT, N., HARRIS, J. L., and GAULT, S. D., Effect of previously injected immune serum and tissue on the survival of tumor grafts in mice. *J. nat. Cancer Inst.* **13**, 847—850 (1953).

—, and SNELL, G. D., The effects of injections of lyophilized normal and neoplastic mouse tissue on the growth of tumor homoiotransplants in mice. *Cancer Res.* **11**, 122—126 (1951).

KANDUTSCH, A. A., Intracellular distribution and extraction of tumor homograft enhancing antigens. *Cancer Res.* **20**, 264—268 (1960).

—, and STIMPFLING, J. H., An isoantigenic lipoprotein from sarcoma 1. *In: Ciba Symposium on transplantation*, p. 72—85. London: J. & A. Churchill 1962.

KOURILSKY, F. M., BLOCH, K. J., BENACERRAF, B., and OVARY, Z., Properties of guineapig 7 S antibodies. V — Inhibition by guinea-pigs γ_1 antibodies of passive immune lysis provoked by $\gamma 2$ antibodies. *J. exp. Med.* **118**, 699—709 (1963).

LINDER, O. E., Induced survival of skin homografts after pretreatment of the adult recipient mice with ovarian grafts of skin donor genotype. *In: Symposium on Mechanisms of immunological tolerance*, p. 359. Prague: Publ. House of the Czechoslovak Academy of Sciences 1962.

MITCHISON, N. A., Studies on the immunological response to foreign tumor transplants in the mouse. I. The role of lymph node cells in conferring immunity by adoptive transfer. *J. exp. Med.* **102**, 157—177 (1955).

—, and DUBE, O. L., Studies on the immunological response to foreign tumor transplants in the mouse. II. — The relation between hemaggluting antibody and graft resistance in the normal mouse and mice pretreated with tissue preparations. *J. exp. Med.* **102**, 179—197 (1955).

MÖLLER, G., *On the role of isoimmune reactions in tissue transplantation*. Stockholm: Tryckeri Balder Ab. 1963.

NEIDERS, M. E., ROWLEY, D. A., and FITCH, F. W., The sustained suppression of hemolysin response in passively immunized rats. *J. Immunol.* **88**, 718—724 (1962).

NELSON, D. S., Immunological enhancement of skin homografts in guinea-pigs. *Brit. J. exp. Path.* **43**, 1—11 (1962).

PATERSON, P. Y., and HARWIN, S. M., Suppression of allergic encephalomyelitis by means of immune serum. *In: Symposium on Mechanisms of immunological tolerance*, p. 507 (M. HASEK, A. LENGEROVA and M. VOJTISKOVA eds.). Prague: Publ. House of the Czechoslovak Academy of Sciences 1962.

PREHN, R. T., The immunity inhibiting role of the spleen and the effect of dosage and route of antigen administration in a homograft reaction. *In: Biological problems of grafting.* Oxford: Blackwell Sc. Publ. 1959.

ROWLEY, D. A., and FITCH, F. W., Homeostasis of antibody formation in the adult rat. *J. exp. Med.* **120**, 987—1005 (1964).

SNELL, G. D., Enhancement and inhibition of the growth of tumor homoiotransplants by pretreatment of the hosts with various preparation of normal and tumor issues. *J. nat. Cancer Inst.* **13**, 719—729 (1952).

— The enhancing effect (or actively acquired tolerance) and the histocompatibility-2 locus in the mouse. *J. nat. Cancer Inst.* **15**, 665—675 (1954).

— The homograft reaction. *Ann. Rev. Microbiol.* **11**, 439—600 (1957).

— CLOUDMAN, A. M., FALLOR, E., and DOUGLASS, P., Inhibition and stimulation of tumor homoiotransplants by prior injections of lyophilized tissue. *J. nat. Cancer Inst.* **6**, 303—316 (1946).

— —, and WOODWORTH, E., Tumor immunity in mice, induced with lyophilized tissue, as influenced by tumor strain, host strain, source of tissue, and dosage. *Cancer Res.* **8**, 429—437 (1948).

— WINN, H. J., STIMPFLING, J. H., and PARKER, S. J., Depression by antibody of the immune response to homografts and its role in immunological enhancement. *J. exp. Med.* **112**, 293—314 (1960).

SNYDER, G., KINSKY, R., and VOISIN, G. A., Evaluation of homograft prolongation methods. *Plast. reconstr. Surg.* **33**, 110—119 (1964).

UHR, J. W., and BAUMANN, J. B., Antibody formation. I. The suppression of antibody formation by passively administered antibody. *J. exp. Med.* **113**, 935—957 (1961).

VOISIN, G. A., Greffes tumorales et facilitation immunologique ("Immunological enhancement"). *Rev. franç. Etud. clin. biol.* **8**, 927—942 (1963).

— Le phénomène de facilitation immunologique, concept élargi du «enhancement phenomenon». *Quatrième Symposium Internat. d'Immuno-Pathologie, Monaco* **1965**, 1 Vol., Schwabe & Co. Publ. Basel/Stuttgart 1966, p. 165.

—, and KINSKY, R., Protection against runting by specific treatment of newborn mice, followed by increased tolerance. *In: Ciba Symposium on Transplantation*, p. 128. London: J. & A. Churchill 1962.

— — and MAILLARD, J., Modification de la maladie homologue des souris nouveau-nées, par facilitation immunologique (enhancement phenomenon) induite passivement et activement. *In:* Colloque C.N.R.S. sur la greffe des cellules hématopoietiques allogéniques, C.N.R.S. édit. Paris 1965, p. 407.

In Vitro and In Vivo Cytostatic Effect of Antiribosome FLS Antisera on Mouse Ascitic Tumour Cells FLS

Fanny Lacour, Claude Verger, and Evelyne Nahon

Institut Gustave-Roussy, 94, Villejuif, France

I would like to present the results of experimental work carried out with Cl. Verger and E. Nahon in the laboratory of Immunology of the Gustave Roussy Institute and also to discuss our findings which indicate that both growth and proliferation of mouse ascitic tumour cells can be modified by an immunological process.

Rabbits and one horse were immunized with ribosomes from mouse ascitic tumour cells FLS. The antiserum thus produced was shown to inhibit or delay the growth of these tumour cells in mice. This effect was obtained either in vitro by pretreating tumour cells with antiserum before these cells were injected intraperitoneally, or in vivo by subcutaneous injection of antiserum after the intraperitoneal injection of tumour cells.

Ribosomes were extracted from the mouse ascitic tumour cells FLS [1]. Electron microscopic examination of the antigen preparations showed their purity (Figs. 1, 2). The average composition of the ribosome preparation was 50% RNA and 50% protein.

Ribosomes used as antigens elicit antibodies reacting not only with ribosomal proteins but also with purified RNA [2]. There is no doubt today that experimental induction of anti RNA antibodies is possible, but this fact was not so obvious a few years ago. Although the immunological response of each immunized animal was quite variable, some of them produced antibodies specifically reacting with purified RNA. If the titer of these antibodies is high enough, an immunoprecipitation is observed with RNA extracted from ascitic cells (Fig. 3) or with RNA from different sources. In the case of our horse antiribosome antiserum, the antibodies fixed the C' in the presence of purified RNA (Fig. 4).

Anti FLS ribosome antibodies react not only with homologous antigen but also cross react with ribosomes from different species (ribosomes extracted from human spleen, hamster tissue and even bacterial ribosomes). RNA itself could be responsible for this cross reaction [3].

Ribosomes playing such an important role in protein synthesis, it seemed interesting to see if antiribosome antibodies were able to influence or modify the biological behaviour of cells.

Antisera did not show any cytotoxicity against ascitic FLS cells. 2×10^7 cells suspended in 3 ml of ClNa 0.14 M pH 7, and 1 ml of antiserum were incubated at 37° C in presence or absence of guinea pig complement. Morphological alterations were not observed after incubation for 1 or 2 hours. After addition of nigrosine 1/1000 or eosine 1/1000 the number of stained cells varied from 5 to

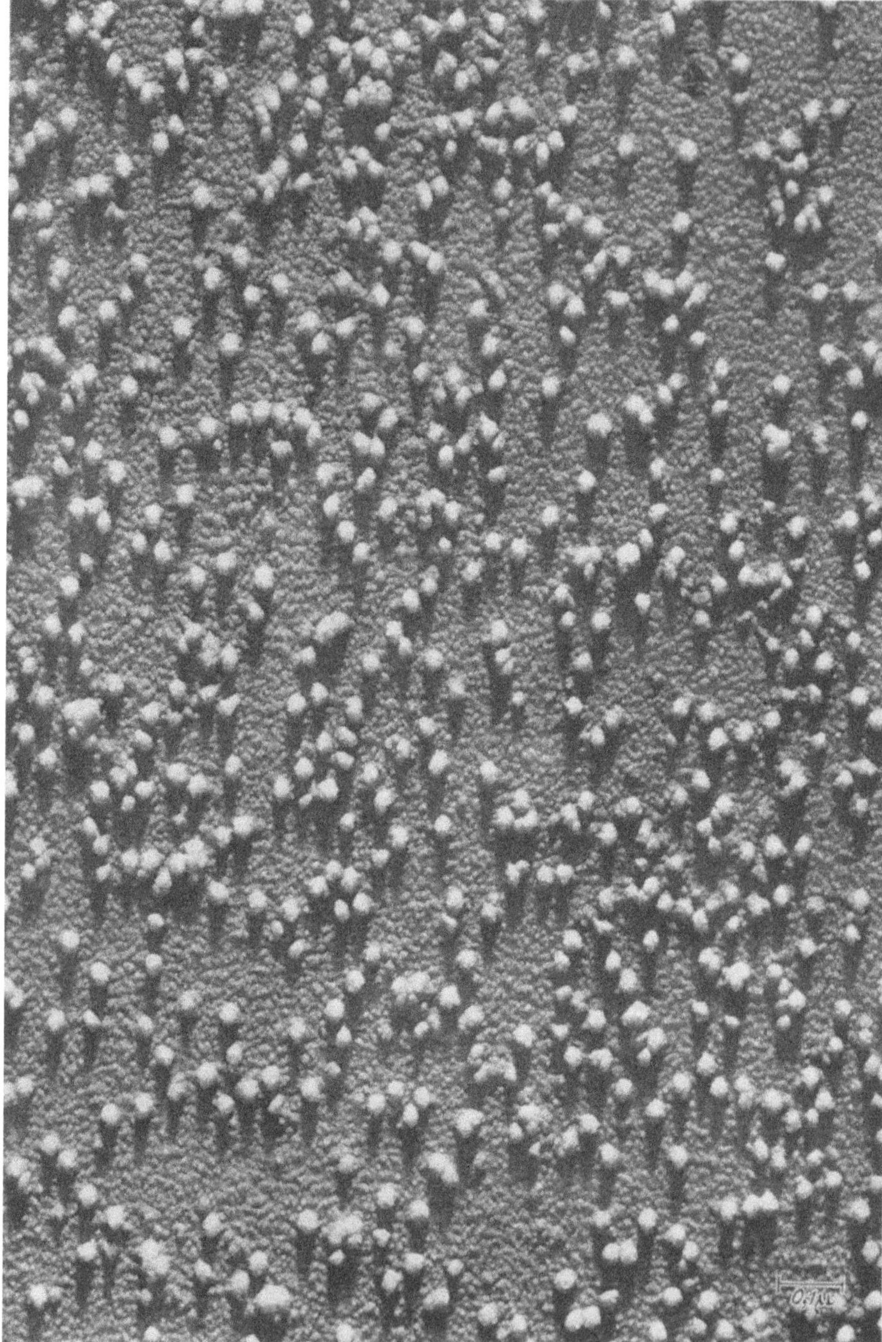

Fig. 1. Electron microscopic picture showing a spread preparation of purified FLS ribosomes shadowed with carbon-platinum ($\times$ 85,000). The fraction consists mainly of monomers

10% as in the control experiments run with normal serum.

However, an inhibition or delaying of growth was observed when the in vitro pretreated cells (with anti ribosome antiserum) were injected in vivo. This cytostatic effect was observed with 3 rabbits and 1 horse antiribosomes FLS

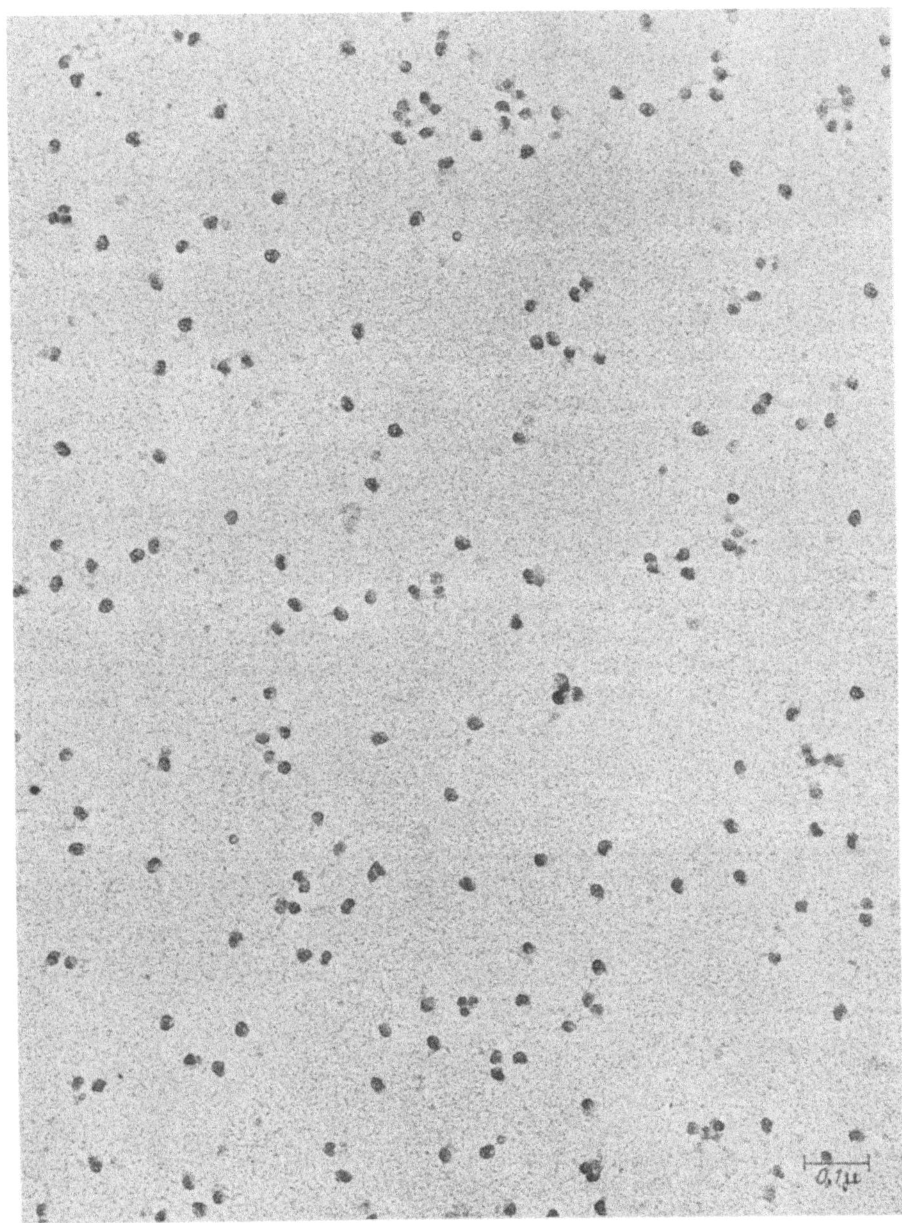

Fig. 2. The same purified ribosomal fraction as in Fig. 1; the spread preparation has been shadowed with carbon-platinum while rotating ($\times 75{,}000$)

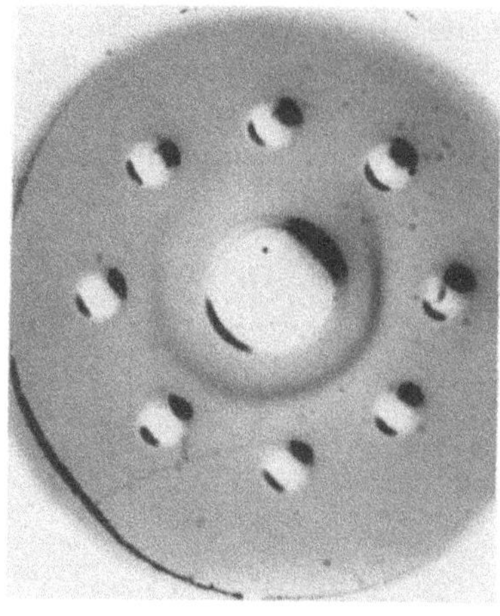

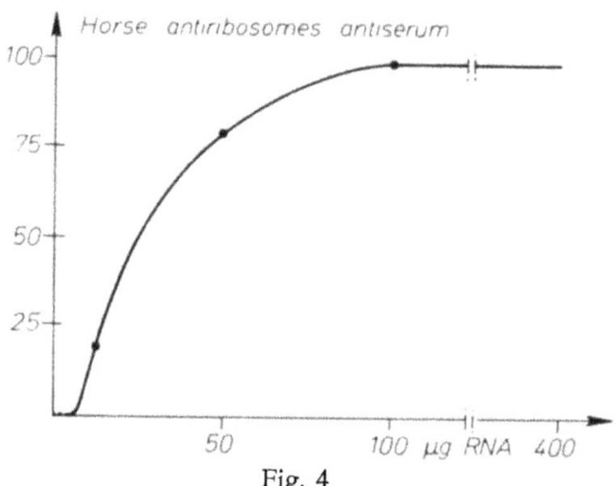

Fig. 4

Fig. 3. Photograph of precipitin reaction in agar double diffusion. Central hole: antiribosome antiserum; peripheral reservoir: purified RNA; dilutions increasing clockwise from 1,6 to 0,01 μg

antisera. Pretreatement in vitro of cells with normal rabbit or horse serum did not affect their growth in vivo.

At this point it was important to determine if we were dealing with an immunological phenomenon. In all our experiments a standardized technique was used:

In Table I we can see that out of the 11 mice injected with FLS cells preincubated with rabbit antiribosome FLS antiserum n° 251, not one died with a tumour (Exp. 1).

This cytostatic effect was not lost by heating the antiserum at 56° C for 30' and was not dependant on the presence of complement (Exp. 2).

2×10^7 ascitic cells were incubated at 37° C with 1 ml of antiserum diluted with 3 ml of NaCl 0.14 M pH 7. Controls were run with normal rabbit serum and normal horse serum. After incubation for 1 h, cells were injected i/peritoneally

Table I. *Cytostatic effect of antiribosomes FLS rabbit antiserum on ascites tumour cells FLS: before and after absorption with ribosomes and RNA*

	Cells incubated with antiserum 251	+/N. total *	Cytostatic effect	Mean survival time of mice bearing ascites (days)
Exp. 1	Cells incubated with antiserum 251	0/11	+++	
Exp. 2	heated at 56° C	0/9	+++	
Exp. 3	absorbed with ribosomes FLS	10/10	—	19,7
Exp. 4	absorbed with RNA	7/10	+	40
Exp. 5	absorbed with RNA (in presence of bentonite)	9/10	±	28
Control	cells incubated with ribosomes	10/10	—	17

* Number of mice dead with ascites tumour over the total number inoculated; each mouse received an inoculum of 1×10^6 cells.

in mice. Each mouse received 1×10^6 cells. In all experiments we used 2 months old Swiss inbred mice.

Table I also illustrates the results of absorption of antibodies with ribosomes or RNA.

In experiment 3, aliquots of antiserum were absorbed with homologous antigens: ribosomes FLS. The samples were centrifuged, the specific precipitate discarded and the cells incubated with the supernatant. All the cytostatic activity disappeared and 10/10 mice injected with cells pretreated with absorbed antiserum died with ascites. When antiserum was absorbed with purified RNA 7/10 mice died with ascites (Exp. 4). In order to avoid enzymatic digestion of RNA by the antiserum ribonuclease, in experiment 5 we added bentonite before absorbing the antibodies with RNA: 9/10 mice injected with cells treated in vitro with the supernatant died with ascites. The cytostatic effect is thus considerably decreased when antiserum is absorbed with RNA and suppressed after absorption with ribosomes. Considering these results it seems logical to think that the antibodies directed against ribosomes and RNA are responsible for the cytostatic effect. We could also follow during immunization the increase of potency of the antiribosome antisera.

In Table II, it can be seen that before immunization rabbit serum 770 has no

Table II. *Increase of the cytostatic effect of the antiribosomes FLS antiserum on cells FLS during immunization*

Cells incubated with rabbit serum 770	+/N. total*	Cytostatic effect
Prior immunization	10/10	—
After first course of immunization	8/10	±
After second course of immunization	1/10	++

* Number of mice dead with ascites tumour over the total number inoculated; each mouse received an inoculum of 1×10^6 cells.

cytostatic effect. After a four week course of immunization with ribosomes growth of the treated tumour cells was inhibited in 2/10 mice. Furthermore growth of tumour cells pretreated with antiserum obtained after a second course of immunization was inhibited in 9/10 mice. The potency of the cytostatic effect increased together with the increase of the antibody titer.

To know if the phenomenon was due to an adsorption of the antibodies on the cells surface or a penetration of the antibodies inside the cells, after incubation with horse antiribosomes FLS antiserum, the cells were washed with NaCl 0.14 M pH 7.

The results of this experiment are suggestive of the fact that we were not dealing with an easily reversible adsorption (table III).

Table III. *Cytostatic effect of antiribosomes FLS horse antiserum on ascites tumour cells FLS*

	+/N. total*	Cytostatic effect	Mean survival time of mice bearing ascites (days)
Cells incubated with horse antiserum	2/10	++	32
Cells washed after incubation in vitro with horse antiserum	4/19	++	29
Control: cells incubated with normal horse serum	20/20	—	22

* Number of mice dead with ascites tumour over/the total number inoculated; each mouse received an inoculum of 1×10^6 cells.

Table III also illustrates that when the growth of tumour cells was not inhibited, it was at least delayed and that the mean time of evolution was longer (32 and 29 days) compared to the evolution time of the controls which received cells pretreated in vitro with normal horse serum (22 days).

We undertook an experiment to see if a direct contact between the cells and the antibodies was indispensable and if it injected with the antiserum 48 h after inoculation of the cells; this perhaps could be explained by the fact that, since we injected the same quantity of antiserum as in other experiments, the dose of antiserum was insufficient: the cells being evidently more numerous since they had been multiplying for 48 h.

Our results show that antiribosome antiserum incubated with tumour cells in vitro, or injected in vivo, is able to

Table IV. *In vivo effect of horse antiribosomes FLS antiserum on tumour cells FLS*

N° of cells injected i/p	First s/c injection after a delay (hours)	Nature of serum injected	+/N. total *	Mean survival time of mice bearing ascites (days)
10^5	3	normal horse serum	10/10	18,2
10^5	3	antiribosomes antiserum	3/10	33
10^5	8	antiribosomes antiserum	7/10	36
5×10^5	16	antiribosomes antiserum	7/10	30
5×10^5	48	antiribosomes antiserum	10/10	19,5
5×10^5		no treatment	10/10	18,2

* Number of mice dead with ascites tumour over total number inoculated.

was possible to obtain a cytostatic effect by injecting the antibodies subcutaneously. Sixty mice were injected intra-peritoneally with 1 to 5×10^5 non treated tumour cells. The animals received a first s/c injection of 0.3 ml of horse antiribosome antiserum within variable periods of time after the cells injection: 3 h, 8 h, 16 h and 48 h. The antiserum injection was repeated in the same way the following two days.

Table IV illustrates the results of this experiment. The same cytostatic effect as in the in vitro experiments was obtained. The tumour cells either did not grow or if they grew, they killed the animal after a much longer period (33 days) than the controls which received normal horse serum (18.2 days) or the controls which were not injected with the antiserum (18.2 days). This cytostatic effect was no longer observed if the mice were delay or inhibit the proliferation of such cells in mice.

This cytostatic effect of the antiserum increases during immunization along with the antibody titer.

Absorption of the antiribosome antibodies with homologous ribosomes or with purified RNA neutralizes the cytostatic effect. With the techniques used, we were not able to show either an immediate lethal effect or a morphological modification visible with a light microscope. However, preliminary experiments (in collaboration with L. Harel and J. Imbenotte) indicate that tumour cell biosynthesis (RNA and proteins) decreases after contact for 1 hour with antiribosome antibodies.

It seemed interesting to us to report these results especially since the cytostatic effect was obtained (in vitro as well as in vivo) with antibodies directed against ribosomes, which are a particularly well defined cellular fraction and whose primordial role in protein synthesis is well known.

Aknowledgement

We are grateful to Pr. L. BENEDETTI, who realized electron microscopic studies of ribosomal preparations.

References

[1] LACOUR, F., LACOUR, J., HAREL, J., and HUPPERT, J., Transplantable malignant tumors in mice induced by preparations containing ribonucleic acid extracted from human and mouse tumors. *J. nat. Cancer Inst.* **24**, 301—319 (1960).

[2] — HAREL, J., et NAHON, E., Etude immunologique de l'acide ribonucleique (RNA) par la microméthode de double diffusion dans l'agar. *C.R. Acad. Sci. (Paris)* **255**, 2322—2324 (1962).

[3] LACOUR, F., HAREL, J., HAREL, L., et HERMET, J., Etude antigènique des ribosomes de cellules de mammifères. *C.R. Acad. Sci. (Paris)* **255**, 1161—1163 (1962).

The Role of Tumour Polypassage at Short Intervals in the Evolution of Experimental Neoplasia

O. Costachel

Oncological Institute, Bucharest, Rumania

Transplantation immunity implies great technical difficulties and its results are hard to apply and reproduce even in experimental practice. Therefore, we have tried to find another method by which to study cancer extension in the organism, with particular reference to metastases.

This method studies the rapid phenomena of the trophicity (minutes, hours, days) and attempts research into the development of neoplasia without implying antibody formation.

Tumour polypassage at short intervals consists in repeated "repiquage", i.e. grafting and taking out of the graft at pre-established intervals (e.g. after the evolutive stages of transplantation reaction) of one or several materials, biological or otherwise (e.g. a tissue graft — tumourous or not — cell or macro-molecular suspensions etc.) on one or several animals or plants.

This method is aimed at interrupting the course of transplantation reaction at selected moments of its evolution in order to accentuate and possibly fix (by eurhythmical polypassing) or repress and possibly suppress (by antirhythmical polypassing) one or several elements of

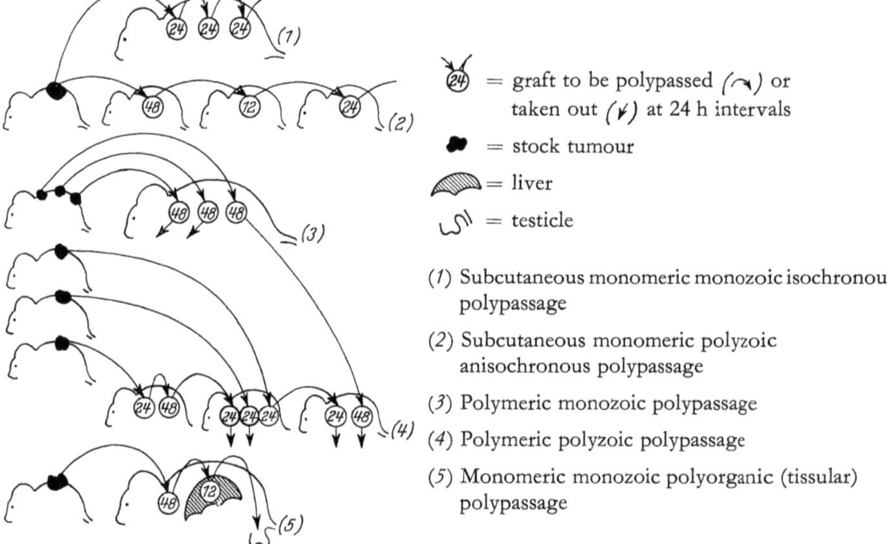

Fig. 1. Some modalities of tumour polypassage

this reaction at the level of grafted materials (e.g. a tissue graft) or of polypassed animals (recipients or donors).

In *transplantation* the polypassage is ntended to study: the rapid trophic

The polypassage may be made: *in vivo, in vitro,* with living or non living materials, mono- or polymeric, mono- or polyzoic, iso- or anisochronous; auto(iso-homo-hetero-)logous etc.

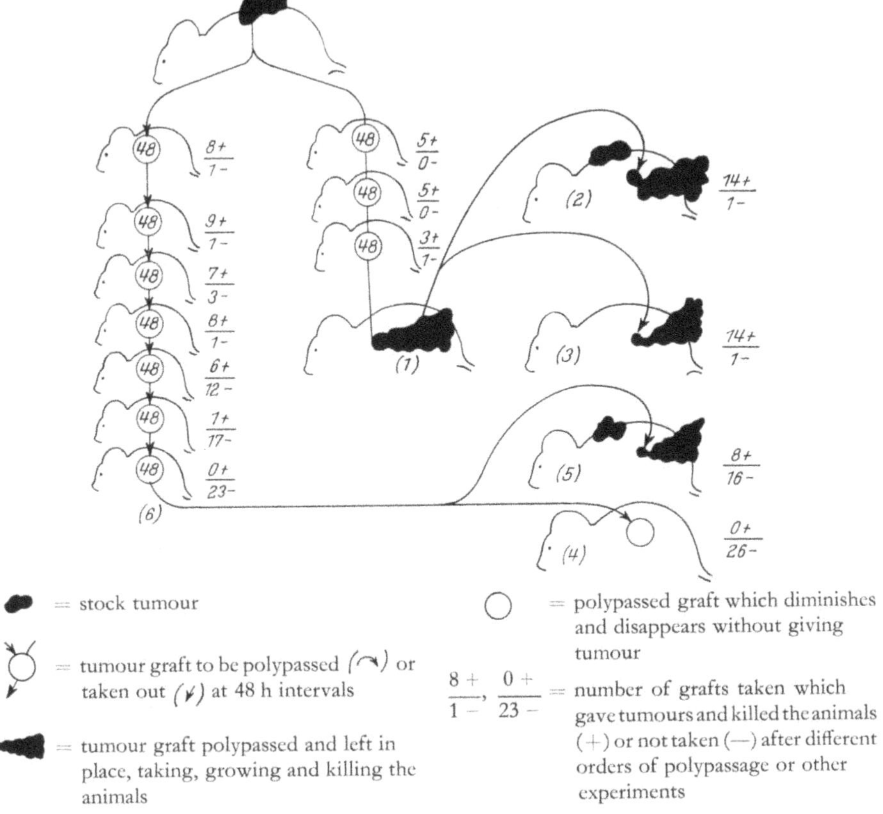

Fig. 2. Progressive loss of taking capacity and differential taking of tumour grafts through polypassage. 1. After three monomeric polyzoic polypassages the graft left in place gives a common tumour, similar to stock tumour (*1*); if this tumour is transplanted to 7 — day tumour-bearing (*2*) or control (*3*) animals, tumours which grow and kill the animals are developing. 2. After 6 polypassages the graft left in place or transplanted to a control animal no longer takes and disappears (*4*); but the same graft (after 6 polypassages) if transplanted to tumour -bearing animals takes, grows and kills them (*5*). 3. Between the 1st and the 6th polypassage, progressive loss of taking capacity of the polyzoic polypassed fragment (*6*) is observed

phenomena of transplantation reaction, biorhythmics, biognosy (reciprocal recognition of biological units) and the trophic phenomena in general at different levels (organisms, organs, tissues, cells, micro-organisms, virus, macromolecules, etc.).

The first significant results obtained in this and other (anterior) works through different models of tumoural polypassage are the following:

1. Differentiation of taking capacity of tumoural grafts (taking only on tumour-bearing animals) [10].

2. Progressive loss of taking capacity of the grafts with the increasing order of polyzoic (at 48 hours) or monozoic (at 24 hours) polypassage [8, 10].

3. The 48-hour interval polypassage is of great importance because of the

the contrary, the 24-hour interval polypassage hinders vascular neoformation and graft development [3, 4, 14, 18, 21].

4. The easy reproducible development *in standard non isologous animals* (non controlled by skin graft) of *resorbable tumours*

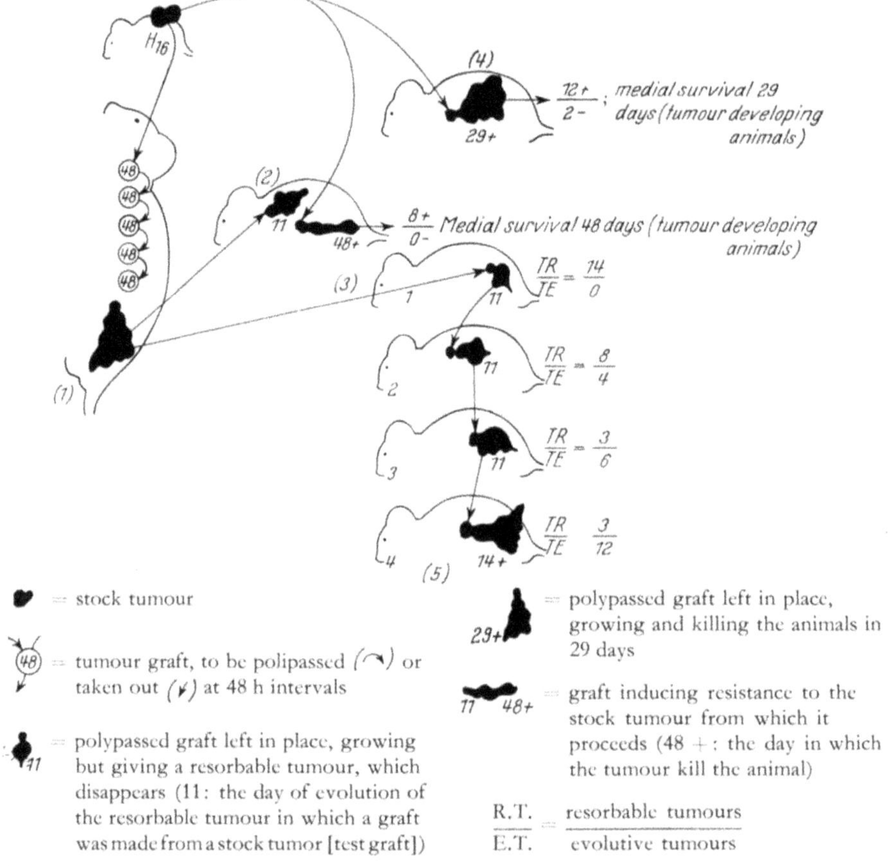

= stock tumour

= tumour graft, to be polipassed (↷) or taken out (↓) at 48 h intervals

= polypassed graft left in place, growing but giving a resorbable tumour, which disappears (11: the day of evolution of the resorbable tumour in which a graft was made from a stock tumor [test graft])

= polypassed graft left in place, growing and killing the animals in 29 days

= graft inducing resistance to the stock tumour from which it proceeds (48 +: the day in which the tumour kill the animal)

R.T. = resorbable tumours

E.T. = evolutive tumours

Fig. 3. Obtaining of resorbable tumours from tumours proceeding from polypassed fragments of stock tumours, left in place after the 5th passage. Obtaining of anti-tumour resistance by passing the resorable tumours. By grafting H 16 tumour developed from the transplant left in place of the 5th monomer monozoic polypassage at 48 hr intervals (*1*), resorbable tumours (*2*) develop, which generate a partial antitumour resistance. The resistance is proved by a test graft, with a fragment of the same stock tumour, made on the 11th day of evolution of the resorbable tumour; the test graft kills the animals in 48 days (*3*) by comparison with the common, stock graft, killing the animals in only 29 days (*4*). The reconversion of the resorbable tumour into stock tumour is achieved after 3—4 passage (*5*)

vascular neoformation which begins before this interval after the first grafting and does not seem to be repressed if the graft is passed again at this interval. On

(from tumours proceeding from standard non isologous tumoural fragments polypassed and left in place at the 5th polypassage [*3*].

5. The easy reproducible enhancement of tumour development through concomitant polypassage of stock or polypassed standard non isologous tumours [9, 17, 22[.

by grafting resorbable tumours obtained as mentioned before [7, 11, 15].

9. The analogous response of adult and new-born animals at certain polypassage models, contradicting in this

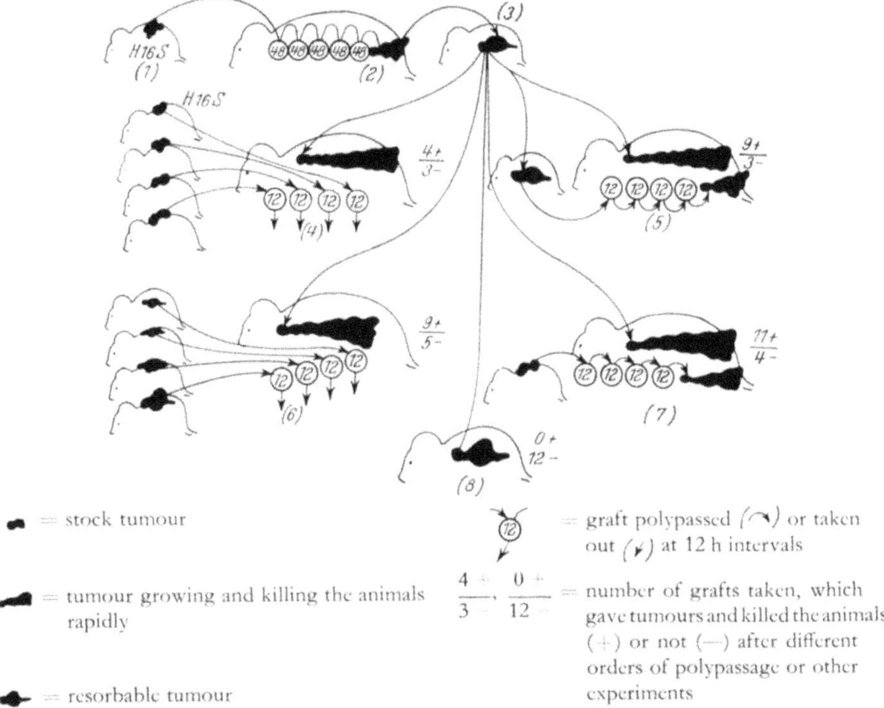

Fig. 4. Enhancement of resorbable tumours by four different types of concomitant polyppassage of H 16s stock and resorbable tumours. A resorbable tumour, obtained by polypassing 5 times and leaving in place a stock H 16s tumour, is passed to 4 experimental lots of animals (4, 5, 6, 7) and to one control lot (8). Concomitant polypassages (monomeric, monozoic, polyzoic, made with grafts of stock or resorbable tumours) enhance the growth of the grafted resorbable H 16s tumours in the experimental lots (4, 5, 6, 7) but increase and disappear in the control lot (8). The concomitant polypassed grafts left in place grow, give tumours and kill the animals after the monomeric monozoic polypassage of the stock tumour (7) and after the monomeric monozoic polypassage of the resorbable tumour (5)

6. Heterograft taking on standard, non isologous, tumour-bearing animals, by polypassing and leaving in place at the 5th polypassage the concomitant heterologous tumoral graft [19].

7. Slow growing tumours by 12-hourly interval polypassages [20].

8. Appearance or increase of the metastasizing capacity of different tumours

manner some aspects of the transplantation immunity [16].

10. The biognosy (reciprocal recognition of biological units — polypassed animals and polypassed graft) and their biorhythmics were studied. Recognition results at very short intervals (e.g. 2 hours) and may be tested by variation of serum glycoproteins after iso-

logous and heterologous grafting [2, 6, 19].

11. Parallel evolution of 2 types of cells in heterologous tumour grafting (obtained as mentioned above):

is obtained. A *decrease* of the percentage rate of caryotype of host cells appears, throughout, and an *increase* of metastasizing capacity of the resulting tumour also follows after intratesticular graft. Tu-

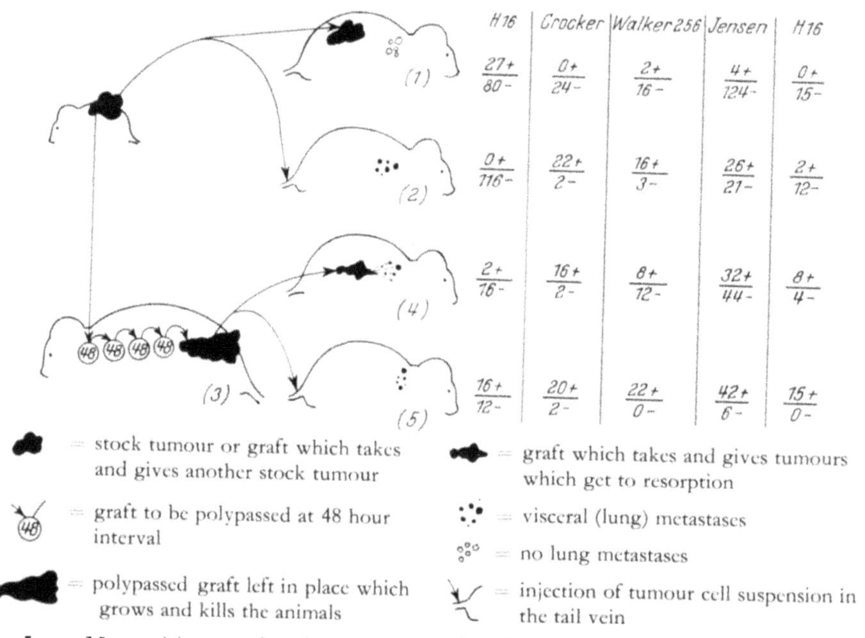

	H 16	Crocker	Walker 256	Jensen	H 16
(1)	$\frac{27+}{80-}$	$\frac{0+}{24-}$	$\frac{2+}{16-}$	$\frac{4+}{124-}$	$\frac{0+}{15-}$
(2)	$\frac{0+}{116-}$	$\frac{22+}{2-}$	$\frac{16+}{3-}$	$\frac{26+}{21-}$	$\frac{2+}{12-}$
(4)	$\frac{2+}{16-}$	$\frac{16+}{2-}$	$\frac{8+}{12-}$	$\frac{32+}{44-}$	$\frac{8+}{4-}$
(3) (5)	$\frac{16+}{12-}$	$\frac{20+}{2-}$	$\frac{22+}{0-}$	$\frac{42+}{6-}$	$\frac{15+}{0-}$

Fig. 5a—c. Metastasizing capacity of tumours proceeding from polypassed grafts. Transplants from the following tumours of: a) Wistar and Sprague-Dawley rats (Walker 256 and Jensen); b) IOB golden *hamsters* (H 10); c) A and H *mice* (H 16s and Crocker); grafted subcutaneously take and give tumours on the grafted place, but no visceral (lung) metastases (*1*). The same injected intravenously (by rats and mice) or in the venous sinus of the orbita (hamsters) produce visceral (lung) metastases (*2*) in variable percentages. By doing a monomeric monozoic subcutaneous polypassage from all the mentioned tumours at 48-hour intervals, and leaving the graft in place at the 5th passage, tumours are obtained which kill the polypassed animals (*3*). But if from each of these tumours a graft is passed subcutaneously to one other animal, the graft generated tumours which are resorbed and disappear, but give metastases in the same animals (*4*). After intraveneous administration of cell suspensions from all the mentioned tumours (proceeding from tumours which became resorbable after polypassage) 2—20 times more visceral (lung) metastases are obtained. The same applies to the stock form administered intravenously in the same conditions (*5*)

Increase of the percentage rate of caryotype of host cells in tumours resulting from polypassed fragments of greater order of polypassage parallel with an *increase* in the metastasizing capacity of the resulting tumours. If fragments are transplanted subcutaneously and also intratesticularly a *decrease* of the percentage rate of caryotype of host cells

mour polygraft was likewise studied [5, 12].

The great number of trophic modifications obtained by tumour fragments after polypassage at short intervals enables us to consider that this new method offers further possibilities in exploring and directing trophicity in general, and biognosy and tumour trophicity in particular.

References

[1] Costachel, O., and Corneci, I., The time factor in the hemocytopoietic tissue graft (unpublished results). Work supported in part by the I.A.E.A., Vienna EB Contract No 226 (1963).

[2] — Dumitrescu, S., Popp, I., and Comisel, V., Biorhythmics of tumor transplantation VII, Conditions of homologation in experimental tumor transplantation. Proceedings of Soc. of Compared Pathology, Bucharest, USSM, 18 June, 1964a.

[3] — Suciu, T., Iliescu, Pl., and Georgescu, D. P., Application of biorhythmics to the rejection reaction in testing tissue compatability. Proceedings of the Soc. of Oncology, Bucharest, August 18, 1964b.

[4] — Mironescu, St., and Stroescu, N., Earlier cellular reactions of the host tissues after an isologous tumoral graft. Proceedings of the Soc. of Oncology, Bucharest, August 18, 1964c.

[5] — Nachtigal, M., and Dumitrescu, S., The chromosome constitution of the mouse H 16 tumor after serial transplantation. Proceedings of the Soc. of Oncology, Bucharest, August 18, 1964d.

[6] — Stroescu, N., and Mironescu, St., Histoenzymatic changes of iso- and heterologous tumor grafts and of recipient animal early after transplantation. Proceedings of the Soc. of Oncology, Bucarest, October 27, 1964e.

[7] — Popp, I., and Dumitrescu, S., Preliminary results in the application of tumor polypassage in experimental model of metastases. *Cult. med. (Roma)* **37**, 139—142 (1964f).

[8] — Dumitrescu, S., and Popp, I., Biorhythmics of tumor transplantation trophic modifications of H 16 s tumor grafts by polypassage at 12 and 48 hr intervals. *Cult. med. (Roma)* **137**, 135—139 (1964g).

[9] — Dumitrescu, S., and Popp, I., Tumoral polypassages, a stimulating factor in restoring the growth capacity on the resorbable form of the IOB H 16 tumor. In: *Oncologia si Radiologia*, vol. III, No 5, p. 402. Bucharest 1964h.

[10] — Popp, I., and Foca-Suciu, N., Comparative trophic changes undergone by tumor fragments in the course of serial passages in one or several animals. In: *Oncologia si Radiologia*, vol. III, No 3, p. 207—208. Bucharest 1964i.

[11] Costachel, O., Dimitrescu, S., and Popp, I., Biorhythmics of tumor transplantation Note XVI. Modifications of the metastasizing capacity of the Jensen tumor obtained by polypassage. Proceedings of the Brasovev Symposium on "Experimental models in Medecine", 25 to 26 Sept., 1964j.

[12] —, and Popp, I., Tumor polypassage at short intervals, a new method in experim. cancer, Arch. immunol. et ther. exp. (in press), 1967.

[13] — Suciu-Foca, N., and Goia, G., Investigations on immunological tumor/host relations in animals poly-grafted with H 16 tumor fragments polypassed pseudoisologously. Proceedings of Biorhythmics Symposium, Bucharest, June 18, 1965a.

[14] — —, and Popp, I., *Trophic modifications of tumor fragments serially transplanted on several animals at intervals of 24, 48, 72 hrs.* Bucharest: Omagiu lui St. G. Nicolau, Ed. Academiei R.S.R. 1965b, p. 343—356.

[15] — Popp, I., and Dumitrescu, S., Metastasizing of Jensen polypassage tumor in normal and graft-tumor-bearing rats. Proceedings of the Soc. of Oncology USSM, Bucharest Jan. 26, 1965c.

[16] — — — Polypassage of the Jensen tumor in adult and new-born rats. Proceedings of the Soc. of Oncology, Bucharest, USSM, Febr. 23, 1965d.

[17] Dumitrescu, S., and Popp, I., Biorhythmics of tumor transplantation Note XVII. Interinfluencing of Lio and H 16 tumors by polypassage. Proceedings of the Brasovev Symposium on "Experimental models in Medicine", Sept. 25—26, 1964.

[18] Dutu, R., and Popp, I., Histopathological modifications of the experimental H 16 tumor obtained by polypassage. *Morfol. norm. si pat.*, 251—257 (1964).

[19] Kitulescu, I., Costachel, O., and Pascu, D., Rhythm of serum mucoprotein variations after iso- and heterologous tumor grafts. In: *Oncologia si Radiologia*, vol. IV, No 1, p. 33—38. Bucharest 1965.

[20] Popp, I., Comparative study of the relation between the host and the evolution of the H 16 tumor polypassed autologously and isologously at 12, 24 and 48 hr intervals. Proceedings of Biorhythmics Symposium, June 18, Bucharest.

[21] — Voiculet, N., Comisel, V., and Costachel, O., Biorhythmics of tumor transplantation, the importance of the 48 hrs interval in comparing grafts of H 16's stock tumor and H 16s tumor rendered isologous by autologous polypassage. Proceedings of the Soc. of Med. Biol. Bucharest, USSM, April 18, 1964.

[22] Popp, I., Nedelescu, P., and Terbea, I., Tumor polygraft. Control method of the interinfluence between the constituted tumor and the induced blastocytemia. Proceedings of the Brasovcov Symposium on "Experimental models in medicine", Sept. 25—26, 1964.

Short-range Factors Affecting Cell Growth and Movement

Michael Stoker

*Institute of Virology, University of Glasgow,
Glasgow, Scotland, Great Britain*

Normal cell populations in culture show certain features which suggest continued operation of some of the regulatory processes which operate in the intact animal. Notable examples are the organised re-aggregation of dispersed cells and the maintenance of cell arrangement by contact inhibition of movement. Tumour cells in culture may show different behaviour which suggests an alteration in these regulatory processes. In addition it is possible to observe a type of invasion with interacting populations of tumour cells and normal cells. Studies of this type obviously have limitations as models of cancer in the animal because transfer to tissue culture may modify, or select, atypical cell populations, and most studies have to be made in two-dimensional systems, or at least on two-dimensional substrates. Indeed it is increasingly clear that characteristics of tumour cells which we study *in vitro* may have little to do with the process of invasion in the intact host. Nonetheless, observations on simplified systems are an initial step towards an understanding of cell regulation and ultimately of cancer itself.

In our laboratory we have been interested in the mechanism of viral carcinogenesis and concerned with the altered state of cells observed soon after neoplastic transformation by viruses and before secondary changes have occurred. Our observations are made with (1) freshly isolated cultures of fibroblastic cells from mouse and hamster embryos or newborn animals, (2) a continuous line of hamster fibroblasts, named BHK21, which is sensitive to viral transformation (Macpherson and Stoker, 1962; Stoker and Macpherson, 1964), and (3) fresh hamster fibroblasts or BHK21 cells recently transformed *in vitro* by polyoma virus (termed "Py cells"). More limited observations have also been made on similar cells transformed by SV40 virus and Rous sarcoma virus.

This paper will be confined to regulatory phenomena in fibroblastic cells, and will deal first with normal cells, second with transformed cells, and third with the interaction between normal and transformed cells respectively. Some of the experimental data are published elsewhere (Stoker, 1964; Stoker and Sussman, 1965).

Interactions Between Normal Cells

Contact Inhibition of Movement. A noticeable feature of cultured fibroblastic cells is their regular arrangement in bundles of parallel cells, each cell contiguous with and probably adherent to its neighbour throughout its length.

This arrangement does not occur in sparse cultures but only when the cells are crowded. It is a manifestation of contact inhibition, which was first described by Abercrombie and his colleagues, who showed that movement ceases at points of contact between normal cells (see Abercrombie and Ambrose, 1962). The general aspects of this important phenomenon and its relationship to the surface will be discussed elsewhere in this symposium by Dr. Abercrombie and Dr. Ambrose. Not only fresh hamster and mouse fibroblasts but also the stable line of BHK21 cells used in our laboratory show evidence of marked contact inhibition of movement, as shown by their regular orientation; and this has been confirmed by time-lapse cinematography (E. J. Ambrose and K. Shepley, personal communication).

Inhibition of Cell Multiplication. When normal cells are cultured on a solid substrate in conditions optimal for growth, there is a short lag phase and then the cell numbers increase logarithmically until the cells cover the substrate. The growth then slows and after the cell layer is confluent division ceases. The maximum cell density (saturation density) for mouse and hamster fibroblasts is about 300,000 to 500,000 cells per sq. cm. substrate. Replenishment of medium during the lag phase or in the stationary phase has no effect on the saturation density once attained. If the cells are suspended and recultured at low density, however, growth starts again.

This inhibition of growth can be distinguished from contact inhibition of movement, because the two are not always co-existent. For example, BHK21 cells show good contact inhibition of movement but lack contact inhibition of growth. Such cells continue to multiply on solid substrates until the saturation density is about five times higher than the maximum reached by freshly isolated fibroblasts. The cells overlap and form piled-up layers five to ten cells thick. We can therefore postulate distinct mechanisms inhibiting movement and growth when cells are in close proximity.

Stimulation of Cell Multiplication. A feature of cell proximity which operates in the opposite way to inhibition of growth, is the feeder effect first described by Puck and Marcus (1955). Normal cells multiply poorly or not at all at very low density (i.e. less than about 1,000 cells per sq. cm.) and to assist the growth of single isolated cells it is necessary to keep them at intermediate densities or on feeder layers of cells which have been X-irradiated to prevent division.

Growth stimulation by feeder layers or increasing cell density is probably a complex phenomenon. Highly enriched medium may partially replace the requirement with some cells. Growth inhibition is also due to a non-dialysable short-range factor released by intact cells which acts with diminishing effect, because of dilution or inactivation, up to distances of 1.5 mm from each cell (Stoker and Sussman, 1965; see also Rubin, H. 1966). Stimulation does not necessarily involve contact because the effect will pass through filters with a pore diameter of $250\,\mu$, which prevent penetration of cell processes. It is possible that at least some of the molecules concerned are essential intracellular substances continuously lost by leakage until the immediate extracellular concentration is in equilibrium (Eagle, 1965).

General Aspects of Regulation in Cultured Normal Cells. Growth stimulation, growth inhibition and movement inhibition are all short-range effects produced by normal cells and they operate on other normal cells in close proximity. Growth stimulation is due to factors which are separable from the cell, growth inhibition involves factors operating at a short distance from the cell surface or actual contact, and movement inhibition apparently depends on contact itself. These effects are summarized diagrammatically in Fig. 1. It will be seen that they provide a homeostatic mechanism to produce and maintain populations of cells at optimal density at least in relation to the underlying substrate. Growth inhibition and stimulation may operate through a class of substances released by cells and subject to very rapid decay. These opposite effects might involve either linked or separate systems of induction or repression and it is possible that a single substance released by cells might act as an inducer at one concentration and a repressor at another.

Dependence on Anchorage. In addition to these homeostatic mechanisms it is necessary to mention one other characteristic of normal cells because it is affected by malignant transformation. Multiplication of many types of normal cells, and of BHK21 cells, is dependent upon attachment of the cell to one or more points on an immobile substrate. When cells are suspended in fluid or a gel such as agar they remain competent for long periods, but cell division only commences after contact with, and anchorage to, fixed points on glass, plastic, or even fibres of cotton wool. The mechanism involved in this process is quite unknown.

Changes in Regulation in Viral-Induced Tumour Cells

Hamster cells transformed by polyoma virus (Py cells) can be obtained from hamster tumours following virus inoculation of newborn animals, or from fresh fibroblasts or BHK21 cells transformed *in vitro*. Similar changes are found in cells from each source; many are

highly transplantable with a minimum tumour-producing dose of 10 to 100 cells and show several other altered characters which distinguish them from normal cells or BHK21 cells. We shall confine ourselves to changes in the regulatory phenomena which are the subject of this discussion.

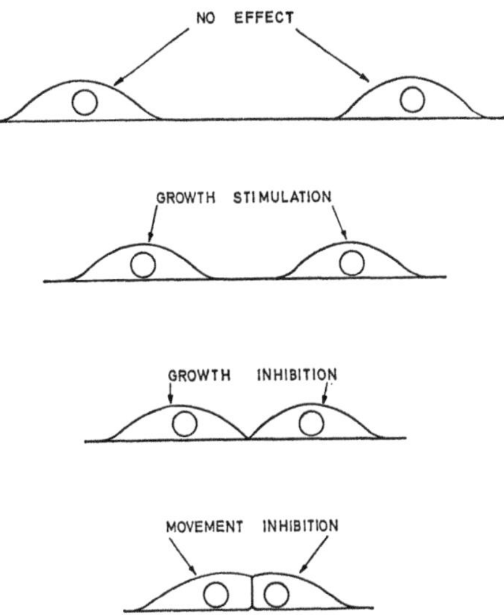

Fig. 1. Diagrammatic representation of some short-range interactions between normal cells in culture

Py cells differ from fresh fibroblasts or BHK21 cells in that they show random orientation and continued active movement when cells are in contact. It appears from time-lapse cinematography that adhesion occurs between cells at localized points rather than continuously over the surface as in fresh fibroblasts or BHK 21 cells. This gives rise to a loose network of actively moving cells with intervening spaces.

Py cells also continue to grow logarithmically to a saturation density about five times that of fresh hamster or mouse fibroblasts (about 2 million cells per sq. cm.). At this density there is a thick felt of cells which usually detaches so it is not known if growth would continue. The Py cells may therefore be insusceptible or less susceptible to the factor which inhibits cell division in contiguous sheets of normal cells.

Isolated Py cells are sensitive to growth promotion by proximity due to density, or by the presence of irradiated feeder cells, but they are less dependent on feeder action than normal cells and

Hamster tumour cells transformed by other viruses have not been examined in detail by us but both Rous sarcoma cells and SV 40 transformed cells show the same growth in suspension, disoriented arrangement, and increased saturation density as Py cells.

Lack of Correlation with Transplantability. Malignant transformation of BHK 21 cells may be produced im-

Table I. *Characteristics of hamster cells*

	HK freshly isolated fibroblasts	BHK 21 original stable line	BHK 21 (T) transplantable variant	HK (Py) BHK 21 (Py) polyoma transformed
Relative transplantability *	0	10^1	10^4	10^4
Mean division time (hr)	24	12	12	12
Saturation density. Cells per sq cm ($\times 10^5$)	4	20	20	20
Colony forming efficiency without feeder layers **	1	20	20	30
Colony forming efficiency suspension in agar ***	1	1	10^2	10^4
Random orientation and movement in contiguous cells	—	—	—	+

* Reciprocal of minimum tumour-producing dose $\times 10^6$.
** Colonies per 100 cells.
*** Colonies per 10^5 cells.

therefore have a higher colony-forming efficiency at low density and in the absence of feeder layers. Irradiated Py cells are themselves efficient as feeders but no precise comparisons have been made with normal cells.

One of the most striking changes following transformation is the loss of dependence on anchorage for cell division. Immediately after transformation by polyoma and other viruses, cells are able to divide in suspension when free from any fixed contact. This is demonstrated by their ability to form colonies with high efficiency in an agar gel (SANDERS and BURFORD, 1964; MONTAGNIER and MACPHERSON, 1964).

mediately by viruses but it may also appear spontaneously after continued cell propagation. Variants appearing spontaneously are as transplantable as Py cells (minimum tumour dose 10 to 100 cells) but in culture they retain the oriented cell arrangement of freshly isolated cells, or early passage BHK 21 cells. Characteristics of these and other hamster fibroblast-like cells are shown in Table I. As pointed out by DEFENDI *et al.* (1963) loss of contact inhibition of movement is not a necessary factor in the acquisition of transplantability. It should also be pointed out that early passage BHK 21 cells, which do not possess the high transplantability of the spontaneous variant, have the same unrestricted growth potential in culture. Therefore the successful growth of cells on transplantation is not due solely to the loss of growth and movement control as studied in culture. This is not surprising in view of the complexity of the whole animal where immunological, hormonal, and other factors play a part. It will be noted from the table that ability to grow without anchorage does show some correlation to transplantability, and it will be important to examine this relationship more thoroughly.

Interaction between Transformed Cells and Normal Cells

Despite the unrestricted growth and movement of Py cells it has been commonly observed that the Py cells in dense colonies avoid contact with any giant cells which are present. These giant cells arise from non-dividing homologous cells or irradiated feeder cells of various types including normal fibroblasts. This suggests that Py cells are not wholly insensitive to contact inhibition and has led to a study of the interaction of Py cells and normal cells.

The following observations were made with hamster Py cells in contact with either freshly isolated mouse or hamster fibroblasts. No species differences were found with the effects observed (STOKER, 1964).

Inhibition of Movement by Contact with Normal Cells. When Py cells labelled with carbon for identification (STOKER, 1964) were allowed to fall on a bare substrate, the cells took up the usual random orientation to one another and this was maintained as the cells multiplied. The same number of cells falling on pre-existing confluent normal cells, however, showed the parallel orientation of the underlying cells and apart from the carbon label were indistinguishable from the normal cells. The arrangement was maintained on continued incubation. It was also observed that colonies of transformed cells developing in intimate mixtures with normal cells took up the oriented arrangement characteristic of a colony of normal cells. The cells in these colonies did not grow at random on top of the normal cells. This orientation of Py cells by contact with normal cells was also seen in mixtures with BHK21 cells.

Thus movement of the transformed cells was apparently inhibited by contact with normal cells but not with other transformed cells. However it was not possible to exclude the suggestion that the cells were subject to contact guidance (WEISS, 1962), and that active movement of the Py cells continued. Subsequently, however, Dr. E. J. AMBROSE and Miss K. SHEPLEY (personal communication) have shown by time-lapse cinematography that carbon-marked Py cells stop active movement when in contact with BHK 21 cells, but not when in contact with other Py cells.

This seemed to conflict with the observations of ABERCROMBIE *et al.* (1957) who showed that advancing sarcoma cells continued to move actively when in contact with normal cells. Polyoma transformed cells may be unusual in sensitivity to movement inhibition, but concurrent studies by BARSKI and BELEHRADEK (1965) have shown that two other types of mouse tumour cell are also subject to arrest of movement by contact with compact sheets of normal mouse embryo cells. Tumour cell types probably vary in their sensitivity to normal contact, and it would be of interest to look for correlation with other characteristics, such as ability to metastasize.

Growth of Py Cells in Contact with Normal Cells. The growth and other aspects of the behaviour of Py cells in relation to normal cells may conveniently be examined by the halfplate method in which petri dish cultures of confluent or sparse cells are prepared so that the cells only occupy part of the substrate. Py cells in small numbers may be seeded evenly over the whole surface and colony development observed at different sites all within the same culture and the same medium. Fig. 2 shows numbers of Py colonies appearing in such cultures.

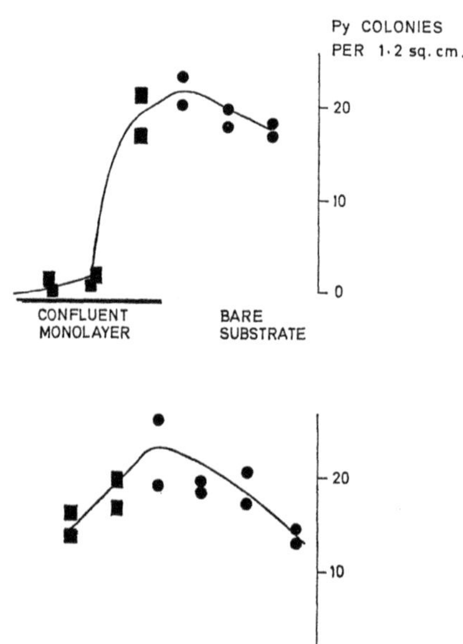

Fig. 2. Colony formation by Py cells on bare substrate, and either confluent or sparse monolayers of normal hamster fibroblasts, occupying half the area of the same petri dish. Round colonies of random cells ○. Elongated colonies of partly oriented cells □

On the bare substrate colonies are relatively small, and the cells are randomly arranged in the usual way. Near the edge of the normal cell sheet the colony size increases presumably due to short-range stimulation.

On the sparse monolayer the number of Py colonies is not markedly affected but they are elongated and composed partly of oriented cells and somewhat resemble colonies of normal cells, though they are distinguishable by their basophilic staining and tendency to pile up. This distortion of the colony is presumably due to contact inhibition of movement by the normal cells which grow from a sparse to almost confluent cell sheet during the experiment. If growth of normal cells is stopped by X-irradiation the Py colonies are not distorted.

On the confluent monolayers, within 2—3 mm from the edge, distorted Py colonies also appear, probably for the same reason. Over the main part of the confluent sheet, however, colony formation by Py cells is inhibited.

It is known from observations of marked Py cells that this is not due to failure of attachment of the cells. It is also known that the Py cells are not killed by the normal cells, because resuspension of the cells and dilution to remove contact allows the Py cells to grow into colonies with normal efficiency. There seem to be two other possible explanations.

First, Py cells may grow unrestrictedly on confluent sheets of normal cells but may be indistinguishable through their loss of active movement and therefore random arrangement. Second, initiation or continued growth of the transformed cells may be completely or partially inhibited by contact with normal cells.

Further experiments have now shown clearly that division of Py cells is inhibited by confluent layers of normal cells at saturation density. Studies on division of carbon-marked Py cells first suggested that growth was inhibited by contact with normal cells, but it was only possible to follow the Py cells for one or two divisions before the carbon was lost. The growth of Py cells was therefore studied by counting colony-forming cells under selective conditions where Py cells but not normal cells will grow. The results also indicated a slower rate of growth of Py cells on normal cells compared to bare substrate. Further studies are in progress but are complicated by variability in the degree of inhibition of growth which can be measured, probably because the growth-promoting effect may predominate with minor changes in experimental conditions. Like the inhibitory action of normal cells on each other, the effect on Py cells seems to be a short-range one and not due to general depletion of medium. It is not at present possible to distinguish, however, between release of short-range inhibitors or local competition for essential growth factors in medium. Local changes in pH might also play an important role.

The sensitivity of transformed cells to inhibition of movement, and perhaps cell division, by close proximity to normal cells, suggested that they were responding to the factors which are responsible for regulation of normal cells. On the other hand transformed cells do not respond to contact with, or proximity to, each other. This apparent paradox led to a hypothesis that transformation by polyoma virus does not affect the ability of a cell to respond to contact or short-range signals, but that it removes or diminishes the production of such signals (STOKER, 1964). In this way, transformed cells would not be subject to inhibition by each other. A similar suggestion has been put forward by BULLOUGH and RYTÖMAA (1965) working with a completely different system involving mitotic inhibition in epidermal cells.

Conclusions

The phenomena described relate to a model system of cells in culture and its main value lies in the preliminary attempt to delineate a few of the many factors which must operate on cells *in vivo*. At this stage the relevance to cancer in the intact animal is conjectural, and the temptation to extrapolate should probably be resisted. The very fact that isolated malignant cells do grow into tumours and penetrate surrounding barriers of normal cells clearly shows that tumour cells *in vivo* are not completely sensitive to the normal contact or proximity control mechanisms which are studied in tissue culture.

One concept which emerges, and which may be generally applicable, is that of critical clone size. If individual cells of some tumours are subject to normal homeostatic mechanisms, a single tumour cell appearing amongst normal cells would not express its altered characteristics of growth and movement while in close proximity or contact with the normal cells. If the daughter cells in the clone remain together, however, they would eventually reach a population of perhaps eight or sixteen adjoining cells. This could be a critical clone size and an entirely new situation would then arise because a few tumour cells would be in the centre of the mass, and shielded from the normal cells so that they could be expected to escape from control. This implies that the behaviour of a tumour cell population would be markedly affected by cell mass, and there might be long periods at subcritical clone size when the tumour cells behaved phenotypically like normal cells.

The suggestion that some tumour cells may be sensitive to normal homeostatic control of movement and perhaps growth should not be too surprising. Transformation into a tumour cell must leave the great majority of regulatory processes in the cell unaltered or else the change would be lethal. Control mechanisms of the type we have discussed which are probably mediated by contact, or short-lived molecules acting near the cell surface, are likely to depend on a complex balance of several opposing factors. The response of an atypical cell to such normal homeostatic mechanisms will depend on the quantitative as well as the qualitative aspects of the abnormality and this may result in the wide variety of invasiveness which we know to be a characteristic of different forms of cancer.

Discussion

Questions put to M. STOKER

Z. Brada: I would like to ask Dr. STOKER a few questions:

1. In what way has it been established that it is not physical influences, but short-range factors that are involved, especially in the direct effect on the cell membranes?

2. Can this effect of stimulation be induced in other cell systems besides the fibroblast system?

3. Do you know the chemical properties of these short-range factors?

G. Barski: You obtained good evidence that in older dense cultures of normal fibroblasts there is a drastic arrest of added transformed malignant cells. Have you done control experiments with normal cells added to these cultures under the same conditions to see whether these additional cells are stopped in the same way?

D. F. H. Wallach: Can you give me a more precise idea of the distances over which growth inhibition by "contact" occurs?

M. Stoker: Firstly, it is at present impossible to distinguish between physical influences and short-range factors. (This also answers your last question, Dr. BRADA, because we cannot yet isolate a factor study.) Secondly, I have not yet studied cells other than fibroblasts. Dr. BARSKI has asked about inhibition between normal cells. We have not yet attempted this, and I confess that I cannot see an easy way to do it without improved cell markers.

I am afraid, Dr. WALLACH, that we cannot estimate the distance involved in the inhibition effect, except to say that it is probably less than a few thousand angstroms.

M. Feldman: I am extremely impressed by the *in vitro* system of cell interactions which you have described, Dr. STOKER. Now I need only to understand it better: you have one type of interaction, whereby the Py cells cannot produce a signal for growth inhibition, but are susceptible to such a signal once it has been produced by normal fibroblasts. I also understand, although you have not discussed it today, that the Py cells do not manifest contact inhibition when interacting among themselves, yet they are susceptible to a signal for contact inhibition produced by normal fibroblasts. The question arises whether there is a causal relationship between the two phenomena — i.e. whether contact inhibition in some way triggers growth inhibition. I suspect that although "contact" is the triggering event in both phenomena, this need not mean that "contact inhibition" is the determining factor. This could perhaps be studied by removing part of a confluent, already growth- and contact-inhibited monolayer of fibroblasts. The cells at the edge of the cut will remain contact-inhibited, yet they will probably now continue to replicate. This may indicate that although the two phenomena involve contact interactions, they are two distinct processes. The question further arises as to whether the growth-controlling factors of a monolayer of fibroblasts, as manifested *in vitro* in growth inhibition, are relevant to the growth control mechanism as realized *in vivo*. If we take a primary sarcoma which, when tested *in vitro,* still shows *contact inhibition,* will it manifest growth inhibition like normal fibroblasts? If it does, this will indicate that cells which do not respond to the *in vivo* control factors respond to the *in vitro* factors; this, in turn, would suggest that the *in vivo* control factors are basically different from the *in vitro* ones.

M. Stoker: There is quite good evidence that inhibition of movement and growth are different phenomena because untransformed BHK 21 cells show good movement inhibition, as seen for example in Dr. AMBROSE's film, but at the same time they grow to high densities like Py transformed cells. In addition, normal fresh fibroblasts show contact inhibition of movement when they reach a thin confluent sheet, but may still continue to divide at least once or twice.

E. J. Ambrose: I was particularly interested in your observations of a time dependence of inhibition effects, Dr. STOKER. I should like to make a few comments on the way in which we think that cell contacts are established between malignant cells and between normal cells in monolayer culture. The initial contact is probably a comparatively non-specific adhesion. In the case of tumours, the active movement of the free regions of the cell is sufficient to break the local adhesions within a short time. With normal cells the adhesions, once formed, are more numerous and therefore maintained for a longer time. Secretion then takes place in the region of the mem-

branes; this takes an extreme form in the desmosomes seen in the electron microscope. Is it possible that it is the time dependence of secretion on contact which affects the production or non-production of contact signals? This might explain the formation of coherent contacts in suspension cultures of malignant cells shown by Prof. HALPERN. The hydrodynamic conditions in the agitated culture may increase the length of time during which contacts can be maintained in the case of the malignant cells.

P. Vigier: In connection with Prof. AMBROSE's comments, it may be of interest to note that normal fibroblasts may still grow slowly when their medium is renewed frequently — for instance, daily — whereas arrest of growth following confluence is more marked when cells are left for a few days without a change of medium. One may therefore speculate as to whether some growth-inhibitory factor could not accumulate on the cells, if not in the medium. This could explain why growth of Py cells seeded on 4-day-old cultures of fibroblasts is more inhibited than that of cells seeded on 1-day-old cultures.

M. Stoker: This is certainly possible. All we know is that no diffusible substance has been detected in the medium.

R. D. Thornes: I would like to ask Dr. STOKER two questions about the short-range growth inhibition he describes.

1. Has he tried to isolate this factor from fibroblasts (normal cells), and, if so, do small amounts of it stimulate growth?

2. Is there any evidence to show that a minute quantity of the short-range inhibitor stimulates growth of Py cells? In other words, does the proximity of fibroblasts stimulate the growth of Py cells outside the range of inhibition?

S. Wood: 1. Does the Py cell contain a virus, either unaltered or altered?

2. Do you regard it as a "viral hyperplasia" or as a true neoplasm — a sarcoma?

3. Upon the inoculation of cell into suitable unconditioned hosts, does it grow and/or metastasize? Is it a true neoplasm?

M. Stoker: In answer, Dr. Thornes, we have not successfully isolated an inhibitory or stimulating factor from normal fibroblasts. There is evidence of a growth stimulation beyond the inhibitory region in cultures, but it is not possible to say if it is due to the same or to a different factor.

The Py cells contain no infectious virus particles, Dr. Wood, but there is evidence that viral information persists.

The tumours formed by polyoma virus have the appearance of anaplastic sarcomas, but they do not metastasize freely. Perhaps someone else could comment on the neoplastic nature of these viral tumours.

K. E. Hellström: I should like to inform Dr. Wood that there is conclusive evidence that the polyoma-virus-induced tumours really consists of autonomously growing tumour cells and are not the symptom of some "viral disease" in the polyoma-infected animal. It has been shown, e.g. by Sjögren (Dept. of Tumour Biology in Stockholm) — that polyoma-induced mouse tumour cells are transplantable and that the tumours appearing after transplantation have the same morphology and karyotype as the tumours which were transplanted. This is independent of whether or not the tumour cells can release the polyoma virus.

References

Abercrombie, M., and Ambrose, E. J., The surface properties of cancer cells — a review. *Cancer Res.* **22**, 525—548 (1962).

— Heaysman, J. E. M., and Karthauser, M. M., Observations on the social behaviour of cells in tissue culture. III. Mutual influence of sarcoma cells and fibroblasts. *Exp. Cell Res.* **13**, 276—291 (1957).

Barski, G., and Belehradek, J., Etude microcinématographique du mécanisme d'invasion cancéreuse en culture de tissu normal associé aux cellules malignes. *Exp. Cell Res.* **37**, 464—480 (1965).

Bullough, W. S., and Rytömaa, T., Mitotic homeostasis. *Nature (Lond.)* **205**, 573—578 (1965).

Defendi, V., Lehman, J., and Kraemer, P., "Morphologically normal" hamster cells with malignant properties. *Virology* **19**, 592—598 (1963).

Eagle, H., Metabolic controls in cultured mammalian cells. *Science* **148**, 42—51 (1965).

Macpherson, I,. and Stoker, M., Polyoma transformation of hamster cell clones — an investigation of genetic factors affecting cell competence. *Virology* **16**, 147—151 (1962).

Montagnier, L., and Macpherson, I., Croissance sélective en gélose de cellules de hamster transformées par le virus du polyome. *C.R. Acad. Sci. (Paris)* **258**, 4171—4173 (1964).

Puck, T. T., and Marcus, P. I., A rapid method for viable cell titration and clone production with HeLa cells in tissue culture: The use of X-irradiated cells to supply conditioning factors. *Proc. Nat. Acad. Sci. (Wash.)*, **41**, 432 (1955).

Rubin, H., The inhibition of chick embryo cell growth by medium obtained from cultures of Rous sarcoma cells. *Exp. Cell Res.* **41**, 149—161 (1966).

Sanders, F. J., and Burford, B. O., Ascites tumours from BHK 21 cells transformed *in vitro* by polyoma virus. *Nature (Lond.)* **201**, 786—789 (1964).

Stoker, M., Regulation of growth and orientation in hamster cells transformed by polyoma virus. *Virology* **24**, 165—174 (1964).

—, and Macpherson, I., Syrian hamster fibroblast cell line BHK 21 and its derivatives. *Nature (Lond.)* **203**, 1355—1357 (1964).

—, and Sussman, M., Studies on the action of feeder layers in cell culture. *Exp. Cell Res.* **38**, 645—653 (1965).

Weiss, P., "Attraction fields" between growing tissue cultures. *Science* **115**, 293—296 (1962).

Amending Statement by Michael Stoker

Since the paper was presented further studies in this laboratory have shown that initiation of growth of Py cells only occurs where contact is made with a non-growing layer of normal cells; contact with growing normal cells permits growth of Py cells (STOKER, SHEARER and O'NEILL, 1966). Thus the transformed cells seem to obey the regulation state present in the normal culture.

It has also been reported recently by EAGLE and LEVINE (1966) that static cultures of human fibroblasts do not inhibit growth of heteraploid human cell lines, and TODARO and GREEN (1966) have shown that normal 3T3 cells only inhibit growth of virus transformed 3T3 cells for a short period after initiation of transformation.

This suggests that escape from growth restriction may vary qualitatively or quantitatively in different cell systems. From the considerations discussed in this paper we would, in fact, predict at least two possible types of changes: loss of ability to initiate growth inhibiting signals, and inability to respond to such signals.

EAGLE, H., and LEVINE, E. M., Growth regulatory effects of cellular interaction. *Nature*, **213**, 1102—1106 (1967).

STOKER, M., SHEARER, M., and O'NEILL, C., Growth inhibition of polyoma-transformed cells by contact with static normal fibroblasts. *J. Cell Sci.*, **1**, 297—310 (1966).

TODARO, G., and GREEN, H., Cell growth and induction of transformation by SV 40. *Proc. Natl. Acad. Sci.*, **55**, 302—307 (1966).

Le Mécanisme de l'Invasion du Cancer en Culture Organotypique

Etienne Wolff

Aucun dispositif n'est plus favorable à l'étude du pouvoir d'invasion des cellules cancéreuses que les associations *in vitro* d'organes embryonnaires et de tumeurs. Cette analyse est encore plus aisée, quand les deux catégories d'explants proviennent de deux espèces très différentes, telles la Poule et l'Homme. Ainsi les cellules malignes se distinguent à la manière d'éléments marqués, des cellules normales de l'autre espèce. Tel est le principe de l'une de nos techniques de culture de cancers *in vitro* (E. Wolff, 1956; E. Wolff, 1958).

Elle présente en outre d'autres avantages. Les tumeurs malignes conservent la structure et les propriétés qu'elles avaient dans l'organisme dont elles proviennent. Ceci est vrai en particulier de leur pouvoir d'invasion, que l'on peut éprouver sur des organes et tissus différents. Enfin, il est à peine besoin de dire que, dans ces conditions, l'organe normal et la tumeur maligne se trouvent directement confrontés, en l'absence de la circulation sanguine et de ses apports, et en l'absence de toute corrélation ou connexion avec aucune autre partie de l'organisme. C'est donc dans des conditions de grande simplicité que les relations entre les cellules normales et les cellules cancéreuses peuvent être étudiées. On peut objecter que, dans ce système, les cellules tumorales ne se trouvent pas dans les conditions habituelles, qu'elles ne sont pas affrontées aux tissus d'un organisme de même espèce qu'elles. Ceci est exact. Cependant, dans l'ensemble, leur comportement ne varie guère d'un organisme à l'autre, les cellules d'un sarcome ou d'un épithelioma conservent leurs proprietés et leur structure spécifique. S'il en était autrement, il serait quand même fort intéressant d'étudier les propriétés spéciales qu'elles manifestent dans de tels systèmes, mais qui n'en sont pas moins révélatrices de leurs potentialités propres.

Matériel et Méthodes

Rappelons brièvement que le milieu sur lequel nous cultivons les organes embryonnaires a la composition suivante:

```
Agar à 1% dans la solution de Gey .  11 parties
Extrait d'embryons dilué à 50% dans
      la solution de Tyrode  . . . . .   4 parties
Serum de cheval . . . . . . . . .   4 parties
Pénicilline . . . . . . . . . . . .   1 goutte
```

A la surface de ce milieu semi-solide, nous déposons les organes embryonnaires de poulet: mesonephros, metanephros, foie, gonades, poumons, peau . . . etc. Ceux-ci sont découpés en grands ou petits morceaux, suivant les organes et les besoins. En général, sauf dans le cas de la peau et des gonades, les organes embryonnaires sont débités en morceaux très fins. C'est entre ces fragments que l'on dispose de petits explants de tumeurs, à peu près de mêmes dimensions que ceux des organes. Les uns et les autres sont enchevêtrés en mosaïque.

Nous avons cultivé ainsi des tumeurs transplantables de souris et de rats (E. Wolff, 1957; 1961), des souches cellulaires malignes de Souris et d'Homme (E. Wolff, 1959), des tumeurs humaines prélevées sur le malade (E. Wolff, 1961). On peut étudier l'évolution de tumeurs différentes sur un même organe, ou le comportement d'une même tumeur dans des organes différents. Nous donnerons quelques exemples tirés de ces expériences.

Nous ajouterons en outre quelques observations qui résultent de l'emploi d'une modalité technique spéciale. Au lieu de cultiver les nodules cancéreux au contact direct des tissus embryonnaires, nous interposons entre les deux types d'explants une membrane filtrante, un morceau de la membrane vitelline de l'oeuf de poule. Ainsi les explants, au lieu de vivre directement en parasites des tissus normaux, sont nourris par les substances qui filtrent à travers la membrane. Il ne s'agit donc pas d'une invasion, car la membrane ne laisse passer aucune cellule. Toutefois ces cultures révèlent certaines propriétés qui peuvent contribuer à éclairer les processus d'invasion.

I. Affrontement de deux Tissus Normaux d'Organes ou d'Espèces Différents

Il n'est pas sans intérêt de se demander comment se comportent deux tissus normaux d'organes ou d'espèces différents, lorsqu'ils sont associés en culture. Nous avons rapproché sur le même milieu deux gonades provenant respectivement d'un embryon de canard et d'un embryon de souris (E. Wolff, 1954). Grâce aux différences frappantes qui existent entre les cellules des deux espèces, on peut observer et suivre avec précision les affrontements qui se produisent entre les deux explants, les associations,

les déplacements éventuels de leurs cellules. On constate que les tissus embryonnaires des deux espèces se tolèrent et qu'ils collaborent à former des structures communes. On peut suivre les migrations importantes des cellules conjonctives de souris dans les tissus de canard. Elles suivent les membranes basales des épithéliums ou des tubes; elles se mêlent aux tissus conjonctifs lâches du partenaire jusqu'à d'assez grandes distances de leur point de départ. D'autre part les tissus propres des organes, tels les épithéliums, tendent à s'associer pour former des structures communes, véritables chimères d'organes. De telles associations se produisent aussi entre des organes différents d'une même espèce (Bresch, 1955) ou d'espèces différentes (Bermann, 1960). Ainsi le poumon et le mesonephros forment des structures chimères, dans lesquelles leurs épithéliums se joignent et se raccordent.

Nous remarquerons que les cellules tumorales associées à un organe embryonnaire ne se comportent pas d'une manière très différente des cellules normales, du moins au début de l'expérience.

II. Evolution de Tumeurs Différentes sur un même Organe

C'est sur le mésonephros que nous cultivons de préférence les tumeurs, de quelque origine qu'elles soient.

Le sarcome S *180* de souris (E. Wolff, 1957) montre, au contact du mesonephros, un pouvoir intense d'invasion. Les cellules du sarcome migrent en grand nombre hors de l'explant initial. Un des caractères les plus remarquables de cette tumeur est que les cellules tendent à essaimer. Elles se répandent individuellement dans les tissus de l'hôte, tout en formant des courants dont les axes matérialisent les directions d'invasion, les régions de plus grande pénétrabilité du mesonephros. C'est dans les tissus conjonctifs, dans les lacunes des tissus que la pénétration est la plus forte. Les parois épithéliales des tubes urinaires, les tissus des glomérules ne sont jamais directement envahis. C'est après un véritable investissement de ces formations que celles-ci sont finalement envahies, mais indirectement. Leurs cellules sont progressivement enserrées, comme étouffées par le sarcome. Elles s'aplatissent, s'amenuisent, et sont en dernier lieu remplacées par les cellules tumorales. Les cellules tumorales se comportent dans l'ensemble comme de grands fibroblastes, dont elles ont l'aspect et le comportement. Mais elles sont douées en outre de malignité.

Un lymphome lymphoïde de souris (POURREAU, 1963) montre des propriétés analogues à celles du sarcome: invasion des tissus conjonctifs par des cellules isolées qui, en se multipliant, ont tendance à former des amas corticaux continus à la périphérie des explants, ou des couches concentriques autour des tubes excréteurs, qu'elles n'envahissent pas.

Une tumeur anaplasique du poumon humain, sans structure définie, et très envahissante, montre des propriétés un peu différentes: c'est la tumeur R 50 caractérisée par des masses confuses de cellules à noyaux en grains d'orge (E. WOLFF, 1962). De petits groupes de cellules ou des émissaires isolés s'en détachent de toutes parts, pénétrant dans tous les tissus, y compris les tubes urinifères, qu'elles entourent, puis envahissent en s'insinuant entre les cellules de l'épithélium.

Les épithéliomas et les adénocarcinomes se comportent généralement d'une manière différente. Il est rare que leurs cellules se dispersent et se multiplient isolément dans les tissus de l'organe embryonnaire. Elles restent groupées et s'insinuent sous forme de lobes pluricellulaires entre les cellules normales;

ceux-ci se scindent parfois de la masse principale, sous forme d'îlots qui se constituent en nodules secondaires. Ainsi certaines tumeurs se fragmentent en petits amas qui deviennent de nouveaux foyers de prolifération. C'est le cas de la tumeur Z 200, métastase hépatique d'une tumeur d'origine digestive (E. WOLFF, 1963). D'autres épithéliomas s'accroissent au contraire sur place, sans s'immiscer entre les tissus de l'hôte. Ils demeurent à l'état de nodules aux contours nets, parfois encapsulés dans une enveloppe composée de cellules cancéreuses ou de cellules des deux explants, cancéreux et normaux. Ces nodules augmentent de volume au détriment des tissus normaux, qu'ils n'envahissent pas directement, mais auxquels ils se substituent après les avoir détruits. Tel est le cas de l'épithélioma gastrique Z 159; cette tumeur forme en culture de curieux glomérules, limités par une enveloppe de cellules aplaties, et contenant un massif de grandes cellules épithéliales reliées par un pédoncule à l'enveloppe.

Les épithéliomas de la première catégorie (ceux qui pénètrent directement dans les tissus de l'hôte) peuvent se comporter de deux manières. Ou bien les groupes de cellules envahissent uniquement les tissus conjonctifs, ou bien ils s'immiscent entre les cellules des épithéliums et pénètrent dans les massifs cellulaires des glomérules. Le premier cas est représenté par la tumeur Z 200, le deuxième par l'épithélioma utérin Z 3. Le pouvoir d'invasion n'est pas forcément moindre dans le premier cas que dans le second, car les cellules tumorales finissent par se substituer, dans les deux éventualités, aux cellules normales.

III. Evolution d'une même Tumeur dans des Organes Différents

On peut étudier le comportement et le pouvoir d'invasion d'une même tumeur dans différents organes embryonnaires. Nous avons fait cette comparaison dans le cas du sarcome de souris S 180 (E. WOLFF, 1957), que nous avons cultivé en présence de mesonephros, de metanephros, de gonades, de foie, de poumon, d'intestin, de peau, de périoste d'embryon de poulet.

D'une façon générale, les organes qui possèdent des tissus conjontifs lâches et lacunaires sont plus facilement envahis que les autres; mais l'invasion se limite souvent à ces tissus. Tels sont le mesonephros, le metanephros, le poumon. Toutefois ce dernier organe n'est pas envahi d'une manière massive; en raison même de la faible densité du tissu conjonctif et de la dispersion des canaux bronchiaux, le milieu pulmonaire doit être faiblement nutritif. Par contre des tissus conjonctifs orientés en faisceaux parallèles ou en couches concentriques sont favorables à la pénétration des cellules du sarcome, pourvu que celles-ci puissent accéder par une brèche au sein de ces tissus. Elles se disposent alors parallèlement à la direction des assises conjonctives, elles forment des courants orientés de grands fibroblastes malins. C'est ce qui se produit dans les tuniques intestinales, dans les mésentères, le long du périoste. Les cellules sarcomateuses longent parfois l'épithélium intestinal, mais elles ne l'envahissent jamais. Dans la peau, les couches profondes du derme sont envahies assez fréquemment, les couches superficielles, plus denses, le sont plus rarement. Les fibroblastes malins longent alors la membrane basale de l'épiderme, dans lequel ils ne pénètrent jamais.

Nous voyons que les épithéliums très structurés, tels l'épiderme, l'épithélium intestinal, et la paroi des tubes urinifères n'offrent jamais de prise à la pénétration du sarcome S 180. Il n'en est pas de même des parenchymes épithé-lioïdes, comme ceux du foie embryonnaire. Les fibroblastes malins se fraient facilement un chemin entre ou à travers les cordons hépatiques. Ils forment de fongues files de cellules allongées, fusiformes, disposées parfois sur plusieurs rangs. Certaines de ces cellules se détachent de la file et pénètrent entre les cellules hépatiques, s'y multiplient fréquemment et propagent ainsi la tumeur. Le parenchyme du foie embryonnaire est donc facilement pénétrable, probablement en raison de la cohésion relativement faible de ses cellules.

Les gonades, mâles ou femelles, prélevées entre 8 et 9 jours d'incubation, offrent aux cellules sarcomateuses des conditions relativement favorables, à condition que celles-ci aient pu pénétrer par une brèche au sein même des tissus. La médullaire testiculaire ou ovarienne, constituée de cordons plus ou moins espacés, est envahie d'une manière massive par des cellules tumorales qui se mêlent aux cellules somatiques et germinales des cordons. Le cortex ovarien est envahi à son tour par les cellules sarcomateuses, venant toujours de l'intérieur de la gonade, car l'épithélium germinatif oppose vers l'extérieur une barrière infranchissable à leur pénétration. Aussi, les gonades n'offrent-elles pas toujours des conditions très favorables à l'invasion. Mais quand les éléments tumoraux ont réussi à s'insinuer par la région du hile dans l'intérieur de la gonade, celle-ci est rapidement envahie: les deux parties de la gonade, cortex et médullaire, sont littéralement truffées de cellules malines.

IV. Tumeurs Séparées du Mesonephros par une Membrane Filtrante

Dans ce système, il ne peut être question d'invasion proprement dite. Mais dans ces conditions, les cellules tumorales manifestent leurs propriétés d'invasion d'une manière un peu différente. Ne pouvant traverser la membrane, elles se pressent contre elle en rangs serrés. Dans le cas des épithéliomas ou des souches cellulaires dérivées d'épithéliomas (HeLa, KB, Fogh), l'assise en contact avec la membrane est souvent une couche régulière de hautes cellules épithéliales (E. WOLFF, 1961). Ces cellules suivent tous les plis de la membrane, la repoussent souvent devant elles, et, se multipliant en grand nombre, elles forment de véritables villosités ou des racines qui, recouvertes par la membrane vitelline, s'enfoncent profondément dans les tissus du mesonephros: c'est une forme de pénétration sans invasion. L'adhérence intime des cellules tumorales à la membrane vitelline, à l'endroit où elle revêt le mesonephros, est un des caractères les plus frappants de ce mode de culture.

Quand on pratique de petits trous dans la membrane, soit en la perforant à l'aiguille, soit en la faisant digérer partiellement par la trypsine, on constate que des cellules malignes ont tendance à se détacher de l'explant, à se frayer un chemin dans les ouvertures, et enfin à s'engouffrer dans le mesonephros. S'agit-il d'une attraction suivie d'une migration active des cellules tumorales? S'agit-il de déplacements passifs dus au hasard de leur situation et aux conditions favorables créées par le passage direct de substances nutritives à travers les pores de la membrane, conditions susceptibles de provoquer localement une multiplication plus active? On ne connaît pas encore la solution de cette question. Mais on peut affirmer que, par un processus actif ou passif, les cellules cancéreuses, séparées par une membrane de dialyse des tissus normaux, se pressent contre elle de manière à assurer le contact le plus intime possible avec le mesonephros.

Conclusions

L'association d'explants cancéreux et de tissus embryonnaires d'espèces différentes permet d'analyser certains processus d'invasion. Les cellules de tumeurs humaines ou de Rongeurs se reconnaissent comme des cellules marquées au milieu des cellules embryonnaires de poulet. L'on peut ainsi suivre tous leurs déplacements. Aucune cellule maligne ne peut échapper à l'observation.

Si l'on compare le comportement des cellules malignes à celui de cellules normales au milieu de tissus normaux étrangers, on constate qu'ils ne sont pas fondamentalement différents. Les tissus conjonctifs sont particulièrement instructifs à cet égard: même pouvoir de migration, mêmes attractions, mêmes modes et mêmes voies d'invasion. Mais les cellules tumorales détruisent les cellules normales au fur et à mesure qu'elles se mêlent à elles, et c'est par là en définitive que se manifeste la différence essentielle entre les unes et les autres. D'autre part, peut-être pour la même raison, elles sont beaucoup plus envahissantes. Quant au mécanisme et aux facteurs des destructions exercées par les cellules malignes sur les tissus embryonnaires en culture, ils ne sont pas encore élucidés, mais les méthodes d'explantation *in vitro* donnent une possibilité d'aborder cette analyse.

Summary

Mechanisms of tumourous invasion can be analyzed by means of *in vitro* associations between malignant tumours and embryonic organs. Those processes become still more evident when explants derive from different species such as mammalian tumours and chick organs. Under these conditions, malignant cells look like labelled cells among host ones. In such a way, we have cultivated transplantable tumours of mice and rats, human malignant strains and human tumours taken directly from patients. It is possible to cultivate the same tumour in association with different embryonic organs, such as mesonephros, metanephros, liver, gonads, etc. It is also possible to cultivate several tumours in association with the same embryonic organ. The invasiveness depends mainly upon the nature of the tumour, but also upon the structure of the embryonic tissues. In the case of mesonephros, some tumours (sarcomas) begin by invading only the connective tissues surrounding the epithelial tubules which are finally also invaded and destroyed. Other tumours (adenocarcinomas, pulmonary carcinomas) penetrate the connective tissues as well as the epithelia. Not all tissues are penetrable by tumours in the same way. So the dense tissues of dermis are not easily invaded by HeLa or KB cells, which form solid clumps, whilst mesonephros or liver are invaded by scattered cells of the same strain.

The behavior of malignant cells does not differ fundamentally from that of normal cells of the same type. Thus, sarcoma cells behave as fibroblasts, following the same paths of penetration into a foreign tissue. The fact that they have a destructive effect on normal cells seems to be the main difference from normal fibroblasts.

Under experimental conditions, embryonic tissues may be separated from the cancerous explants by a thin dialyzing membrane, the vitelline membrane of the yolk of the hen's egg. In such a way there is no direct contact between both kinds of explants; the tumourous explants are fed and stimulated by substances which pass through the membrane. Further, malignant cells press themselves against the membrane in very dense layers and show tendencies to form roots and villosities which depress the membrane and to break into the embryonic tissues when holes are accidentally or intentionally made in the membrane.

Discussion

Questions put to E. WOLFF

M. Feldman: Dr. WOLFF, your experiments have added an important parameter to our discussions. We have so far analysed here *in vitro* interactions of tumour and normal cells, in systems of cell-monolayers, where the cell-glass surface is an important factor. Your *in vitro* system, Dr. WOLFF, which is an organ culture system, avoids this "artificial" factor. It would then be of great interest to test how tumour cells, which are inhibited — in terms of movement and *growth* — by fibroblasts in monolayers — will behave when interacting with normal cells in organ cultures.

B. Kellner: 1. Have you observed a change in the type of growth following prolonged cultivation?

2. When cultivating benign tumours or atypical epithelium, did you observe a change in the type of growth?

E. Wolff: There is no contact inhibition between normal cells in organotypical culture — at least, between cells of *two different species* (birds and mammals). The essential difference between malignant and normal cells is that malignant cells posses a greater invasive capacity.

G. Barski: How do, cells of the normal histiocyte-macrophage type, behave in association with the mesonephros in organotypical cultures?

E. Wolff: The technique for the organotypical culture of malignant tumours was mentioned in my paper. It is a second-degree culture on embryonic organs, such as the mesonephros, which are themselves cultivated *in vitro*.

Benign tumours are less easy to cultivate than malignant tumours. Generally speaking, they penetrate rapidly without multiplying.

J. Harel: May I ask Prof. WOLFF one brief question in this connection. Some of your pictures of invasion of the mesonephros by malignant cells reveal a considerable destructive effect; have you ever seen normal histiocytes exert a destructive effect?

M. Feldman: Dr. ABERCROMBIE, what I meant in my comment to Prof. WOLFF is this: I was impressed by Dr. STOKER's demonstration that this transformed Py hamster cells — once interacting with normal fibroblasts in monolayers — are inhibited in terms not only of contact inhibition, i.e. of movement, but in terms of growth. Had Prof. WOLFF tested the same cells, in normal organ cultures, and had he found that under his conditions the same cells are not growth-inhibited when in contact with normal organ culture cells, I would have found myself slightly confused.

M. Abercrombie: I would like to suggest that there is not necessarily a contradiction between the results of organ culture, in which Prof. WOLFF has found a good deal of invasion by normal cells, and those of monolayer culture, in which contact inhibition occurs to a marked extent. A possible explanation of the apparent discrepancy is that Prof. WOLFF's cultures, being maintained for a longer time, give greater opportunities for deficiencies of contact inhibition of

low degree to show themselves. Prof. WOLFF does find a difference between normal and malignant cells in the amount of invasion in organ culture, and I would regard this as an expression of quantitative differences in contact inhibition.

O. Costachel: I should like to mention one aspect of invasiveness which cannot be reproduced *in vitro*, but should nevertheless be born in mind even in this type of experiment.

If a stock tumour (JENSEN) is transplanted, it takes and grows locally without giving rise to metastases. But if the fragments are first passaged five times at 48-hourly intervals, the tumour no longer takes locally and pulmonary metastases appear.

This means that apart from contact inhibition there is another factor controlling invasiveness — a factor with at least two different aspects: *local* growth (at the site of inoculation) and *remote* growth in the lungs (no local tumour being produced).

The role played by the karyotype of a tumour is demonstrated by another model.

If a heterologous hamster tumour (H 16 H) is passaged several times in the rat (as has been done at the Oncological Institute in Bucharest), the percentage of the two karyotypes (of the host and of the tumour) changes as follows: during the first few passages the percentage of cells possessing the karyotype of the tumour exceeds 90%; this percentage then gradually diminishes with succeeding passages until at the sixth only 4% of the cells have the karyotype of the tumour, while 96% have the karyotype of the host.

In parallel with this development the metastasizing capacity of the heterologous tumour also increases.

E. Wolff: There ist not necessarily any correlation between the metastasizing capacity of tumours and their invasive capacity in organ cultures *in vitro*. But these two properties are often found together.

Bibliography

BERMANN, F., Associations xénoplastiques d'organes embryonnaires: étude de quelques structures mixtes obtenues *in vitro* et *in vivo*. *C.R. Soc. Biol. (Paris)* **154**, 911—914 (1960).

BRESCH, D., Recherches préliminaires sur les associations d'organes embryonnaires de poulet en culture *in vitro*. *Bull. Biol.* **89**, 179—188 (1955).

POURREAU-SCHNEIDER, N., BERNARD, C., BOIRON, M. et WOLFF, ET., Comportement de la moelle osseuse humaine normale et leucémique associée au rein embryonnaire de Poulet en culture organotypique. *Exp. Cell Res.* **32**, 51—58 (1963).

WOLFF, ET., et SCHNEIDER, N., Sur l'association d'une tumeur de Souris et d'organes embryonnaires de Poulet en culture *in vitro*. *C.R. Soc. Biol. (Paris)* **150**, 845—846 (1956).

— — La culture d'un sarcome de Souris sur des organes de Poulet explantés *in vitro*. *Arch. Anat. micr. Morph. exp.* **46**, 173—197 (1957).

—, et SIGOT, M. F., Comportement de différents types de tumeurs de Rongeurs associés à du rein embryonnaire de poulet en culture *in vitro*. *C.R. Soc. Biol. (Paris)* **155**, 265—267 (1961).

—, et WENIGER, J. P., Recherches préliminaires sur les chimères d'organes embryonnaires d'Oiseaux et de Mammifères en culture *in vitro*. *J. Embryol. exp. Morph.* **2**, 161—171 (1954).

WOLFF ET., et WOLFF, EM., Les résultats d'une nouvelle méthode de culture de cellules cancéreuses *in vitro*. *Rev. franç. Étud. clin. biol.* **3**, 945—951 (1958).

— — Sur le comportement de souches cancéreuses humaines en association avec des organes embryonnaires de poulet cultivés *in vitro*. *C.R. Soc. Biol. (Paris)* **153**, 1898—1900 (1959).

— — Peut-on associer, en culture organotypique, des cancers humains fraîchement prélevés à des tissus embryonnaires de poulet? *C.R. Acad. Sci. (Paris)* **252**, 1873—1875 (1961a).

— — Cultures de cellules cancéreuses humaines sur des organes embryonnaires de poulet explantés *in vitro*. *Coll. intern. C.N.R.S.*, Nogent 1960, 199—208 (1961b).

— — Sur la culture de longue durée d'un cancer humain *in vitro*. *C.R. Acad. Sci. (Paris)* **256**, 1173—1174 (1963).

— — et RENAULT, P., Sur la culture organotypique de carcinomes humains très proliférants, en présence de mesonephros d'embryon de Poulet. *Path. et Biol.* **10**, 1161—1169 (1962).

Induced Dissociation of Walker Tumour 256 into its "Carcinomatous" and "Sarcomatous" Patterns of Growth *

Joseph Leighton, Richard M. Iammarino, and Raymond Mark

Department of Pathology, School of Medicine, University of Pittsburgh, Pittsburgh, Pa., U.S.A.

The Walker tumour of the rat, a characteristically bimorphic tumour (Stewart *et al.*, 1959), grows on the chorioallantois of the chick embryo after topical inoculation with a different microscopic architecture depending on the temperature of incubation of the egg (Leighton *et al.*, 1963). In our studies an inoculum consisting of two or three drops of Walker tumour ascites fluid, was placed on the dropped chorioallantoic membrane of eight- or nine-day-old chick embryos. The embryos were maintained as before at the normal temperature of incubation, 38° C. On the eleventh day of embryonic life the inoculated eggs were candled. Of the viable eggs 10% were harvested for histologic study while the remaining ones were divided into three equal groups. One group was returned to the normal temperature of incubation, the second group was placed at 32° C, and the third group at 42° C. On the eighteenth day of incubation all of the transplant sites were removed for histologic examination. The predominant microscopic picture of the tumours from the group at the normal temperature, 38° C, was that of an anaplastic carcinoma consisting of tumour cells growing in open alveolar patterns (Fig. 1). The cells were spherical or polyhedral and were in loose association with one another. At the low temperature of 32° the microscopic pattern was that of a densely cellular tumour, in some areas composed of predominantly spindle-shaped cells (Fig. 2) At the high temperature, 42° C, alveolar patterns occurred but many of the tumour cells were gigantic with bizarre nuclei (Fig. 3). Mitotic figures were seen at all three temperatures.

We have since found that the metastatic growth of the Walker tumour after intravenous inoculation in the chick is also modified depending upon the temperature of incubation, both as to the distribution of metastases and their architecture. For these studies an inoculum consisting of 0.025 ml of fresh ascites fluid was injected with the use of a one quarter ml tuberculin syringe and a 27 guage disposable needle. The eggs were inoculated on the eleventh day of incubation and the tissues examined on the eighteenth day. Following inoculation the eggs were divided into three groups, one placed at the normal temperature of 38° C, another at 32° C and the third at 42° C.

In eggs incubated at 38° C the chorioallantoic membrane frequently showed

* This work was supported by Research Grant No. Ca-02800 from the U.S.P.H.S., National Cancer Institute.

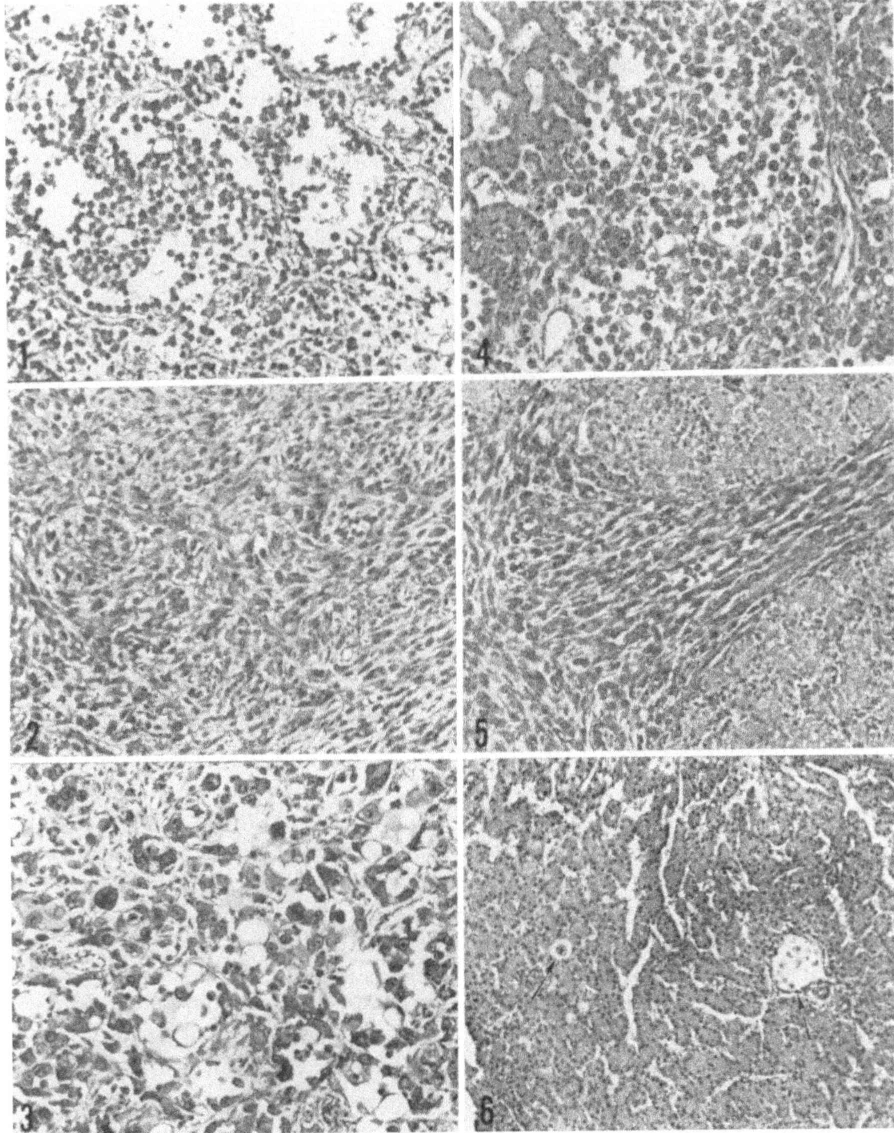

Figs. 1, 2, and 3. Microscopic sections of tumours produced following topical inoculation of the chorioallantois on the eighth day of incubation. On the eleventh day the embryos were divided and incubated at three different temperatures. Transplants were harvested on the eighteenth day. Hematoxylin and eosin. × 80. — Fig. 1. 38° C, the normal temperature. The tumour is composed of loosely adherent spherical cells which in many areas form an open alveolar pattern. The walls of the alveolar structures are composed of chick connective tissue. — Fig. 2. 32° C. The tumours are densely cellular and compact. Most of the neoplastic cells are spindle-shaped, and arranged in ill-defined whorls. — Fig. 3. 42° C. The tumour grows in an alveolar epithelial pattern; many of the tumour cells are bizarre, giant cell forms

Figs. 4, 5, and 6. Microscopic sections of tumour growth in the liver. Eleven-day-old embryos were inoculated intravenously with a suspension of cells, and incubated at the three temperatures. The embryos were examined on the eighteenth day. Hematoxylin and eosin. × 80. — Fig. 4. 38° C, the normal temperature. The pattern in the liver resembles that seen in the chorioallantois after topical inoculation. See Fig. 1. — Fig. 5. 32° C. The pattern resembles that seen in the chorioallantois at this temperature. See Fig. 2. — Fig. 6. 42° C. Rare solitary tumour cells are seen in the liver (left arrow). At this temperature in both tumour-bearing and uninoculated eggs many vessesls contain acid mucopolysaccharide material in which mononuclear cells are embedded (right arrow) a fine, gray stippling representing colonies of Walker tumour cells. The livers were enlarged and friable. Microscopic examination disclosed massive involvement of the liver, brain, meninges, chorio-allantoic membrane and mesonephros. Moderate involvement was seen in the lungs, gonads, adrenals, lumbar voluntary muscles, heart, and spleen. Lesions were of minimal number and size in the metanephros and in the gastrointestinal tract. Occasional tumour cells could be seen in the bursa of Fabricius but not in the thymus. In embryos incubated at 32° C extensive involvement with tumour was seen in the liver and brain. Tumour was seen in lesser amounts in the mesonephros and chorioallantoic membrane. At 42° C no tumour growth was seen in any organ, although in the liver and occasionally in the mesonephros and chorioallantoic membrane single tumour cells were seen (Leighton, 1963).

The extent of growth as metastases in the organs at the three different temperatures paralleled that seen on the chorioallantois following topical inoculation (Figs. 4, 5 and 6). Furthermore the microscopic pictures observed at the three temperatures on the chorioallantois were reproduced with particular clarity in the liver. Growth at the normal temperature in the liver was voluminous and was composed of cells in a predominantly epithelial pattern with an alveolar arrangement. Growth at 32° C in the liver was less, generally in association with the larger vessels. The tumour cells were predominantly spindle-shaped. At the high temperature of incubation, 42°, occasional tumour giant cells were seen near large vessels.

Discussion

The significance of the observations reported here may be considered from two points of view. The dissociation of the microscopic architecture of the Walker tumour into either an epithelial or a connective tissue tumour pattern may be an expression of two phenotypes, or it may represent genetic selection. The reaction of the tumour may be a specific example of a neoplasm responding as an indicator or end organ to systemic alterations in the host (Leighton et al., 1964).

Summary

The Walker carcinosarcoma 256 of the rat is readily transplanted to the chick embryo. Following topical inoculation on the chorioallantois, a large tumour nodule develops. After intravenous inoculation metastases arise in many organs in the embryo, with massive involvement of the liver. The normal bimorphic appearance of the tumour in the rat can be dissociated in the chick egg by varying the temperature of incubation. At 38° C, the normal temperature of incubation, the tumour grows predominantly as an alveolar, anaplastic carcinoma; at 32° C as a sarcoma. The response of the tumour to the temperature of incubation may be secondary to the effect of the abnormal temperatures on the host.

Discussion

Questions put to J. Leighton

P. Sträuli: I should expect you to find the same wide range of chromosome numbers within the two growth patterns of the Walker carcinosarcoma as in the tumour as a whole. It might be assumed that the cells of this highly anaplastic tumour have a range of phenotypic expression which comprises every one of the three functional states of undifferentiated cells formulated by WILLMER epitheliocyte, mechanocyte and amoebocyte.

J. Leighton: Your suggestion that this tumour may include elements of each of the three cell types proposed by WILLMER for growth *in vitro* is actually substantiated by the information now available. Epitheliocytes and amoebcyte (or fibroblasts) have already been illustrated. In the peritoneal fluid from the rat one sees many definite tumour cells that have red blood cells in their cytoplasm. This is presumably the result of phagocytosis, which is one of the attributes of the amoebocyte. Perhaps, in the case of the Walker tumour, all these patterns may be exhibited by cells of the same genetic constitution or of distinctly different constitution. We are trying to answer this question now. My guess is that these changes will not prove to be genotypic selection but phenotypic expression.

Incidentally, a number of other rodent tumours have been examined for evidence of temperature-dependent histotypic changes. We have found no tumour as yet whose microscopic architecture responds to the temperature of incubation as does the Walker tumour. Our use of the Walker tumour as the first one studied was fortuitous.

F. Lacour: What were the biological characteristics of the two tumours transplanted together on to the chorio-allantoic membrane? One of the tumours was apparently of viral origin (the mammary carcinoma of the C3H mouse) and I presume that the second was not of viral origin.

You have shown that there was a very considerable stromal reaction following transplantation of these two tu-

mours. Was there also a change in the rhythm of growth or time of development of these transplants?

J. Leighton: Both tumours came from C3H mice. The mammary adenocarcinoma, C3HBA, has a long experimental history. It was develop by MORRIS K. BARRETT, of the National Cancer Institute, and I believe that it contains the Bittner milk factor. The squamous-cell carcinoma of the uterine cervix was developed by my colleague, Dr. ROBERT H. FENNELL jr., of the University of Pittsburgh, by inserting a thread previously impregnated with methylcholanthrene in the cervical canal. Both tumours transplant readily in the C3H mouse and on the chorio-allantois of the chick. C3HBA grows a little faster than does the cervical cancer when passed in the mouse. The two tumours grow equally well on the chorio-allantois.

The conjugal tumour has so far been studied only in original passage in mice and on the chorio-allantois of the chick. I am planning studies in which these new tumours will be serially passed in mice and in chicks to see whether both components persist, or if only one is maintained. We will have to be alert to a number of possibilities and be prepared to recognize the unexpected — for example, the possibility that a somatic mating will occur *in vivo*. We must become familiar enough with distinctive markers of each tumour type to be able to recognize the products of such mating. If the duality of the conjugal tumours persists in serial passage, we will have good experimental material with which to invent techniques for separating the tumour into its two original elements. Afterwards, the application of analytic methods of this kind to naturally occurring tumours in which a conjugal character is suspected may permit us to examine in isolation the individual clonal lineages that we postulate as the complex ecologic system existing in some naturally occurring tumours.

J. Huppart: The fact that the two growth types are dependent on the incubator temperature puts one in mind of the bacterial mutants studied in recent years, in which some enzymes are thermolabile. Did you try to re-incubate the low-temperature type of cells at the normal temperature after a long series of passages at a low temperature? If they did not grow, this would indicate a mutation.

J. Leighton: In one experiment tumour tissue from the chorio-allantois of the low temperature-sarcoma pattern and the normal temperature-carcinoma pattern was inoculated into rats. The tumours grew rapidly in the rats and were indistinguishable on microscopic examination.

We have considered long-term experiments in which tumours would be serially passed in two groups — a normal group and a low-temperature group — with the thought that distinct cryophilic and thermophilic variants might be selectively isolated and characterized.

B. Kellner: What are the possibilities that the growth that looks like connective tissue is actually epithelium? Do the two forms exhibit a different pattern with silver staining for reticulum? Have you examined the two cell types from tumours in the embryo with the aid of the electron microscope? You know that in many human carcinomas some of the tumour cells are elongated, resembling connective tissue cells.

J. Leighton: With reticulum stains in areas that are purely sarcomatous almost every spindle-shaped cell is in intimate contact with reticular fibres. In the tumours in which the epithelial alveolar pattern predominates, these areas have reticular fibres restricted to their stromal components, the connective tissue of the walls of the alveolar spaces.

Preliminary studies of the two cell types with the electron microscope indicate significant differences, especially in the cytoplasmic organelles. My limited competence with electron microscopy prevents me from saying more.

G. Barski: Dr. Leighton, have you tried to do similar experiments by inoculating intravenously into chick embryos normal, heterologous embryo or *in vitro* adapted malignant or non-malignant cell cultures?

J. Leighton: Suspensions of chick embryonic cells bearing an endogenous physiological marker, the ability to produce pigment, were inoculated intravenously into non-pigmented varieties of chick embryos by Weiss and Andres years ago. They used embryos younger than those which I inoculated. They found that the recipients had pigmented feathers here and there, reflecting the seeding and participation of these cells in tissue of their own kind. In occasional small foci elsewhere in the embryo, macrophages containing pigment were the only residue of the inoculum. These reflected implantation in incompatible ectopic sites.

I have injected several human cell lines both topically and intravenously into the chorio-allantois. In the case of the intravenous route, a suspension of HeLa cells gave rise to a fine stippling of the chorio-allantois with minute nodules. There were marked alterations in vascular patterns, and occasional ghosts of HeLa cells were seen in the edematous stroma of these foci.

A thorough systematic examination of cell lines following intravenous inoculation in the chick embryo has yet to be made.

References

LEIGHTON, J., The appearance of disseminated minute tumor nodules in the chorioallantoic membrane of the chick following intravenous inoculation of ascites tumor cells. *Cancer Res.* **23**, 148—152 (1963a).

— A method for the comparison of the fate of intravascular tumor cell emboli *in vivo* and in organ culture. *Nat. Cancer Inst. Monograph* **11**, 157—179 (1963b).

— MERKOW, L., and JUSTH, G., Temperature-dependent histotypic changes in Walker carcinosarcoma in the chorioallantois. *Science* **141**, 1181—1182 (1963).

LEIGHTON, J., MERKOW, L., and LOCKER, M., Alteration in size of the heart of late chick embryos after incubation at varied temperatures. *Nature (Lond.)* **201**, 198—199 (1964).

STEWART, H. L., SNELL, K. C., DUNHAM, L. J., and SCHLYEN, S. M., Transplantable and transmissible tumors of animals. Atlas tumor path., sect. XII, fasc. 40. *U.S. Armed Forces Inst. Path.* 261—271 (1959).

UICC Publications

Kaposi's Sarcoma. S. Karger AG., Basle (Switzerland) — New York (1963).

Cancer of the urinary bladder. S. Karger AG., Basle (Switzerland) — New York (1963).

Prognosis of malignant tumours of the breast. S. Karger AG., Basle (Switzerland) — New York (1963).

The lymphoreticular tumours in Africa. S. Karger AG., Basle (Switzerland) — New York (1964).

Cellular control mechanisms and cancer. Elsevier Publishing Company, Amsterdam — London—New York (1964).

Illustrated Tumor Nomenclature. Springer-Verlag, Berlin — Heidelberg — New York (1965).

Structure and control of the melanocyte. Springer-Verlag, Berlin — Heidelberg — New York (1966).

Public education about cancer; cancer education programmes in various countries. UICC, Geneva (1966).

Cancer incidence in five continents. Springer-Verlag, Berlin — Heidelberg — New York (1966).

Choriocarcinoma. Springer-Verlag, Berlin — Heidelberg — New York (1967).

Cancer detection. Springer-Verlag, Berlin — Heidelberg — New York (1967).

Public education about cancer; research findings and theoretical concepts. Springer-Verlag, Berlin — Heidelberg — New York (1967).

Tumour specific antigens. Munksgaard, Copenhagen (1967).

Cancer of the nasopharynx. Munksgaard, Copenhagen (1967).

Potential Carcinogenic Hazards from Drugs. Springer-Verlag, Berlin — Heidelberg — New York (1967).

Treatment of Burkitt's Tumor. Springer-Verlag, Berlin — Heidelberg — New York (1967).

Proceedings of the Ninth International Cancer Congress — Congress Lectures and Official Spreeches. Springer-Verlag, Berlin — Heidelberg — New York (1967).

Proceedings of the Ninth International Cancer Congress — Panel discussions. Springer-Verlag, Berlin — Heidelberg — New York (1967).

Ovarian Cancer. Springer-Verlag, Berlin — Heidelberg — New York (1967).

GPSR Compliance
The European Union's (EU) General Product Safety Regulation (GPSR) is a set
of rules that requires consumer products to be safe and our obligations to
ensure this.

If you have any concerns about our products, you can contact us on

ProductSafety@springernature.com

In case Publisher is established outside the EU, the EU authorized
representative is:

Springer Nature Customer Service Center GmbH
Europaplatz 3
69115 Heidelberg, Germany

www.ingramcontent.com/pod-product-compliance
Ingram Content Group UK Ltd.
Pitfield, Milton Keynes, MK11 3LW, UK
UKHW052352070726
473059UK00009B/2688